Chronic Immune Thrombocytopenia

Guest Editor

HOWARD A. LIEBMAN, MD

HEMATOLOGY/ONCOLOGY CLINICS OF NORTH AMERICA

www.hemonc.theclinics.com

December 2009 • Volume 23 • Number 6

SAUNDERS an imprint of ELSEVIER, Inc.

W.B. SAUNDERS COMPANY
A Division of Elsevier Inc.

1600 John F. Kennedy Blvd. ● Suite 1800 ● Philadelphia, PA 19103-2899

http://www.theclinics.com

HEMATOLOGY/ONCOLOGY CLINICS OF NORTH AMERICA Volume 23, Number 6
December 2009 ISSN 0889-8588, ISBN 13: 978-1-4377-1228-5, ISBN 10: 1-4377-1228-2

Editor: Kerry Holland
Developmental Editor: Donald Mumford

Hematology/Oncology Clinics (ISSN 0889-8588) is published bimonthly by Elsevier Inc., 360 Park Avenue South, New York, NY 10010-1710. Months of issue are February, April, June, August, October, and December. Business and Editorial Offices: 1600 John F. Kennedy Blvd., Ste. 1800, Philadelphia, PA 19103–2899. Customer Service Office: 3251 Riverport Lane, Maryland Heights, MO 63043. Periodicals postage paid at New York, NY and at additional mailing offices. Subscription prices are $306.00 per year (domestic individuals), $483.00 per year (domestic institutions), $152.00 per year (domestic students/residents), $347.00 per year (Canadian individuals), $591.00 per year (Canadian institutions) $413.00 per year (international individuals), $591.00 per year (international institutions), and $206.00 per year (international and Canadian students/residents). International air speed delivery is included in all *Clinics* subscription prices. All prices are subject to change without notice. **POSTMASTER:** Send address changes to *Hematology/Oncology Clinics of North America*, Elsevier Health Sciences Division, Subscription Customer Service, 3251 Riverport Lane, Maryland Heights, MO 63043. Customer Service (orders, claims, online, change of address): Elsevier Health Sciences Division, Subscription Customer Service, 3251 Riverport Lane, Maryland Heights, MO 63043. Tel: 1-800-654-2452 (U.S. and Canada); 314-447-8871(outside U.S. and Canada). Fax: 314-447-8029. E-mail: journalscustomerservice-usa@elsevier.com (for print support); journalsonlinesupport-usa@elsevier.com (for online support).

Reprints. For copies of 100 or more, of articles in this publication, please contact the Commercial Reprints Department, Elsevier Inc., 360 Park Avenue South, New York, New York 10010-1710; Tel.: 212-633-3813, Fax: 212-462-1935, E-mail: reprints@elsevier.com.

Hematology/Oncology Clinics of North America is covered in *MEDLINE/PubMed (Index Medicus), EMBASE/ Excerpta Medica, and BIOSIS.*

Printed and bound by CPI Group (UK) Ltd, Croydon, CR0 4YY

Transferred to Digital Print 2011

Contributors

GUEST EDITOR

HOWARD A. LIEBMAN, MD
Professor of Medicine and Pathology, University of Southern California–Keck School of Medicine; Jane Anne Nohl Division of Hematology, Department of Medicine and Pathology Norris Comprehensive Cancer Center, Los Angeles, California

AUTHORS

DANIEL G. ARKFELD, MD
Division of Rheumatology and Immunology, University of Southern California–Keck School of Medicine, Los Angeles, California

CAROLYN M. BENNETT, MD, MSc
Assistant Professor of Pediatrics, Aflac Cancer Center and Blood Disorders Service, Emory University School of Medicine and Children's Healthcare of Atlanta, Atlanta, Georgia

JAMES B. BUSSEL, MD
Professor, Department of Pediatrics, Department of Obstetrics-Gynecology, and Department of Medicine, Weill Medical College of Cornell University, New York, New York

ERIC CHEUNG, MD
Jane Anne Nohl Division of Hematology, Department of Medicine, Norris Comprehensive Cancer Center, University of Southern California-Keck School of Medicine, Los Angeles, California

DOUGLAS B. CINES, MD
Department of Medicine and Pathology, University of Pennsylvania, Philadelphia, Pennsylvania

NICHOLA COOPER, MA, MD, MRCP, MRCPath
Consultant Haematologist and Honorary Senior Lecturer, Department of Haematology, Hammersmith Hospital, Imperial Health Care NHS Trust, London, United Kingdom

PATRICK F. FOGARTY, MD
Associate Professor of Clinical Medicine, Division of Hematology/Oncology, Department of Medicine, University of California, San Francisco, San Francisco, California

TERRY B. GERNSHEIMER, MD
Professor of Medicine, University of Washington; Puget Sound Blood Center, Seattle, Washington

EDWARD C. GORDON-SMITH, MD
Department of Haematology, St George's Hospital, London, United Kingdom

DAVID J. KUTER, MD, DPhil
Professor of Medicine, Harvard Medical School; Chief, Division of Hematology,
Massachusetts General Hospital, Boston, Massachusetts

HOWARD A. LIEBMAN, MD
Professor of Medicine and Pathology, University of Southern California–Keck School
of Medicine, California; Jane Anne Nohl Division of Hematology, Department of Medicine
and Pathology, Norris Comprehensive Cancer Center, Los Angeles, California

KEITH R. McCRAE, MD
Professor of Medicine and Pathology, Division of Hematology-Oncology, Case Western
Reserve University School of Medicine, Cleveland, Ohio

ROBERT McMILLAN, MD
Professor Emeritus, Division of Molecular and Experimental Medicine, The Scripps
Research Institute, La Jolla, California

FRANCESCO RODEGHIERO, MD
Division of Hematology, Department of Cell Therapy and Hematology, San Bortolo
Hospital, Vicenza, Italy

JOHN W. SEMPLE, PhD
Director of Transfusion Medicine Research, Keenan Research Centre, Li Ka Shing
Knowledge Institute, St Michael's Hospital; Department of Pharmacology, Department of
Medicine, Department of Laboratory Medicine and Pathobiology, University of Toronto;
Canadian Blood Services, Toronto Platelet Immunobiology Group, Toronto, Ontario,
Canada

MURIEL S. SHANNON, MD
Department of Haematology, St George's Hospital, London, United Kingdom

ROBERTO STASI, MD
Department of Haematology, St George's Hospital, London, United Kingdom

EVI STAVROU, MD
Division of Hematology-Oncology, Case Western Reserve University School of Medicine,
Cleveland, Ohio

MICHAEL TARANTINO, MD
Professor of Pediatrics and Medicine, University of Illinois College of Medicine-Peoria,
Peoria, Illinois

CARLO VISCO, MD
Division of Hematology, Department of Cell Therapy and Hematology, San Bortolo
Hospital, Vicenza, Italy

ILENE C. WEITZ, MD
Division of Hematology, University of Southern California–Keck School of Medicine,
Los Angeles, California

FENELLA WILLIS, MD
Department of Haematology, St George's Hospital, London, United Kingdom

Contents

This article presents a brief history of immune thrombocytopenia (ITP) from the first clinical description written in 1735, through years of controversy about the nature and causes of what was first known as idiopathic thrombocytopenia purpura, then immune thrombocytopenic purpura, and, finally, ITP. Current understanding of ITP's primary and secondary forms and the effect of diverse defects in immune self tolerance that result in the development of antiplatelet antibodies is described. This overview is followed by a narrative list of other articles in this issue on topics ranging from a comprehensive review of the role of antiplatelet antibodies in platelet destruction and production to a review of classic treatment modalities and newer approaches to initial treatment.

Chronic immune thrombocytopenia (ITP) is an autoimmune disorder manifested by immune-mediated platelet destruction and suppression of platelet production. Chronic ITP characteristically has an insidious onset, usually requires therapy, and is most commonly seen in adults. The diagnosis of chronic ITP is one of exclusion and is based on the American Society of Hematology Guidelines: The patient's history, physical examination, and peripheral blood film must be consistent with the diagnosis and other causes of thrombocytopenia must be ruled out. This article reviews the role of antiplatelet autoantibody in adult chronic ITP.

In the last 20 years, many publications have shed new light on the complex immunopathogenesis of immune thrombocytopenic purpura. They are associated with 3 interrelated areas of environmental autoimmunity, for example, infectious influences, antigen-presenting cell (APC) function, and T-cell abnormalities, particularly tolerance induction. This article highlights the recent literature and argues that infectious agents and platelets can significantly modulate APCs, which create an environment that dysregulates autoreactive T cells, leading to the production of autoantibodies.

agents can simultaneously improve concurrent thrombocytopenia. The best evidence to date would support the targeting of treatment to the connective tissue disorder, expecting a simultaneous improvement in the platelet count. Due to the frequent relapses associated with many of the connective tissue disorders and the frequent use of immunosuppressant agents, splenectomy should be undertaken only in highly refractory patients. Differentiating the varying immunopathic etiologies that contribute to development of connective tissue disorders may lead to a better understanding of the mechanisms of thrombocytopenia in a subset of these patients. The use of target therapies to treat connective tissue disorders has the potential of reducing the risk of the development of ITP or, conversely, inducing the development of immune thrombocytopenia.

The literature regarding an association between thyroid disease and immune thrombocytopenic purpura (ITP) suggests that autoimmune thyroid disease is a frequent finding in patients with ITP. A strong association between other systemic autoimmune diseases and autoimmune thyroid diseases is also well documented. Therefore, the combination of autoimmune thyroid disease and ITP could reflect a more significant defect in the immune self-tolerance of these patients compared with those who have primary ITP alone. Such defects may characterize an ITP patient population as more refractory to standard ITP therapy. Screening patients for antithyroid antibodies would identify a patient population at greater risk of developing overt thyroid disease. These patients may be further screened with a thyroid-stimulating hormone assay to detect subclinical thyroid disease.

Lymphoproliferative disorders are recognized as a common cause of secondary immune thrombocytopenia (ITP). The mechanisms involved in the pathogenesis of ITP associated with lymphoproliferative disorders are heterogeneous and often linked to the presence and activity of the malignant clone. A better understanding of the responsible mechanisms leading to ITP in each disease may allow for targeted treatment decisions, avoiding unwarranted immunosuppression and bleeding complications.

Persistent thrombocytopenia may be the consequence of chronic infections with hepatitis C virus (HCV), human immunodeficiency virus (HIV), and *Helicobacter pylori*, and should be considered in the differential diagnosis of primary immune thrombocytopenia (ITP). Studies have shown that on diagnosis of infections, treatment of the primary disease often results in substantial improvement or complete recovery of the thrombocytopenia. In patients with thrombocytopenia due to HCV-related chronic liver disease, the use of eltrombopag, a thrombopoietin receptor agonist, normalizes platelet levels, thereby permitting the initiation of antiviral therapy. Antiviral therapy with highly active antiretroviral therapy for HIV has aided in platelet recovery, with a corresponding decrease in circulating viral load. Thrombocytopenia in the absence of other disease symptoms requires screening for *H. pylori*, especially in countries such as Japan, where there is a high prevalence of the disease and the chances of a platelet response to eradication therapy are high.

Management of immune thrombocytopenia in pregnancy can be a complex and challenging task and may be complicated by fetal-neonatal thrombocytopenia. Although fetal intracranial hemorrhage is a rare complication of immune thrombocytopenia in pregnancy, invasive studies designed to determine the fetal platelet count before delivery are associated with greater risk than that of fetal intracranial hemorrhage and are discouraged. Moreover, the risk of neonatal bleeding complications does not correlate with the mode of delivery, and cesarean section should be reserved only for obstetric indications.

Intravenous immunoglobulin and intravenous anti-D are common therapies in the management of patients with immune thrombocytopenia (ITP). Both are pooled plasma products and both result in an increase in the platelet count in approximately 60% to 70% of patients with ITP. Despite immediate increases in the platelet count, the duration of response is limited, with platelet increments lasting between 2 and 4 weeks. Infusion reactions are common but adverse events rare. Although responses are similar, human and murine data suggest that the mechanisms of action of these treatments are complex and likely different.

Diagnosis and management of chronic ITP requires experience and the appropriate use of the laboratory despite the absence of a diagnostic test for ITP. Consideration of secondary ITP is important because identification of immunodeficiency infections or of lymphoproliferative disorders would change the management approach to a given patient. The development of newer therapies such as rituximab and the thrombopoietic agents has had a major impact on the management of ITP. In the future, combinations of agents may be a critical approach although the schedule and dosing remains difficult to establish. Finally, current studies to augment therapy in newly diagnosed ITP patients to prevent chronic disease may lessen the number of patients in chronic disease category.

THE CLINICS ARE NOW AVAILABLE ONLINE!

Access your subscription at:
www.theclinics.com

Preface

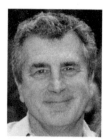

Howard A. Liebman, MD
Guest Editor

When I was a medical student and young house medicine officer, idiopathic thrombo-cytopenic purpura (ITP) was a disease easily understood. I knew that thrombocyto-penia in patients with ITP was the result of antiplatelet antibodies leading to rapid clearance of the platelets in the spleen. The clearance of the antibody-coated platelets easily overwhelmed any attempt of the bone marrow to compensate for the thrombo-cytopenia. Corticosteroids were effective in inhibiting platelet phagocytosis and reducing the amount of antiplatelet antibody. If patients failed corticosteroid treatment, they could be cured with splenectomy. The few patients who failed splenectomy simply made too much antibody, causing platelet clearance in the liver.

This was a beautifully simple story, but like most things in medicine, the truth was much more complex. The full story of ITP is still unknown. However, in the last decade, with our growing understanding of normal immune regulation, we have seen how complex the immunology and pathogenesis of "immune thrombocytopenia" is. The disease involves an intricate interaction of antigen-presenting cells, antibody-producing B lymphocytes, and regulatory thymic lymphocytes. Over 20% of patients with ITP have other immune disorders or chronic infections. ITP must now be considered a syndrome with a common phenotype of thrombocytopenia, with or without bleeding manifesta-tions. In this issue of *Hematology/Oncology Clinics*, we have been fortunate enough to bring together many of the investigators who have made important contributions to our growing understanding of the ITP syndrome. As the editor of this issue, I am sincerely grateful to all my coauthors for their excellent reviews, which I believe will provide a more comprehensive and contemporary picture of the ITP syndrome.

Howard A. Liebman, MD
University of Southern California-Keck School of Medicine
Jane Anne Nohl Division of Hematology
Norris Comprehensive Cancer Center
Rm 3466, 1441 Eastlake Avenue
Los Angeles, CA 90033-0800, USA

E-mail address: liebman@usc.edu

Hematol Oncol Clin N Am 23 (2009) xi
doi:10.1016/j.hoc.2009.09.005
0889-8588/09/$ – see front matter © 2009 Elsevier Inc. All rights reserved.

The Immune Thrombocytopenia Syndrome: A Disorder of Diverse Pathogenesis and Clinical Presentation

Douglas B. Cines, MD[a], Howard A. Liebman, MD[b],*

KEYWORDS

• Thrombocytopenia • ITP • Immune tolerance

Two young girls with symptoms of epistaxis and purpura are seen by a German physician. Later, one young patient has a spontaneous remission while the second suffers from repeated relapses. This report by Paul Gottlieb Werlhof[1] in 1735 is believed to be the first clinical description of a patient with immune thrombocytopenia (ITP).

Nearly 150 years passed before this disorder was determined to be due to a deficiency in blood platelets.[2] Controversy soon emerged regarding the pathologic mechanisms responsible for the thrombocytopenia. In 1915, Frank[3] proposed that the thrombocytopenia resulted from toxic suppression of the megakaryocyte by a substance produced in the spleen. A year later, Kaznelson,[4] a Viennese medical student, reported on the beneficial effect of splenectomy in this disorder. In contrast to Frank, he proposed that thrombocytopenia resulted from increased platelet destruction in the spleen.

The controversy continued as to whether this disorder, now termed idiopathic thrombocytopenia purpura, resulted from increased platelet destruction, defective production, or both. Dameshek and Miller,[5] in a study of bone marrow specimens from patients with ITP, found an increase in the total number of megakaryocytes in the bone marrows, but the majority of cells appeared not to be producing platelets. Effective platelet production appeared to increase after splenectomy. In 1951, a series of reports appeared to firmly document an immunologic role for accelerated platelet

[a] Department of Medicine and Pathology, University of Pennsylvania, Philadelphia, PA, USA
[b] Jane Anne Nohl Division of Hematology, Department of Medicine and Pathology, Norris Comprehensive Cancer Center, University of Southern California–Keck School of Medicine, Room 3466, 1441 Eastlake Avenue, Los Angeles, CA 90033-0800, USA
* Corresponding author. Jane Anne Nohl Division of Hematology, Department of Medicine and Pathology, Norris Comprehensive Cancer Center, University of Southern California–Keck School of Medicine, Room 3466, 1441 Eastlake Avenue, Los Angeles, CA 90033-0800.
E-mail address: liebman@usc.edu (H.A. Liebman).

Hematol Oncol Clin N Am 23 (2009) 1155–1161
doi:10.1016/j.hoc.2009.09.003
0889-8588/09/$ – see front matter © 2009 Elsevier Inc. All rights reserved.

destruction.[6,7] Evans and colleagues[6] reported an association between Coombs test-positive hemolytic anemia and ITP—suggesting an autoimmune mechanism for the thrombocytopenia. Harrington and colleagues[7] clearly demonstrated a humoral factor responsible for the rapid clearance of the thrombocytopenia. With these publications, "idiopathic" thrombocytopenic purpura became "immune" thrombocytopenic purpura. Subsequent studies by a number of investigators confirmed that the "humoral anti-platelet factor" was an antibody directed against platelet glycoproteins.[8–10]

In the early 1980s, the dogma of ITP as a disorder of accelerated platelet destruction alone was again challenged by several groups of investigators.[11–13] Using platelet kinetic studies with indium-111 labeled autologous platelets, these investigators found evidence of increased platelet clearance in addition to impaired platelet production. These studies were initially viewed with a good deal of skepticism. However, additional studies performed in the last decade have demonstrated inhibition of in vitro megakaryocyte growth and maturation by antibodies from ITP patients.[14,15] In addition, more recent studies have strongly supported an important role for the thymic lymphocyte in the initiation, progression, and response to treatment in ITP.[16–18]

The recognition that a number of other medical conditions can be associated with development thrombocytopenia that is clinically indistinguishable from classic ITP has lead to a separation of the disease into a primary (idiopathic) and secondary forms.[2,19,20] An increasing recognition of the secondary forms of ITP, such as observed with the recent reports of *Helicobacter Pylori*-associated disease,[20,21] has lead to the impression that primary ITP may be a less common disorder and that many cases are secondary to other conditions. The significant variability in the natural history, clinical presentation, and response to treatment in patients with ITP would suggest that the disorder results from diverse genetic or environmental perturbations of the immune system.

The authors have previously proposed that ITP, in its primary and secondary forms, be considered an autoimmune syndrome resulting in a common phenotype of thrombocytopenia with clinical manifestations of mucocutaneous bleeding.[22] In an attempt to provide an immunologic context to this disorder, the authors have proposed that diverse defects in immune self tolerance result in the development of antiplatelet antibodies in patients with ITP. These immune defects can be roughly divided into three categories: those resulting from defects in early immune development (central tolerance defects), differentiation blocks with abnormalities of peripheral B and T lymphocyte subsets, and peripheral tolerance defects resulting from immune stimulation (**Fig. 1**).[22] Response to treatment, the authors believe, may be in large part dependent on the nature of the checkpoint defect in immune tolerance (**Fig. 2**).

This issue of the *Hematology/Oncology Clinics of North America* attempts to present a contemporary overview of the ITP syndrome emphasizing its immunologic and clinical diversity. The pathogenic role of antiplatelet antibodies in the development of thrombocytopenia has expanded beyond the simple-model increased platelet clearance as proposed by Harrington and colleagues. Dr Robert McMillan provides a comprehensive review of the role of antiplatelet antibodies in platelet destruction and production in patients with ITP. Central to the development of ITP is a loss of self-tolerance, which involves a complex interaction between antigen presenting cells, antibody-producing B lymphocytes, and thymic lymphocytes. Quantitative or qualitative defects in $CD4^+CD25^+Foxp3^+$ regulatory T lymphocytes (Tregs) may play an important role in the loss of self-tolerance in patients with ITP and the persistence of disease. Recovery of Treg number and function appears to correlate with successful treatment of ITP. The role of the thymic lymphocyte in the induction of chronic ITP, its persistence and response to treatment is reviewed by Dr John Semple.

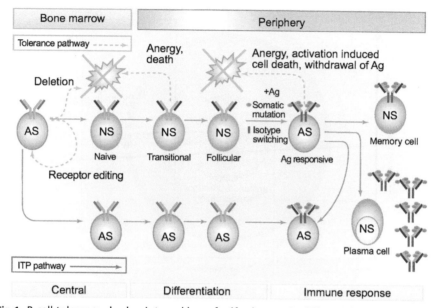

Fig. 1. B-cell tolerance checkpoints and loss of self-tolerance in different forms of secondary ITP. Tolerance pathways are denoted by green dashed lines. Solid blue lines represent normal B-cell developmental stages. Where failures in central and peripheral B-cell tolerance might occur in secondary forms of ITP are shown by the solid pink lines. Central B-lymphocyte tolerance checkpoints operate during primary cell maturation in the bone marrow and include clonal deletion and receptor editing. Cross-linking of membrane-bound antibodies on immature B cells leads to apoptosis. Antigen receptor specificity is also revised by receptor editing, that is, the continuation or reinitiation of antibody gene rearrangement, usually at light chain loci, in lymphocytes that already have functional antibody. Receptor editing can change a self-reactive light chain (shown in pink) to a non–self-reactive light chain (shown in purple). Peripheral tolerance checkpoints monitor and alter the repertoire in lymphocytes that have exited from primary lymphoid organs. Even if central tolerance is perfect, there is a need to regulate peripheral tolerance because somatic mutation can randomly generate autoreactive specificities. Somatic mutations are shown as pink circles on the heavy and light chain V-regions. Heavy-chain isotype switching (which usually accompanies somatic mutation during an immune response) is shown by the change in color of the heavy chain constant region from green to blue. Anergy and death of lymphocytes after an immune response also contribute to peripheral tolerance. Immune stimulation with a pathogen that mimics self-antigen (molecular mimicry) can also lead to a loss of peripheral tolerance and feed into the antiself ITP pathway. Peripheral AS cells in ITP can arise either primarily, through a defect in central or early tolerance checkpoints, or secondarily because of immune stimulation. Autoreactive peripheral B lymphocytes in ITP can include memory cells and plasma cells. Because of space constraints, only the activated cell arising from an immune response for the ITP pathway (not the plasmablast, memory cell, or plasma cell) is shown. AS, antiself (autoreactive); Ag, antigen; NS, non–self-reactive. Cines DB, Bussel JB, Liebman HA, et al. The ITP Syndrome: a diverse set of disorders with different immune mechanisms. Blood 2009;113:6511–21. Copyright © 2009 the American Society of Hematology.

Chronic ITP is a disorder of both increased platelet destruction and inadequate production. Platelet kinetic studies in this disease clearly demonstrate an inadequate bone marrow response to peripheral platelet destruction in many, if not most, patients. In patients with chronic ITP, the megakaryocyte also appears to be a target of antibody and cytoxotic T-lymphocyte injury resulting in ineffective thrombopoiesis. Unlike

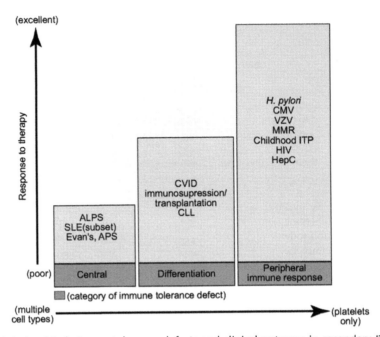

Fig. 2. Relationship between tolerance defects and clinical outcome in secondary ITP. The abscissa indicates whether platelets are the sole hematopoietic lineage affected (*right*) or whether there is often concurrent hemolytic anemia and immune neutropenia (*left*). The ordinate indicates responsiveness to treatment of the inciting infection or underlying disease. The proposed corresponding tolerance checkpoint defects are given in shaded boxes at the base of the figure. Cines DB, Bussel JB, Liebman HA, et al. The ITP Syndrome: a diverse set of disorders with different immune mechanisms. Blood 2009;113:6511–21. Copyright © 2009 the American Society of Hematology.

the normal physiologic response to anemia, which results in increased erythropoietin production, thrombocytopenia does not result in a compensatory increase in thrombopoietin (TPO) and, in patients with ITP, blood TPO levels are not increased. Dr David Kuter and Dr Terry Gernsheimer's article on the platelet production in patients with chronic ITP and the role of TPO in normal megakaryopoiesis provides an essential background to the use of newly approved TPO-receptor agonists in the treatment of patients with persistent and refractory ITP.

Dr Patrick Fogarty reviews the epidemiology and clinical presentation of adult chronic ITP. This article clearly shows that previous epidemiologic studies on ITP suffer from a lack of a uniform definition of the disease that would allow for reasonable comparisons between published studies. This may explain the widely different estimates of ITP prevalence in the population ranging from 5.6 to 20 per 100,000. Future epidemiologic studies will be greatly helped by the recent publication of international consensus guidelines for terminology and definitions in ITP.[23] Recent studies find an increased incidence with advancing age, with a female predominance among younger patients, and no sex predominance in older patients. This increasing incidence observed in the older patient population most likely results from age-related abnormalities in immune regulation. In contrast to the adult population, the majority of children with ITP have spontaneous remission of their disease within 1 year and chronic disease develops in less than 10% of children. Drs Carolyn Bennett and Michael

Tarantino review ITP in children and emphasize the need to evaluate carefully children who develop chronic disease for associated immune abnormalities, including autoimmune disorders or inherited immunodeficiency syndromes such as common variable immunodeficiency (CVID) or autoimmune lymphoproliferative syndrome (ALPS). The development of chronic ITP in children most likely reflects a central or differentiation defect in immune self-tolerance.

Primary ITP is a diagnosis of exclusion in which nonimmune causes of thrombocytopenia must first be excluded. A number of other disorders can result in the development of antiplatelet antibodies with ITP as a secondary event. These secondary forms of ITP can occur with autoimmune connective tissue diseases, lymphoproliferative disorders, and acute and chronic infections. Mild-to-moderate thrombocytopenia is frequently reported in patients with systemic lupus erythematosus, although severe thrombocytopenia is rare. In addition, there are a number of case reports and case series describing ITP in patients with other autoimmune connective tissue and rheumatologic disorders including Sjögren's syndrome, rheumatoid arthritis, and the antiphospholipid antibody syndrome. The differential diagnosis of ITP in these patients can be complicated by associated vasculitis; treatment-related bone marrow suppression or drug-induced thrombocytopenia. The difficulties associated with the diagnosis and management of ITP in patients with autoimmune connective tissue disorders and the antiphospholipid antibody syndrome are reviewed by Dr Daniel Arkfeld and Dr Ilene Weitz. These authors also note that many of these patients frequently express more than one autoimmune disorder characteristic of a central defect in immune regulation.

Many patients with chronic ITP develop additional antibodies targeting other tissues and organ systems. The most common secondary autoantibody target organ in patients with ITP appears to be the thyroid gland. Antibodies directed against thyroid tissue may be detected in up to 40% of ITP patients. Nearly 25% of ITP patients in some studies develop symptomatic or subclinical hyperthyroidism or hypothyroidism. Hyperthyroidism appears to be associated with accelerated platelet clearance independent of antiplatelet antibodies. Therefore, the development of hyperthyroidism in patients with ITP can result in disease refractory standard therapies. The association and clinical effect of thyroid disease in patients with ITP is reviewed by Dr Eric Cheung and Dr Howard Liebman.

Lymphoproliferative disorders have on been recognized as a common cause of secondary ITP. While the majority of ITP cases have been reported in patients with chronic lymphocytic leukemia (CLL), case reports have also documented the development of ITP in patients with Hodgkin's disease and non-Hodgkin's lymphoma. In patients with CLL, the development of ITP may also be a surrogate marker for an unmutated lymphocyte clone predicting a worse CLL prognosis. Dr Carlo Visco and Dr Francesco Rodeghiero provide a comprehensive overview of the immune regulatory defects that may account for the higher prevalence of ITP in CLL. Their article also suggests that standard ITP therapy in patients with CLL may be less effective and treatment should be directed toward the CLL.

ITP in children is frequently preceded by a febrile illness suggesting a possible infectious initiation of the thrombocytopenia. Unlike adults, nearly 90% recover a normal platelet count within a year. The role of an infectious agent in the induction of adult chronic ITP was only speculative until the first reports of ITP in patients with HIV infection in the early 1980s. Recent studies have provided evidence that chronic infections with H pylori and hepatitis C can also initiate ITP. In particular, the study of the infectious causes of ITP has provided new insights into the role of antigenic mimicry in autoimmune disorders, infection-induced Fc receptor modulation of phagocytosis, and the role of the thymic lymphocyte repertoire in persistence of disease. Dr Roberto Stasi and colleagues review the epidemiology, clinical presentation, pathogenesis, and management of infection-related chronic ITP.

There have been significant recent advances in the treatment of ITP that result in less patient morbidity and improved treatment outcomes. However, there are clinical situations in which treatment options may be limited and one such situation is the pregnant patient with ITP. ITP in pregnancy is not rare and may complicate 2 in 1000 pregnancies, indicating the need for a standard treatment algorithm. Dr Evi Stavrou and Dr Keith R. McCrae provide a comprehensive review of the clinical manifestations, diagnosis, and management of ITP in pregnancy, emphasizing that the vast majority of pregnancies result in safe and satisfactory outcomes for both the mother and child.

Treatment of the ITP patient can be separated into three general phases: initial treatment of the patient with very low platelet counts and bleeding manifestations, treatment directed toward maintenance of a safe platelet count with minimal toxicity, and treatment of the refractory patient. Intravenous immunoglobulin and anti-RhD, when combined with corticosteroid treatment, provide a safe and effective modality to rapidly raise the platelet count in the first phase of ITP treatment. The use of these therapeutic agents, their mechanisms of action, and potential toxicities are reviewed by Dr Nichola Cooper. Dr James Bussel reviews the classic treatment modalities and the newer approaches to the initial treatment of patients with ITP. The use of pulse dexamethasone and anti-CD20 therapy used early in the management of the newly diagnosed patient with ITP may produce a higher number of patients with unmaintained remissions and reduce the number requiring splenectomy. The TPO-receptor agonists have proven highly effective in the treatment of refractory patients and may be considered the agents of choice in the refractory postsplenectomy patient.

REFERENCES

1. Werlhof PG. Disquisitio medica et philologica de variolis et anthracibus. Hannover, 1735 [in Latin].
2. Mueller-Eckhardt C. Idiopathic thrombocytopenic purpura (ITP): clinical and immunologic considerations. Semin Thromb Hemost 1977;3:125.
3. Frank E. Die Essentielle Thrombopenia (Konstitutionelle purpura-Pseudohamophilie). I. Klinische Bild. H. Pathogenese. Berl Klin Wochenschr 1915;52:454 [in German].
4. Kaznelson P. Verschwinden der hamorrhagischen diathese bei einem Falle von "essentieller Thrombopenie" (FRANK) nach Milzexstirpation. Splenogene thrombolytische Purpura. Wien Klin Wochenschr 1916;29:1451 [in German].
5. Dameshek W, Miller EB. The megakaryocytes in idiopathic thrombocytopenic purpura, a form of hypersplenism. Blood 1946;1:27.
6. Evans RS, Takahashi RT, Duane RT, et al. Primary thrombocytopenic purpura and acquired hemolytic anemia: evidence for a common etiology. Arch Intern Med 1951;87:48–65.
7. Harrington WJ, Minnich V, Hollingworth JW, et al. Demonstration of a thrombocytopenic factor in the blood of patients with thrombocytopenic purpura. J Lab Clin Med 1951;38:1–10.
8. Shulman NR, Marder V, Weinrach R. Similarities between known antiplatelet antibodies and the factor responsible for thrombocytopenia in idiopathic thrombocytopenic purpura. Physiologic, serologic and isotopic studies. Ann N Y Acad Sci 1965;124:499–542.

9. Harrington WJ, Sprague C, Minnich V, et al. Immunologic mechanism in idiopathic and neonatal thrombocytopenic purpura. Ann Intern Med 1953;38:433–8.
10. Fujisawa K, Tani P, O'Toole TE, et al. Different specificities of platelet-associated and plasma autoantibodies to platelet GPIIb-IIIa in patients with chronic immune thrombocytopenic purpura. Blood 1992;79:1441–6.
11. Stoll D, Cines DB, Aster RH, et al. Platelet kinetics with idiopathic thrombocytopenic purpura and moderate thrombocytopenia. Blood 1985;65:584–8.
12. Ballem PJ, Segal GM, Stratton JR, et al. Mechanisms of thrombocytopenia in chronic autoimmune thrombocytopenic purpura. Evidence of both impaired platelet production and increased platelet clearance. J Clin Invest 1987;80: 33–40.
13. Gernsheimer T, Stratton J, Ballem PJ, et al. Mechanisms of response to treatment in autoimmune thrombocytopenic purpura. N Engl J Med 1989;320:974–80.
14. McMillan R, Wang L, Tomer A, et al. Suppression of in vitro megakaryocyte production by antiplatelet autoantibodies from adult patients with chronic ITP. Blood 2004;103:1364–9.
15. Chang M, Nakagawa PA, Williams SA, et al. Immune thrombocytopenic purpura (ITP) plasma and purified ITP monoclonal autoantibodies inhibit megakaryocytopoiesis in vitro. Blood 2003;102:887–95.
16. Kuwana M, Kaburaki J, Ikeda Y. Autoreactive T cells to platelet GPIIb-IIIa in immune thrombocytopenic purpura. Role in production of anti-platelet autoantibody. J Clin Invest 1998;102:1393–402.
17. Semple JW. Pathogenic T-cell responses in patients with autoimmune thrombocytopenic purpura. J Pediatr Hematol Oncol 2003;25(Suppl 1):S11–3.
18. Stasi R, Cooper N, Del Poeta G, et al. Analysis of regulatory T-cell changes in patients with idiopathic thrombocytopenic purpura receiving B cell-depleting therapy with rituximab. Blood 2008;112:1147–50.
19. Cines DB, Blanchette VS. Immune thrombocytopenic purpura. N Engl J Med 2002;346:995–1008.
20. Liebman HA, Stasi R. Secondary immune thrombocytopenic purpura. Curr Opin Hematol 2007;14:557–73.
21. Stasi R, Sarpatwari A, Segal JB, et al. Effects of eradication of Helicobacter pylori infection in patients with immune thrombocytopenic purpura: a systematic review. Blood 2009;113:1231–40.
22. Cines DB, Bussel JB, Liebman HA, et al. The ITP syndrome: a diverse set of disorders with different immune mechanisms. Blood 2009;113:6511–21.
23. Rodeghiero F, Stasi R, Gernsheimer T, et al. Standardization of terminology, definitions and decisional criteria in immune thrombocytopenic purpura (ITP) in adults and children. Report from an International Working Group. Blood 2009; 113:2386–93.

Antiplatelet Antibodies in Chronic Immune Thrombocytopenia and Their Role in Platelet Destruction and Defective Platelet Production

Robert McMillan, MD[a,b],*

KEYWORDS

- Thrombocytopenia • Autoimmune • Autoantibody
- Immune thrombocytopenia

Chronic immune thrombocytopenia (ITP) is an autoimmune disorder manifested by immune-mediated platelet destruction and suppression of platelet production. Chronic ITP characteristically has an insidious onset, usually requires therapy, and is most commonly seen in adults. In children, there are two forms of ITP: acute ITP, the most common form, which often follows a viral illness and in most cases remits spontaneously either with or without therapy; and a chronic form, occurring in about 10% to 15% of children, which is similar to adult chronic ITP. The diagnosis of chronic ITP is one of exclusion and is based on the American Society of Hematology Guidelines[1]: The patient's history, physical examination, and peripheral blood film must be consistent with the diagnosis and other causes of thrombocytopenia must be ruled out. This article reviews the role of antiplatelet autoantibody in adult chronic ITP.

HISTORY

The classic studies of Harrington and colleagues[2] provided the first evidence for an antiplatelet factor in chronic ITP. These investigators infused blood or plasma from

[a] Division of Molecular and Experimental Medicine, The Scripps Research Institute, 10550 North Torrey Pines Road, La Jolla, CA 92037, USA
[b] 203 12th Street, Del Mar, CA 92014, USA
* Corresponding author.
E-mail address: robtmcmillan@sbcglobal.net

Hematol Oncol Clin N Am 23 (2009) 1163–1175
doi:10.1016/j.hoc.2009.08.008
0889-8588/09/$ – see front matter © 2009 Elsevier Inc. All rights reserved.

ITP patients into normal subjects, which resulted in thrombocytopenia in 16 (61.5%) of the 26 recipients. In the 1960s, the ITP plasma infusion studies of Shulman and colleagues[3] showed that the effect of this plasma factor was dose-dependent; the factor could be adsorbed from ITP plasma by preincubation with platelets; and that it was localized in the IgG-rich fraction. The factor reacted with heterologous and autologous platelets and a larger volume of plasma was required to produce the same effect in patients who had undergone splenectomy. Both groups concluded that the antiplatelet factor was an antiplatelet antibody.

MEASUREMENT OF ANTIPLATELET AUTOANTIBODY

Early attempts to measure autoantibody, using platelet agglutination, complement activation, or platelet lysis were unsuccessful because of the lack of sensitivity or specificity. In the 1970s, several groups reported that platelet-associated IgG was increased in approximately 90% of chronic ITP patients. Subsequent studies showed a high percentage of positive results in patients with nonimmune types of thrombocytopenia,[4,5] however, and these assays were abandoned because of their lack of specificity.

In 1982, van Leeuwen and colleagues[6] reported that antibody, eluted from ITP platelets, binds to platelets from normal subjects (42 of 42) but to only a small percentage of platelets from patients with Glanzmann's thrombasthenia (10 [23.8%] of 42), which are known to be severely deficient in glycoprotein (GP) IIb-IIIa. They postulated that some ITP patients have antibodies against this platelet surface complex. Subsequently, several laboratories have demonstrated autoantibodies to a variety of platelet surface proteins, most commonly against GPIIb-IIIa or GPIb-IX. The detection of antibodies against more than one GP is not uncommon.

Of the reported approaches, there are two antigen-specific capture assays that can be easily adapted to the clinical setting: the immunobead assay[7] and the monoclonal antibody-specific immobilization of platelet antigen (MAIPA) assay.[8] These two assays are technically easy to perform, capable of measuring both platelet-associated and plasma autoantibodies, and give similar results.

Three large prospective studies have been published using these antigen-specific assays. In the descriptions that follow, "sensitivity" is the percentage of ITP patients with a positive assay and "specificity" is the percentage of patients with non-ITP with negative assays.

Brighton and colleagues[9] studied 81 patients with ITP (66 with acute or chronic ITP and 15 with secondary ITP) using the direct MAIPA assay. They noted a sensitivity of 49% (ITP 52% and secondary ITP 40%) and a specificity of 78%. The authors acknowledged that two factors may have affected their results: 13 additional patients with severe ITP could not be assayed because their platelet counts were too low for testing; and they included patients, in their "nonimmune" group, with disorders that may have associated ITP (eg, lymphoproliferative disorders).

Warner and colleagues[10] studied 56 ITP patients and 26 patients with non-immune ITP and noted 66% sensitivity and a 92% specificity. They obtained identical results with the MAIPA assay and an antigen-capture assay.

McMillan and colleagues[11] reported on 282 adult chronic ITP patients and 289 patients with other illnesses associated with thrombocytopenia (**Table 1**). Patients with ITP were separated into four groups: (1) presplenectomy ITP, mild (ITP-premild) patients with platelet counts greater than 50,000/μL who required no therapy; (2) presplenectomy ITP, severe (ITP-presevere) patients with platelet counts less than 30,000/μL who required therapy, but not splenectomy, because they developed a spontaneous remission, safe platelet counts on treatment, or either refused or

Table 1
Prospective immunobead autoantibody assay study in ITP patients

Patient Group[a]	No. Patients (%)	No. Positive (%)	No. Negative (%)
Total ITP patients	282	159 (55)[b]	128 (45)
ITP-premild	77 (27.3)	24 (31)	53 (69)
ITP-presevere	61 (21.6)	26 (43)	35 (57)
ITP-CR/PR[c]	46 (16.3)	23 (50)	23 (50)
ITP-ref	98 (34.8)	86 (88)	12 (12)
Other types of thrombocytopenia	289	45[d]	242

[a] ITP subgroups: ITP-premild, platelet count <50,000/μL and required no therapy; ITP-presevere, platelet count <30,000/μL who required therapy but not splenectomy because of either safe platelet counts on therapy, development of a spontaneous remission, refusal of surgery or was not a splenectomy candidate; ITP-CR/PR, postsplenectomy platelet count >30,000/μL and required no further therapy; ITP-ref, no response to splenectomy or relapsed after surgery.
[b] Anti–GPIIb-IIIA, 66%; anti–GPIb-IX, 17%; both antigens, 17%.
[c] CR, complete remission; PR, partial remission; all studied before surgery.
[d] Includes 25 patients with documented secondary immune thrombocytopenia (12 chronic lymphocytic leukemia, 5 non-Hodgkins lymphoma, 5 myeloproliferative disorder, 2 myelodysplasia, 1 chronic granulocytic leukemia); 9 patients with possible secondary immune thrombocytopenia; 5 patients with false-positive tests; and 6 patients lost to follow-up.
Data from McMillan R, Wang L, Tani P. Prospective evaluation of the immunobead assay for the diagnosis of adult chronic immune thrombocytopenic purpura (ITP). J Thromb Haemost 2003;1:485–91.

were not a candidate for splenectomy; (3) ITP postsplenectomy with a complete or partial remission who had platelet counts greater than 30,000/μL after surgery and required no further therapy (ITP-CR/PR); and (4) ITP postsplenectomy refractory (ITP-ref) patients who were nonresponsive or relapsed after splenectomy and required further therapy. Positive antibody results in these ITP patient groups were: total ITP group, 56.4%; ITP premild, 31.1%; ITP presevere, 42.6%; ITP complete or partial remission, 50%; and ITP ref, 87.8%. The refractory ITP patients also had a higher degree of positivity when compared with the other three groups. Autoantibodies were directed to GPIIb-IIIa (67.9%); GPIb/IX (17.6%); or to both complexes (14.5%). Of the 289 patients with other types of thrombocytopenia, 244 were negative (84%) and 45 patients were positive (16%). On chart review, 25 of the positive patients had ITP, 9 patients had possible ITP that could not be definitely documented, 5 were false-positives, and 6 patients were lost to follow-up. If all 20 patients without definite ITP are assumed to be false-positives, there is 93% specificity.

There are several possible explanations for ITP patients with negative assays: (1) the patient may not have ITP (eg, older patients with mild thrombocytopenia who never require therapy or patients with early myelodysplasia); (2) other platelet antigens or Ig subtypes, which were not examined, may be involved; (3) patients may have received treatment before assay, which suppressed autoantibody levels[12]; and (4) other mechanisms may be involved that are independent of autoantibody, such as T lymphocyte–dependent platelet cytotoxicity.[13]

A positive antigen-specific antibody assay provides strong evidence for the presence of ITP but a negative assay does not rule it out.

Autoantibodies as a Prognostic Factor

Fabris and colleagues[14] studied 50 consecutive ITP patients; 25 patients had detectable autoantibodies and 25 did not. They defined "clinical worsening" as the need to either begin or modify treatment because of either progressive thrombocytopenia or hospital admission for bleeding symptoms. Patients with autoantibodies had a higher probability ($P < .004$) of clinical worsening (18 of 25 patients) than antibody-negative patients (8 of 25 patients). The median time to clinical worsening was 27.7 months for antibody-negative patients and 2.1 months for antibody-positive patients. It was concluded that the assay of antigen-specific autoantibodies may be a useful prognostic tool.

AUTOANTIGENS IN CHRONIC ITP
Antigenic repertoire

The following studies provide evidence that the antigenic repertoire in chronic ITP is limited: (1) there is significantly less binding of the murine monoclonal anti-GPII antibody (3B2) to ITP platelets than to normal platelets[15]; (2) F(ab')$_2$ fragments from two serum anti–GPIIb-IIIa antibodies blocked the binding of seven other serum ITP antibodies to GPIIb-IIIa[16]; (3) Fab fragments from two human monoclonal anti–GPIIb-IIIa antibodies inhibited the binding of 8 of 12 platelet-associated autoantibodies from other ITP patients[17]; (4) a common idiotype, present in 18 of 23 ITP patients with anti-GPI/IX antibodies, was absent in 16 normal plasmas and 258 plasmas from patients with other types of thrombocytopenia[18]; (5) 6 of 16 serum anti–GPIb-IX antibodies from ITP patients reacted with the GPIb amino acid sequence TKEQTTFPP[19]; and (6) ITP patients have been shown to have light chain restriction of both serum and platelet-associated antibodies, which is consistent with antibody clonality.[20]

Further support for a limited repertoire is provided by the studies of Roark and colleagues[21] who used repertoire cloning to evaluate autoantibody genetics in ITP. They constructed phage display libraries from the splenic cells of two ITP patients and isolated multiple unique platelet-specific antibodies. Platelet-reactive Fabs from both patients used nearly exclusive rearrangements of the VH3-30 IgG heavy-chain variable gene despite variability among antigen specificities. A limited number of B-cell clones produced the antiplatelet antibodies as the result of antigen-driven somatic mutation. Antibody reactivity with platelets was highly dependent on specific heavy- and light-chain pairings. The author's conclusions were that antibody development in ITP is driven by "an encounter with diverse platelet antigens through the clonal expansion of B cells using genetically restricted and highly specific combinations of heavy- and light-chain gene products."

Epitopes in Chronic ITP

Epitopes may be either linear (defined by sequential amino acids) or nonlinear (amino acids involved in the epitope are contiguous because of protein folding). Fujisawa and McMillan[22] showed that many ITP autoantibodies against GPIIb-IIIa bind to cation-dependent epitopes. They preincubated ITP autoantibody, eluated from patient platelets, with purified intact GPIIb-IIIa, EDTA-dissociated GPIIb-IIIa, GPIIIa, or GPIIb and then assayed residual unbound antibody. Of the 15 platelet-associated autoantibodies tested, the intact GPIIb-IIIa complex, in every instance, caused greater inhibition of antibody binding than the EDTA-dissociated complex. No inhibition was noted using either purified GPIIb or GPIIIa. Kosugi and colleagues[23] confirmed the importance of cations for epitope stability in ITP.

Epitope Localization

Because autoantigens on GPIIb-IIIa and GPIb-IX are the most common, only these two complexes are discussed.

GPIIb-IIIa

To determine whether GPIIb-IIIa antigens are localized on GPIIIa, Bowditch and colleagues[24] synthesized five recombinant peptides that spanned the GPIIIa molecule and used these as targets to study the binding of ITP autoantibody. Of the 33 platelet-associated autoantibodies tested, only one showed convincing binding to any of these GPIIIa peptides. As controls, antibodies against known GPIIIa epitopes (anti-PI^{A1} allo-antibody, anti-LIBS2 monoclonal antibody, and anti-GPIIIa c-terminus autoantibody) bound to the appropriate peptide. The authors concluded that most GPIIb-IIIa epitopes were not present on GPIIIa.

McMillan and colleagues[25] evaluated the reactivity of ITP platelet-associated antibodies with CHO cell lines expressing either GPIIb-IIIa ($\alpha_{IIb}\beta_3$), the vitronectin receptor ($\alpha_v\beta_3$), or α_{IIb}-$\alpha_v\beta_3$ chimeras where a segment of α_{IIb} (amino acids 1-459, 1-223 or 223-459) was substituted for that portion of α_v. Of the 17 platelet-associated anti-$\alpha_{IIb}\beta_3$ ITP antibodies that were studied, 16 bound to CHO cells expressing $\alpha_{IIb}\beta_3$ but not to CHO cells expressing $\alpha_v\beta_3$. Because these GP complexes share the same beta chain, the antigenic epitopes must depend on the presence of α_{IIb}. The remaining eluate bound to CHO cells expressing either $\alpha_{IIb}\beta_3$ or $\alpha_v\beta_3$, indicating that either the major epitope for this antibody was localized on β_3 or that multiple antibodies were present. Eluted anti-PI^{A1} alloantibodies, as expected, bound to both $\alpha_{IIb}\beta_3$ and $\alpha_v\beta_3$-transfected CHO cells because both cell lines express β_3, whereas platelet eluates from normal subjects or patients with anti–GPIb-IX antibodies did not bind to either CHO cell line. These findings, showing that most autoantigens are localized on GPIIb, are consistent with those of Varon and Karpatkin[15] who noted reduced binding of a murine anti-GPIIb monoclonal antibody to ITP platelets, and of Tomiyama and colleagues[26] who reported on two ITP patients whose sera, in the immunoblot studies, bound to GPIIb.

Fifteen of the ITP eluates, whose epitope was dependent on the presence of α_{IIb}, were further tested against CHO cells expressing the α_{IIb}-$\alpha_v\beta_3$ chimeras. Eleven of the 15 bound to α_{IIb} (aa1-459)-$\alpha_v\beta_3$ showing that ITP autoepitopes are often localized to the N-terminal region of GPIIb.[27] In addition, each of the autoantibodies binding to α_{IIb} (aa1-459)-$\alpha_v\beta_3$ also bound to CHO cells expressing either α_{IIb} (aa1-223)-$\alpha_v\beta_3$ and α_{IIb} (aa223-459)-$\alpha_v\beta_3$. The other four eluates bound to CHO cells expressing $\alpha_{IIb}\beta_3$ but to none of the chimeras, suggesting that these epitopes are distal to amino acid 459. Because the autoantibodies bind to the chimera expressing α_{IIb} amino acids 1-459, and to chimera's expressing α_{IIb} amino acids 1-223 and 223-459, the results are compatible with either multiple autoantibodies with epitopes on either side of amino acid 223, or epitopes with contact points on either side of amino acid 223. Adsorption study results were most compatible with the second hypothesis.

The studies of Kosugi and colleagues[28] provide further support for the importance of this GPIIb region in autoepitope formation. They compared the binding of 34 ITP platelet-associated antibodies with the following GPIIb-IIIa recombinants expressed by 293 cells: wild type; GPIIb-IIIa with the ligand-binding defects of either the K0 thrombasthenic variant (2 amino acid insertion [R-T] between GPIIb residues 160 and 161) or the CAM thrombasthenic variant (GPIIb-IIIaD119Y); or to GPIIbD163A-IIIa. Of these antibodies, 11 (34%) showed diminished antibody binding to the K0 GPIIb variant, and decreased binding to GPIIbD163A-IIIa. Antibody binding to the CAM GPIIIa variant did not differ from normal GPIIb-IIIa. The ligand-mimetic monoclonal antibody OP-G2 inhibited binding of the antibodies that showed diminished binding to the K0 variant GPIIb-IIIa; small ligand binding antagonists, such as the RGDW peptide, did not. Many of the autoantibodies also inhibited fibrinogen binding to GPIIb-IIIa, particularly those showing impaired binding to the K0 variant. The authors concluded that some ITP autoantibodies bind to epitopes near the GPIIb ligand-binding site.

GPIb-IX

He and colleagues[19] incubated 16 serum anti–GPIb-IX antibodies with either glycocalicin or with two recombinant peptides: peptide one (amino acids 1-247) or peptide 2 (amino acids 240-485). Six of the 16 antibodies bound to both glycocalicin and peptide 2. Further studies showed that each of these six sera, and platelet eluates from two of these ITP patients, bound to a small peptide in this region (amino acids 326-346). Epitope scanning with overlapping synthetic peptides localized the epitope to GPIbα amino acids 333-41.

AUTOANTIBODY PRODUCTION SITES

The initial antigenic recognition in ITP patients should occur either in the spleen, which monitors the intravascular space, or in the bone marrow where intramedullary platelets or megakaryocytes could conceivably stimulate the immune system. Animal studies show that the spleen is the major lymphoid organ that responds to intravascular antigens, whereas the bone marrow assumes major importance later in the immune response. Lymph nodes, although of primary importance in the response to subcutaneous antigens, are minimally involved in the response to intravascular antigens.[29] In chronic ITP, the spleen is a major autoantibody production site as shown by in vitro studies where cultured ITP splenic cells produce IgG that binds to either autologous or homologous platelets,[30–32] and to megakaryocytes.[33] Because in some ITP patients autoantibody persists after splenectomy, there must be additional production sites. In vitro studies show that ITP bone marrow cells can also produce IgG that binds to platelets[34] and this organ is the most likely site of residual autoantibody production.

THE ROLE OF AUTOANTIBODY IN ITP PATHOGENESIS
Platelet Destruction

Platelet destruction is, without a doubt, an important mechanism in many ITP patients. Infusion of ITP blood or plasma into normal subjects results in thrombocytopenia in about two thirds of the recipients. In addition there is reduced survival of both homologous and autologous radiolabeled platelets in essentially all ITP patients as shown by the combined results of five large studies, which show reduced intravascular platelet survival in 117 of 119 ITP patients.[35–39] Two mechanisms of platelet destruction have been reported: antibody-mediated destruction and lysis of platelets caused by cytotoxic T lymphocytes.[13]

After the binding of autoantibody to platelets, they can be removed from the circulation either by phagocytosis or complement-mediated platelet lysis; there is experimental evidence supporting both mechanisms. Platelet phagocytosis has been demonstrated morphologically[40,41] and by in vitro studies[42,43] and may be triggered by either the Fc portion of IgG with or without antibody-mediated C3b fixation to the platelet surface. The Fc mechanism is clearly crucial in some ITP patients as demonstrated by the effect of Fc receptor blockade by either red blood cell stroma[44] or monoclonal anti-Fc receptor antibody infusion.[45] In addition, an ITP patient has been reported[46] with high-titer platelet-bound IgG4 autoantibody (IgG4 is poorly recognized by phagocytic cells) who had a normal platelet count but a severe bleeding diathesis caused by interference with platelet function by the autoantibody. Activation of the complement pathway by autoantibody may play a role in some patients. Increased levels of platelet-associated C3, C4, and C9 have been demonstrated on platelets from some ITP patients[47,48] and in vitro studies have demonstrated binding of C4 and C3 followed by platelet lysis after incubation of normal platelets with selected ITP serum autoantibodies.[49]

The major site for platelet destruction is almost certainly the spleen because about one third of the circulating platelet mass is present in this organ at all times and the local antibody production subjects intrasplenic platelets to high antibody concentrations. These antibody-sensitized platelets then circulate slowly through the spleen, which is rich in phagocytic cells. The liver, although an efficient phagocytic organ, produces no antibody locally, has a rapid circulation, and no intraorgan platelet pool. The liver assumes importance in patients with severe ITP where platelets are heavily sensitized. The bone marrow has both a resident platelet and megakaryocyte population, may produce autoantibody, and contains an RE system. Because autoantibody binds to both platelets and megakaryocytes, it is possible that intramedullary platelet destruction may occur.

Suppression of Platelet Production

There are multiple lines of evidence showing that platelet production is suppressed in many ITP patients.

Morphologic

Early light microscopy studies of ITP bone marrow showed normal or increased numbers of megakaryocytes with a shift to younger forms lacking cytoplasmic granularity or platelet formation and manifesting nuclear and cytoplasmic degenerative changes.[50,51] These findings were confirmed by phase-contrast studies, which also showed that these megakaryocytic abnormalities could be produced in healthy control subjects by infusion of ITP plasma.[52] Early electron microscopy studies showed extensive damage to 50% to 75% of megakaryocytes, and monocytes attached to the damaged cells in the process of phagocytosis.[53] More recently, ultrastructural studies by Houwerzijl and colleagues[54] confirmed these extensive megakaryocytic abnormalities and showed that they were present in a significant percentage of all stages of ITP megakaryocytes: 37% ± 37% of stage I (immature) megakaryocytes; 65% ± 37% of stage II (maturing) megakaryocytes; and 84% ± 16% of stage III (mature) megakaryocytes. Of all megakaryocytes, 78% ± 14% showed morphologic abnormalities. The abnormal cells showed features of para-apoptosis, including mitochondrial swelling with cytoplasmic vacuolization, distention of demarcation membranes, and condensation of nuclear chromatin. Many of the abnormal megakaryocytes were surrounded by either neutrophils or macrophages, some in the process of phagocytosis. There was also evidence of apoptotic features in stage III megakaryocytes in some marrow specimens. Para-apoptotic changes could be induced in megakaryocytes, produced in culture from CD34$^+$ stem cells, in the presence of ITP plasma. The authors suggested that autoantibody may initiate the cascade of programmed cell death.

Platelet turnover studies

Heyns and colleagues[55] in 1982, used autologous platelet survival studies to calculate platelet turnover as a measure of platelet production. They noted that many ITP patients had platelet turnover rates that were normal or reduced rather than increased as is expected if platelet destruction were the only thrombocytopenic mechanism. These results have been confirmed by several other investigators.[37–39] Of 55 ITP patients studied in these four reports, 21 patients (38.2%) had decreased turnover, 24 (43.6%) had normal turnover, and only 10 (18.2%) had increased turnover. These results are consistent with an impaired response of the ITP bone marrow to ongoing platelet destruction.

In vitro suppression of megakaryocyte production and maturation by ITP antibody

McMillan and colleagues[56] evaluated the effect of ITP plasma on the in vitro production and maturation of megakaryocytes (**Fig. 1**). Enriched CD34$^+$ cells from normal donors were cultured for 10 days in medium containing marrow growth and development factor and 10% plasma from either control subjects or ITP patients. Of the 18 ITP plasmas tested, 12 suppressed in vitro megakaryocyte production without affecting the number of nonmegakaryocytic cells. The percent suppression ranged from 26% to greater than 90%. Of the 12 positive plasmas, 6 had antibody against GPIIb-IIIa, 3 against GPIb-IX, and 3 against both complexes. Suppression was also noted using purified IgG from positive ITP plasmas and there was reduced suppression if the antibody was preadsorbed with immobilized antigen. ITP plasmas that suppressed megakaryocyte production reduced not only the total number of megakaryocytes produced but also impaired maturation, as manifested by a reduction in the percentages of 4N, 8N, and 16N megakaryocytes, an effect not noted after antibody adsorption with

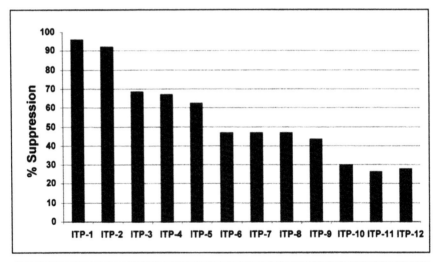

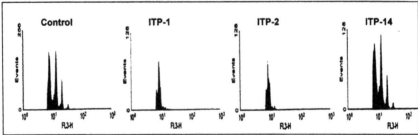

Fig. 1. The effect of ITP plasma on in vitro megakaryocyte production and maturation. (*Top*) Percent suppression of in vitro megakaryocyte production by 12 of the 18 ITP plasmas tested when compared with control plasmas. (*Bottom*) Histograms of the cell ploidy distribution of CD34$^+$-rich cells cultured for 10 days in the following plasmas (left to right): control, ITP-1, ITP-2, and ITP-14. Cells cultured in control or ITP-14 plasma (no suppression of in vitro megakaryocyte production) show four distinct peaks (2N, 4N, 8N, and 16N), whereas cells cultured in ITP-1 or ITP-2 plasma (both suppressed in vitro megakaryocyte production) show primarily 2N cells.

immobilized antigen. ITP plasmas that did not suppress megakaryocyte production did not affect ploidy distribution.

Similar results were noted by Chang and colleagues[57] in their studies of childhood ITP, although there were some differences. Umbilical cord blood (as a source of $CD34^+$ cells) was incubated in the presence of thrombopoietin and plasma from either ITP patients (44 with acute ITP and 9 with chronic ITP) or healthy donors. They noted reduced production of megakaryocytes when $CD34^+$ cells were cultured in ITP plasmas containing either antibody against GPIb-IX alone or antibody against both GPIb-IX and GPIIb-IIIa but no suppression in cultures containing control plasma, patient plasma with no detectable antibodies, or only anti–GPIIb-IIIa. There was no evidence of shifts in ploidy distribution. The major differences between the adult and childhood studies were the absence of suppression by plasmas with only anti–GPIIb-IIIa (only five were studied) and the lack of an ITP plasma effect on megakaryocyte maturation. The disparities noted between the adult and pediatric studies probably reflect differences in pathogenic mechanisms between adult and pediatric ITP.

Effect of thrombopoietic growth factors in chronic ITP

There is solid evidence that many ITP patients respond to the thrombopoietin mimetics that have been recently used for therapy.[58,59] If platelet destruction were the only mechanism in ITP, the bone marrow should be maximally activated and further stimulation should not be possible. The response of ITP patients to these agents provides further support that suppression of platelet production is an important mechanism in some ITP patients.

From the in vitro studies, it is clear that autoantibody is capable of suppressing marrow production of megakaryocytes in some ITP patients. Possible mechanisms to explain the suppression of platelet production in ITP include any of the following: (1) antibody-induced destruction of megakaryocytes by phagocytic cells, (2) antibody-induced complement activation with subsequent megakaryocytic lysis, or (3) autoantibody-induced induction of apoptosis. Because there is evidence that T lymphocytes may induce platelet lysis in ITP,[13] it is probable that T lymphocyte–mediated effects on megakaryocytes may also play a role in ITP.

SUMMARY

This article discusses autoantibodies and their epitopes in patients with chronic ITP and how these autoantibodies are involved in the pathogenesis of ITP. It has been shown that autoantibodies are involved in both platelet destruction and in the suppression of platelet production. The relative importance of these two mechanisms almost certainly varies among ITP patients. Future studies are required to clarify the relative importance of these two mechanisms in individual patients.

REFERENCES

1. George JN, Woolf SH, Raskob GE, et al. Idiopathic thrombocytopenic purpura: a practice guideline developed by explicit methods for the American Society of Hematology. Blood 1996;88:3–40.
2. Harrington WJ, Sprague CC, Minnich V, et al. Immunologic mechanisms in idiopathic and neonatal thrombocytopenic purpura. Ann Intern Med 1953;38: 433–69.

3. Shulman NR, Marder VJ, Weinrach RS. Similarities between known antiplatelet antibodies and the factor responsible for thrombocytopenia in idiopathic purpura: physiologic, serologic, and isotopic studies. Ann NY Acad Sci 1965;124:499–542.

4. Kelton JG, Powers PJ, Carter CJ. A prospective study of the usefulness of the measurement of platelet-associated IgG for the diagnosis of idiopathic thrombocytopenic purpura. Blood 1982;60:1050–3.

5. Mueller-Eckhardt C, Kayser W, Mersch-Baumert K, et al. The clinical significance of platelet-associated IgG: a study on 298 patients with various disorders. Br J Haematol 1980;46:123–31.

6. van Leeuwen EF, van der Ven JTH, Engelfriet CP, et al. Specificity of autoantibodies in autoimmune thrombocytopenia. Blood 1982;59:23–6.

7. McMillan R, Tani P, Millard F, et al. Platelet-associated and plasma anti-glycoprotein autoantibodies in chronic ITP. Blood 1987;70:1040–5.

8. Kiefel V, Santoso S, Weisheit M, et al. Monoclonal antibody-specific immobilization of platelet antigens (MAIPA): a new tool for the identification of platelet-reactive antibodies. Blood 1987;70:1722–6.

9. Brighton TA, Evans S, Castaldi PA, et al. Prospective evaluation of the clinical usefulness of an antigen-specific assay (MAIPA) in idiopathic thrombocytopenic purpura and other immune thrombocytopenias. Blood 1996;88:194–201.

10. Warner MN, Moore JC, Warkentin TE, et al. A prospective study of protein-specific assays used to investigate idiopathic thrombocytopenic purpura. Br J Haematol 1999;104:442–7.

11. McMillan R, Wang L, Tani P. Prospective evaluation of the immunobead assay for the diagnosis of adult chronic immune thrombocytopenic purpura (ITP). J Thromb Haemost 2003;1:485–91.

12. Fujisawa K, Tani P, Piro L, et al. The effect of therapy on platelet-associated autoantibody in chronic immune thrombocytopenic purpura. Blood 1993;81: 2872–7.

13. Olsson B, Andersson P, Jernas M, et al. T-cell-mediated cytotoxicity toward platelets in chronic idiopathic thrombocytopenic purpura. Nat Med 2003;9:1123–4.

14. Fabris F, Scandellari R, Ruzzon E, et al. Platelet-associated autoantibodies as detected by a solid-phase modified antigen capture ELISA test (MACE) are a useful prognostic factor in idiopathic thrombocytopenic purpura. Blood 2004;103: 4562–4.

15. Varon D, Karpatkin S. A monoclonal antiplatelet antibody with decreased reactivity for autoimmune thrombocytopenic platelets. Proc Natl Acad Sci U S A 1983;80:6992–5.

16. Hou M, Stockelberg D, Kutti J, et al. Glycoprotein IIb/IIIa autoantigenic repertoire in chronic idiopathic thrombcytopenic purpura. Br J Haematol 1995;91:971–5.

17. Escher R, Muller D, Vogel M, et al. Recombinant human natural autoantibodies against GPIIb/IIIa inhibit binding of autoantibodies from patients with AITP. Br J Haematol 1998;102:820–8.

18. Nugent DJ. Human monoclonal antibodies in the characterization of platelet antigens. In: Kunicki T, George JN, editors. Platelet immunobiology: molecular and clinical aspects. Philadelphia: Lippincott; 1989. p. 273–90.

19. He R, Reid DM, Jones CE, et al. Extracellular epitopes of platelet glycoprotein Ibα reactive with serum antibodies from patients with chronic idiopathic thrombocytopenic purpura. Blood 1995;86:3789–96.

20. McMillan R, Lopez-Dee J, Bowditch R. Clonal restriction of platelet-associated anti-GPIIb/IIIa autoantibodies in patients with chronic ITP. Thromb Haemost 2001;85:821–3.

21. Roark JH, Bussel JB, Cines DB, et al. Genetic analysis of autoantibodies in idiopathic thrombocytopenic purpura reveals evidence of clonal expansion and somatic mutation. Blood 2002;100:1388–98.

22. Fujisawa K, McMillan R. Platelet-associated antibody to glycoprotein IIb/IIIa from chronic immune thrombocytopenic purpura patients often binds to divalent cation-dependent antigens. Blood 1993;81:1284–9.

23. Kosugi S, Tomiyama Y, Shiraga M, et al. Platelet-associated anti-glycoprotein (GP) IIb-IIIa autoantibodies in chronic immune thrombocytopenic purpura mainly recognize cation-dependent conformations: comparison with the epitopes of serum autoantibodies. Thromb Haemost 1996;75:339–45.

24. Bowditch RD, Tani P, McMillan R. Reactivity of autoantibodies from chronic ITP patients with recombinant glycoprotein IIIa peptides. Br J Haematol 1995;91:178–84.

25. McMillan R, Lopez-Dee J, Loftus JC. Autoantibodies to aIIbb3 in patients with chronic immune thrombocytopenic purpura bind primarily to epitopes on aIIb. Blood 2001;97:2171–2.

26. Tomiyama Y, Kurata Y, Mizutani H, et al. Platelet glycoprotein IIb as a target antigen in two patients with chronic immune thrombocytopenic purpura. Br J Haematol 1987;66:535–8.

27. McMillan R, Wang L, Lopez-Dee J, et al. Many aIIbb3 autoepitopes are localized to aIIb between amino acids L1 and Q459. Br J Haematol 2002;118:1132–6.

28. Kosugi S, Tomiyama Y, Honda S, et al. Platelet-associated anti-GPIIb-IIIa autoantibodies in chronic immune thrombocytopenic purpura recognizing epitopes close to the ligand-binding site of GPIIb. Blood 2001;98:1819–27.

29. Askonas BA, Humphrey JH. Formation of specific antibodies and g-globulin in vitro: a study of the synthetic ability of various tissues from rabbits immunized by different methods. Biochem J 1958;68:252–61.

30. McMillan R, Longmire RL, Yelenosky R, et al. Immunoglobulin synthesis in vitro by splenic tissue in idiopathic thrombocytopenic purpura. N Engl J Med 1972;286:681–4.

31. Karpatkin S, Strick N, Siskind GW. Detection of splenic anti-platelet antibody synthesis in idiopathic autoimmune thrombocytopenic purpura (ATP). Br J Haematol 1972;23:167–76.

32. McMillan R, Longmire RL, Yelenosky R, et al. Quantitation of platelet-binding IgG produced in vitro by spleens from patients with idiopathic thrombocytopenic purpura. N Engl J Med 1974;291:812–7.

33. McMillan R, Luiken GA, Levy R, et al. Antibody against megakaryocytes in idiopathic thrombocytopenic purpura. JAMA 1978;239:2460–2.

34. McMillan R, Yelenosky RJ, Longmire RL. Antiplatelet antibody production by the spleen and bone marrow in immune thrombocytopenic purpura. In: Battisto JR, Streinlein JW, editors. Immunoaspects of the spleen. Amsterdam: North Holland Biomedical Press; 1976. p. 227–37.

35. Harker LA. Thrombokinetics in idiopathic thrombocytopenic purpura. Br J Haematol 1970;19:95–104.

36. Branehog I, Kutti J, Weinfeld A. Platelet survival and platelet production in idiopathic thrombocytopenic purpura (ITP). Br J Haematol 1974;27:127–43.

37. Stoll D, Cines DB, Aster RH, et al. Platelet kinetics in patients with idiopathic thrombocytopenic purpura and moderate thrombocytopenia. Blood 1985;65:584–8.

38. Heyns AP, Badenhorst PN, Lotter MG, et al. Platelet turnover and kinetics in immune thrombocytopenic purpura: results with autologous 111-In-labeled and homologous 51- Cr-labeled platelets differ. Blood 1986;67:86–92.

39. Ballem PJ, Segal GM, Stratton JR, et al. Mechanisms of thrombocytopenia in chronic autoimmune thrombocytopenic purpura: evidence for both impaired platelet production and increased platelet clearance. J Clin Invest 1987;80: 33–40.

40. Handin RI, Stossel TP. Phagocytosis of antibody-coated platelets by human granulocytes. N Engl J Med 1974;290:989–93.

41. Zucker-Franklin D, Karpatkin S. Red-cell and platelet fragmentation in idiopathic autoimmune thrombocytopenic purpura. N Engl J Med 1977;297:517–23.

42. McMillan R, Longmire RL, Tavassoli M, et al. In vitro platelet phagocytosis by ITP splenic leukocytes in idiopathic thrombocytopenic purpura. N Engl J Med 1974; 290:249–51.

43. Tsubakio T, Kurata Y, Kanayama Y, et al. In vitro platelet phagocytosis in idiopathic thrombocytopenic purpura. Acta Haematol 1983;70:250–6.

44. Shulman NR, Weinrach RS, Libre EP, et al. The role of the reticuloendothelial system in the pathogenesis of idiopathic thrombocytopenic purpura. Trans Assoc Am Physicians 1965;78:374–90.

45. Clarkson SB, Bussel JB, Kimberly RP, et al. Treatment of refractory immune thrombocytopenic purpura with anti-Fcg-receptor antibody. N Engl J Med 1986;314:1236–9.

46. McMillan R, Bowditch R, Tani P, et al. A non-thrombocytopenic bleeding disorder due to an IgG4-kappa anti-GPIIb/III a autoantibody. Br J Haematol 1996;95: 747–9.

47. Hauch TW, Rosse WF. Platelet-bound complement (C3) in immune thrombocytopenia. Blood 1977;50:1129–36.

48. Kurata Y, Curd JG, Tamerius JD, et al. Platelet-associated complement in chronic ITP. Br J Haematol 1985;60:723–33.

49. McMillan R, Martin M. Fixation of the third component of complement (C3) to platelets in vitro by antiplatelet antibody for patients with ITP. Br J Haematol 1981;47:251–6.

50. Dameshek W, Miller EB. The megakaryocytes in idiopathic thrombocytopenic purpura, a form of hypersplenism. Blood 1946;1:27–52.

51. Pisciotta AV, Stefanini M, Dameshek W. Studies on platelets. X. Morphologic characteristics of megakaryocytes by phase contrast microscopy in normals and in patients with idiopathic thrombocytopenic purpura. Blood 1953;8:703–23.

52. Diggs LW, Hewlett JS. A study of the bone marrow from thirty-six patients with idiopathic hemorrhagic (thrombopenic) purpura. Blood 1948;3: 1090–104.

53. Stahl CP, Zucker-Franklin D, McDonald TP. Incomplete antigenic cross-reactivity between platelets and megakaryocytes: relevance to ITP. Blood 1986;67:421–8.

54. Houwerzijl EJ, Blom NR, van der Want JJL, et al. Ultrastructural study shows morphological features of apoptosis and para-apoptosis in megakaryocytes from patients with idiopathic thrombocytopenic purpura. Blood 2004;103:500–6.

55. Heyns AP, Lotter MG, Badenhorst PN, et al. Kinetics and sites of destruction of 111-Indium-oxine-labeled platelets in idiopathic thrombocytopenic purpura: a quantitative study. Am J Hematol 1982;12:167–77.

56. McMillan R, Wang L, Tomer A, et al. Suppression of in vitro megakaryocyte production by antiplatelet autoantibodies from adult chronic ITP patients. Blood 2004;103:1364–9.

57. Chang M, Nakagawa PA, Williams SA, et al. Immune thrombocytopenic purpura (ITP) plasma and purified ITP monoclonal autoantibodies inhibit megakaryocytopoiesis in vitro. Blood 2003;102:887–95.

58. Bussel JB, Kuter DJ, Pullarkat V, et al. Safety and efficacy of long-term treatment with romiplostim in thrombocytopenic patients with chronic ITP. Lancet 2009;113: 2161–71.

59. Bussel JB, Provan D, Shamsi T, et al. Effect of eltrombopag on platelet counts and bleeding during treatment of chronic idiopathic thrombocytopenic purpura: a randomized, double-blind, placebo-controlled trial. Lancet 2009;373:641–8.

Infections, Antigen-Presenting Cells, T Cells, and Immune Tolerance: Their Role in the Pathogenesis of Immune Thrombocytopenia

John W. Semple, PhD[a,b,c,d,e,f],*

KEYWORDS

- Autoimmunity • Platelets • Thrombocytopenia
- T lymphocytes • Immune tolerance

The mammalian immune system has evolved to produce an extraordinary potential for making receptors that sense and neutralize any foreign entity entering the body. Inevitably, some of these receptors recognize components of our own body, and so cellular mechanisms have evolved to control the activity of these "forbidden" receptors and to achieve immunologic self-tolerance. Thus, autoimmunity is present in everyone to some extent, but it is usually harmless and probably a universal phenomenon of vertebrate life. Autoimmunity, however, can be the cause of a broad spectrum of human illnesses and occurs when there is progression from benign autoimmunity to pathogenic autoimmunity. This progression is determined by at least 3 major mechanisms: genetic influences, immune dysregulation, and environmental triggers. Autoimmune diseases can strike any part of the body, and thus symptoms vary widely and

[a] Keenan Research Centre, Li Ka Shing Knowledge Institute, St Michael's Hospital, 30 Bond Street, Toronto, Ontario M5B 1W8, Canada
[b] Department of Pharmacology, University of Toronto, Toronto, Ontario, Canada
[c] Department of Medicine, University of Toronto, Toronto, Ontario, Canada
[d] Department of Laboratory Medicine and Pathobiology, University of Toronto, Toronto, Ontario, Canada
[e] Canadian Blood Services, Toronto, Ontario, Canada
[f] Toronto Platelet Immunobiology Group, Toronto, Ontario, Canada
* Keenan Research Centre, Li Ka Shing Knowledge Institute, St Michael's Hospital, 30 Bond Street, Toronto, Ontario M5B 1W8, Canada.
E-mail address: semplej@smh.toronto.on.ca

Hematol Oncol Clin N Am 23 (2009) 1177–1192
doi:10.1016/j.hoc.2009.08.007
0889-8588/09/$ – see front matter © 2009 Elsevier Inc. All rights reserved.

diagnosis and treatments are often difficult. Some autoimmune diseases can be life threatening unless properly diagnosed and treated. Chronic autoimmune disorders affect up to 7% of the human population and create heavy burdens not only on patients' families but also on the society. Understanding the immunopathogenesis of autoimmunity is a critical step in designing effective therapeutic modalities to reduce the burden caused by these chronic illnesses.

Immune thrombocytopenia (ITP) is an autoimmune bleeding disorder characterized by the production of autoreactive antibodies against one's own platelets, resulting in increased platelet destruction by phagocytic macrophages in the reticuloendothelial system. It is also recognized that in ITP, platelet autoantibodies are primarily of the IgG3 and IgG1 isotypes, although less prevalent IgM and IgA autoantibodies targeted against glycoprotein (Gp) IIb/IIIa and GpIb-IX also exist.[1-7] The age-adjusted prevalence of ITP has been estimated to be 9.5 per 100,000 persons in the United States, whereas its annual incidence is estimated to be 2.68 per 100,000 in Northern Europe (at a cut off platelet count<100 $\times$ 10^9/L).[8]

ITP used to be distinguished into 2 forms, acute and chronic, but an international working group of recognized experts convened a consensus conference in October 2007 and significantly revised the definitions and recommendations of the clinical diagnosis of ITP.[9] Primary ITP is now defined as an autoimmune disorder characterized by isolated thrombocytopenia (peripheral blood platelet count<100 $\times$ 10^9/L) in the absence of other causes or disorders that may be associated with thrombocytopenia.[9] The phases of ITP are divided based on the time since diagnosis; newly diagnosed ITP occurs within 3 months from diagnosis, persistent ITP occurs between 3 and 12 months from diagnosis, and chronic ITP is now defined as thrombocytopenia lasting for more than 12 months.[9] The term "severe ITP" is reserved for conditions where there are bleeding symptoms at presentation or the occurrence of new bleeding symptoms requiring therapeutic intervention.[9] The term "acute," which was used to describe a self-limited form of the disease (eg, secondary to viral illness in children), was avoided because of its vagueness and its post hoc or retrospective definition.[9]

Newly diagnosed and persistent ITP in children often occurs after a viral or bacterial infection and usually spontaneously resolves within 6 months of diagnosis, but in approximately 10% of children, the disease progresses to the chronic form.[1-9] In contrast to childhood ITP, chronic ITP is predominantly found in adults, with more women being affected than men.[1-9] Although both childhood ITP and adult ITP are immune mediated, the pathophysiologic mechanisms may be different.[10-13] This article discusses the infectious nature of childhood and adult ITP and primarily focuses on the autoreactive T-cell abnormalities that appear to be responsible for breaking immune tolerance and for initiating the autoimmune attack against platelets.

THE INFECTIOUS NATURE OF NEWLY DIAGNOSED AND CHRONIC ITP

Relatively little research has focused on the cellular immunology of ITP in children.[10-13] However, because this form of the disease often follows an infectious event, it suggests that childhood ITP may be associated with the immune mechanisms stimulated by the preceding infection. For example, in children with ITP associated with varicella-zoster virus (VZV) infection, Wright and colleagues[14] demonstrated that the patient's serum IgM and IgG antiplatelet autoantibodies could be purified on affinity columns conjugated with VZV Gps and that the eluted IgG molecules were cross reactive with normal group O-positive platelets. At the T-cell level, however, antiplatelet reactive T-cell activity in these children with VZV-associated ITP was no different from what was observed in healthy individuals, which suggested that T cells in this disorder were not necessarily directed against platelet antigens.[10,11,14] Analogous findings were found with HIV Gps and sera from patients with immune thrombocytopenia associated with HIV infection.[15] Taken together, these initial reports suggested a hypothesis that at least in some children with ITP, antiplatelet antibodies are simply a result of molecular mimicry mechanisms, antiviral antibodies cross reacting with the patient's own platelets. This may explain why the thrombocytopenia in most children (eg, due to antigenic mimicry) spontaneously resolves by itself; as the antiviral immune response subsides or affinity matures toward the virus, the cross-reactive antiplatelet antibody response is lost.

Using a similar approach, Takahashi and colleagues[16] suggested a role for molecular mimicry in 20 Japanese patients with chronic ITP associated with *Helicobacter pylori* infection. Patients who completely responded to *H pylori* eradication therapy showed increased platelet counts concomitantly with significant declines in platelet-associated IgG (PAIgG) levels. Platelet eluates from 12 of the patients recognized *H pylori* cytotoxin-associated gene A (CagA) protein. The cross reactivity between PAIgG and *H pylori* CagA protein suggested that molecular mimicry by CagA may play a key role in the pathogenesis of a subset of chronic ITP patients.

Molecular mimicry has also been shown in patients with immune thrombocytopenia associated with HIV and hepatitis C infection. Nardi and colleagues[17,18] showed in a series of elegant experiments that HIV-associated ITP was associated with the production of a particular IgG antibody that reacted with an epitope composed of amino acid residues 49 to 66 of the platelet GpIIIa molecule. Binding of the antibody caused a GpIIIa conformational change that stimulated the platelet's 12-lipoxygenase system to produce 12(S)-hydroxyeicosatetraenoic acid, which then stimulated nicotinamide adenine dinucleotide phosphate oxidase to generate superoxide that subsequently mediated platelet fragmentation. Zhang and colleagues[19] have demonstrated that hepatitis C infection can also lead to the generation of antibodies that recognize the GpIIIa 49 to 66 amino acid sequence, and binding of these antibodies also leads to platelet fragmentation via superoxide production. The reasons why these antibodies induce platelet fragmentation are unknown, but the same group has suggested that antibody binding requires a specific conformation of GpIIIa that stimulates the subsequent fragmentation.[20] It is intriguing that 2 different viruses can stimulate antibodies of identical antiplatelet specificity; however, the significance of this phenomenon is not clear. In contrast, however, Peterson and colleagues[21,22] and Aster[23] have previously shown that IgG antibodies from patients with quinine-induced immune thrombocytopenia can also recognize the same peptide sequence (GpIIIa 49–66), yet the quinine-dependent antibodies appear not to be capable of inducing platelet fragmentation. Why the autoantibodies identified by Zhang and colleagues[19] have this unusual property is not fully understood, but further studies of this process at the molecular level could lead to characterization of a new mechanism for immune-mediated cytopenia.[23]

On the other hand, in some patients with chronic ITP, infections are associated with an exacerbation of thrombocytopenia, and this has also been demonstrated in a mouse model of immune thrombocytopenia.[24] Alternatively, eradication of the gram-negative bacterium *H pylori* in patients with ITP increases platelet counts, although this has not been observed in some studies.[25–27] It is possible that, in susceptible individuals, infectious agents in the presence of antiplatelet antibodies affect platelet-monocyte interactions and alter platelet destruction. Pathogens are first encountered by toll-like receptors (TLRs) on phagocytes.[28–30] TLRs are germline-encoded proteins that bind various infectious molecular structures and are critical for stimulating innate immune mechanisms.[28–30] The seminal studies of Janeway and colleagues[28] elegantly showed that TLRs are responsible for focusing infectious agents to antigen-presenting cells (APCs) for their presentation to the T cells of the adaptive immune system, the critical link between innate and adaptive immune defenses.[28–30] TLRs are also expressed on many cell types including platelets,[31–40] and platelet TLR4 expression, at least, seems responsible for mediating lipopolysaccharide (LPS)-induced thrombocytopenia in vivo.[34,35] Using an in vitro phagocytosis assay, the authors demonstrated that LPS together with IgG autoantibodies bound to human platelets significantly enhanced Fc-mediated platelet phagocytosis by mononuclear phagocytes.[41] These in vitro observations were subsequently confirmed in vivo when mice injected with antiplatelet antibody together with only picogram doses of LPS became profoundly thrombocytopenic compared with control mice injected with only the antiplatelet antibody.[42] Intravenous immunoglobulin treatment of the LPS/antibody-treated mice was ineffective in raising the platelet counts in contrast to antibody-treated control mice.[42] Perhaps more importantly, Asahi and colleagues[43] demonstrated that the improvements in platelet counts in patients with ITP after initiating H pylori eradication therapy were associated with decreased platelet phagocytosis and modulation of the inhibitory Fcγ receptor IIB in peripheral blood monocytes. Taken together, these results suggest that infectious agents in combination with an already established antiplatelet antibody response can significantly affect platelet destruction in vitro and in vivo. This may be at least 1 explanation of why thrombocytopenia worsens in some patients with chronic ITP during infections and, alternatively, resolves in other patients with chronic ITP who are treated with bacterial eradication therapy.[41]

Thus, it seems that infectious agents play a significant role in either initiating the immune mechanisms responsible for platelet destruction or affecting immune platelet destruction by an already established antiplatelet immune response (**Fig. 1**). Infectious agents may also significantly influence how innate immune responses, for example, antigen processing and presentation, affect the autoimmune adaptive immune system and alter autoimmune platelet attack.

GENETIC STUDIES IN ITP

Expression of certain human leukocyte antigen (HLA) molecules is known to be associated with many autoimmune diseases and may predispose the host to autoimmunity.[44] This predisposition is probably because of how polymorphic HLA molecules present antigens to autoreactive T helper (T_H) cells. For certain autoimmune diseases, it has been possible to identify short stretches of amino acids within the polymorphic regions of HLA molecules that appear to play a major role in disease susceptibility and/or resistance.[45] Although early studies in Caucasian patients suggested that ITP may be associated with HLA class I and class II molecules,[46–49] subsequent studies failed to show any HLA association with ITP.[50,51] These apparent inconsistencies may be because of the small number of patients studied or also because of differing autoimmune causes that may exist within populations of ITP patients. Further studies with large patient populations are needed to ascertain which HLA molecules (if any) may be associated with chronic ITP. In contrast, examination of HLA serotypes and alleles in Japanese patients with ITP have suggested an association of HLA with antiplatelet antibody production.[52,53] Given the distinctive HLA diversity across the major ethnic groups,[54] differences in disease associations between HLA genes and phenotypes with ITP might be expected. For example, the distribution of HLA alleles within the Caucasian population is more heterogeneous than that in the Japanese population, and hence, HLA association studies may be more difficult to demonstrate. Nonetheless, it seems that to date, there is no firm evidence of HLA association within patients with ITP.

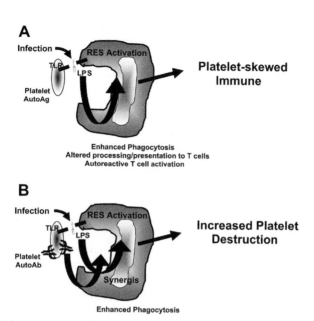

Fig. 1. Potential mechanism of how infectious events can alter platelet immunity and/or destruction. (A) In newly diagnosed ITP, an infectious particle (LPS [lipopolysaccharide]) binds to the platelet toll-like receptors (TLRs) and as the platelet traverses the spleen, presents the LPS to TLR-expressing macrophages. This event could affect several processes, such as the kinetics of platelet phagocytosis, altered platelet autoantigen (autoAg) processing, and potential presentation to autoreactive T cells, leading to their activation. These events could ultimately lead to a skewing toward an antiplatelet autoreactive response. (B) In patients with chronic ITP, the presence of platelet autoantibodies (autoAb) maintains a level of enhanced platelet destruction via FcR-mediated phagocytosis. On infection, the autoAb opsonized platelets can additionally present infectious particles (LPS) to the macrophages, causing a synergistic response between FcR and TLR intracellular signaling mechanism, which can ultimately result in greater platelet phagocytosis and destruction, leading to even lower platelet counts. As the infection subsides, the platelet phagocytosis is reset to preinfection levels, and platelet counts rise again.

Fc receptor (FcR)-mediated destruction of antibody-sensitized platelets is the primary immune pathophysiology of ITP, and allelic variants exist for some FcRs. The variants represent single nucleotide polymorphisms, leading to functional differences in the ability of APCs to bind IgG subclasses. Studies have attempted to understand if these variants may have a role to play in ITP. For example, a comparison of cytokine and low-affinity $Fc\gamma R$ polymorphisms revealed an association between the proinflammatory cytokines tumor necrosis factor α and lymphotoxin A with $Fc\gamma R3A$ and $Fc\gamma R3B$.[55] It was suggested that variant genotypes of $Fc\gamma Rs$ and cytokines might contribute to the pathogenesis of chronic ITP. However, it remains to be determined whether these associations are important for the initiation of the disease or for the perpetuation of the disorder. In a subsequent study, the genotypic frequencies for 2 FcR single nucleotide polymorphisms, FcRIIa-131 arginine (A) versus histidine (H) and FcRIIIa-158 valine (V) versus phenylalanine (F), were examined in 98 children diagnosed with ITP and the genotype frequencies were compared with those of 130 healthy subjects.[56] It was determined that the FcRIIa-131H and the FcRIIIa-158V were significantly overrepresented in the children with ITP than in the control subjects.

However, there was no statistical difference between children who later developed chronic ITP and children with newly diagnosed ITP, suggesting that additional factors may be responsible for the development of the chronic form of the disease.[56]

To search for novel mechanisms that might contribute to the pathophysiology of ITP, Sood and colleagues[57] used DNA microarrays and determined the whole blood gene expression profile in 5 patients with ITP. They found 176 cDNAs that were strongly correlated with ITP, which included a cluster of interferon-regulated genes and TLR7, and many less-well-characterized genes. These types of studies may likely yield new insights into the understanding of the molecular pathophysiology of ITP; however, genetic studies in ITP are still not complete compared with those performed for other autoimmune diseases.

APCS IN CHRONIC ITP

Chronic ITP seems to be a true organ-specific autoimmune disorder. It rarely remits spontaneously. There is usually no previous history of an infectious event, and it almost always requires some form of immunosuppressive therapy.[58,59] The antibody specificities are directed against several platelet Gp epitopes.[1–7] Since 1991, many investigators have demonstrated that the chronic form of the disorder is associated with T-cell–related and cytokine abnormalities, which appear to be responsible for the production of IgG antiplatelet autoantibodies.[10–13]

All IgG responses, including autoreactive IgG, against protein antigens are initiated by activated T_H cells that recognize their cognate antigens on APCs, such as major histocompatibility complex (MHC) class II positive dendritic cells (DCs) or macrophages.[60–70] APCs function to internalize protein antigens and proteolytically process them into small peptides so that they can be inserted into the antigen-binding groove of MHC molecules and then reexpressed on the APC surface membrane.[61,62] The MHC-peptide complex is then examined by various T cells that migrate through either the spleen or the lymph nodes.[61,62] T cells having sufficient TcR-MHC/peptide affinity together with appropriate APC-dependent costimulatory events (eg, CD28-CD80/86 interaction and cytokine production) become activated and mediate immune effector functions, such as immunoglobulin class switching from IgM to, for example, IgG or initiation of cytotoxic T lymphocyte (CTL) activation.[65–68]

Several reports have described a role for platelets in affecting antigen processing and presentation events within APCs and also how platelets may affect APCs derived from patients with ITP.[71–78] For example, several publications have suggested that platelets can interact with potent APCs, such as DCs, and affect their activation and differentiation.[71–78] In particular, Catani and colleagues[71] studied CD14-derived DCs from 29 patients with chronic ITP and demonstrated that platelets from the ITP patients, either fresh or aged in vitro, showed increased apoptosis (with low levels of activation) in comparison with their normal counterparts.[71] Furthermore, when patients' DCs were prepulsed with either autologous or allogeneic platelets, they were able to efficiently stimulate autologous T-cell proliferation compared with DCs derived from healthy donors.[71] This observation correlated with upregulated expression of the costimulatory molecule CD86 on DCs from ITP patients.[71] It was concluded that DC dysfunction, together with increased propensity of platelets to undergo apoptosis, may play a significant role in the stimulation of autoimmunity in patients with ITP. This underscores the importance of focusing on how the innate immune responses involving APCs could significantly affect an autoimmune platelet-specific environment.

A BRIEF OVERVIEW OF THE HISTORY OF T-CELL INVOLVEMENT IN CHRONIC ITP

T-cell abnormalities in ITP have been reported since the early 1970s, although most of the early reports either did not recognize the association of ITP with T cells or were early phenotypic studies.[10–13] Nonetheless, these early studies were the beginnings of what has become an important and intriguing area of research in ITP pathogenesis. In 1991, the authors reported that chronic ITP was associated with a CD4$^+$ T_H-cell defect in which peripheral blood T cells could secrete interleukin (IL) 2 on stimulation with platelets.[79] This suggested that chronic ITP may be the result of an abnormal T_H-cell defect that could direct autoreactive B cells to differentiate and secrete IgG autoantibodies. These results were subsequently confirmed by Ware and Howard[80] and, since then, many reports have been published describing various T-cell and cytokine abnormalities in patients with chronic ITP.[10–13] Filion and colleagues[81] reported that healthy individuals contained anergic T_H cells, which could be activated in vitro after incubation with platelet GpIIb-IIIa and exogenous IL-2; once this tolerance was broken, however, the T_H cells could secrete their own IL-2 on stimulation with GpIIb-IIIa. These results were the first to suggest that T-cell tolerance against platelet autoantigens was somehow broken in the pathogenesis of ITP, and this may involve the posttranscriptional regulation of IL-2 expression. Subsequently, Shimomura and colleagues[82] demonstrated that in the peripheral blood of patients with chronic ITP, there was an oligoclonal accumulation of CD4$^+$ T_H cells that frequently used Vβ3, 6, 10, 13.1 and 14 genes for their T-cell receptors. This group concluded that distinctive T-cell clones accumulated in patients with chronic ITP and were related to the disease pathogenesis.[82] Subsequently, the authors and other investigators reported that children and adults with chronic ITP have a serum cytokine profile suggesting a T_H0/T_H1 (IL-2/IL-10/interferon gamma) activation pattern.[83–88] Taken together, these results were the beginnings of a movement that suggested that chronic ITP is associated with abnormal autoreactive T-cell activation that may have resulted from a breakdown in tolerance mechanisms and that may be defective in its regulatory functions.

T CELLS AND ITP IN THE NEW MILLENNIUM

Building on the early results, Kuwana and colleagues[89] demonstrated that T cells from Japanese patients with chronic ITP could proliferate in vitro in response to disulfide-reduced GpIIb-IIIa or the molecule's tryptic peptides. This suggested that autoreactive CD4$^+$ T_H cells in chronic ITP need to recognize a modified GpIIb-IIIa molecule, implying that antigen processing mechanisms within recipient APCs may be required to present GpIIb-IIIa autoantigens in the context of self-HLA-DR molecules. Subsequently, they attempted to map the antigen specificity of the T_H cells by using 6 large (approximately 200 amino acid residues) recombinant fragments encoding different portions of the GpIIbα and GpIIIa chains.[90] They demonstrated that the T cells from patients with ITP recognized primarily the amino terminal portion of the 2 Gp chains (GpIIbα18-259 and GpIIIa22-262) and that these molecules also stimulated the production of antiplatelet autoantibodies.[90] Sukati and colleagues,[91] who published the first report of the fine specificity of CD4$^+$ T_H cells from Caucasian patients with chronic ITP, used 15-mer peptides of the GpIIIa chain. This work revealed that several immunodominant peptides spanning the entire breadth of the GpIIIa molecule stimulated T cells. It was intriguing that despite a lack of HLA association observed in Caucasian patients with ITP,[50–53] some patients in the peptide mapping study apparently recognized common elements on the GpIIIa molecule.[91] Although preliminary, this may suggest that either a host (eg, antigen processing) or an environmental factor (eg, infection) could be responsible for generating a common autoepitope that is presented to T cells across different HLA. If this were true, it would be an efficacious way of developing peptide antigen-specific T-cell therapies for autoantibody production and subsequent platelet destruction in ITP. Collectively, these studies have clearly linked the T-cell abnormalities in chronic ITP with the processing and presentation pathways of platelet antigens within APCs, and further research is warranted to better understand the detailed nature of these pathways in an attempt to identify novel therapeutic targets for the disorder.

In addition to the T-cell recognition studies, there have also been several exciting concepts related to T-cell abnormalities in patients with ITP. Since the turn of this century, perhaps the most important discovery in ITP has been that of Olsson and colleagues,[92] who elegantly demonstrated that in patients with ITP, devoid of platelet autoantibodies, thrombocytopenia can be mediated by CD8[+] T cells. Patients with active disease had peripheral blood CTL that could bind to platelets in vitro and cause significant lysis of the platelets, whereas those patients in remission had little antiplatelet CTL reactivity.[92] This seminal observation was confirmed in a large clinical study reported by Zhang and colleagues.[93] Furthermore, Sabnani and Tsang[94] studied a small population of patients with chronic ITP who failed various treatment regimens for ITP, including steroids, gamma globulins, splenectomy, and rituximab. They found a limited T-cell clonopathy in the patients with persistent chronic ITP and concluded not only that ITP has heterogeneous biologic mechanisms but also that patients should be evaluated for T-cell clonality and those failing standard therapies should be considered for treatment options that are directed against cytotoxic T cells. Thus, in those patients with chronic ITP who do not have any detectable autoantibodies and who fail standard treatment options, platelets and/or megakaryocytes may be destroyed or inhibited by T-cell–mediated mechanisms in the spleen and/or the bone marrow respectively. These results might suggest that different therapeutic strategies need to be developed to combat these different reactions.

Perhaps the newest concept of immune dysregulation in autoimmunity is that tolerance-inducing regulatory T cells (Tregs) are usually reduced in number and function in several autoimmune conditions.[95–108] Tregs are the critical lymphocytes that are essential in maintaining peripheral tolerance, preventing autoimmune disease, and limiting chronic inflammatory diseases.[95] Tregs have a unique surface expression profile, including CD25, CD62L, and specific CD45 isoforms, and a Treg-cell–specific transcription factor termed Foxp3.[95–104] There are several subpopulations of Treg cells, such as CD4[+]CD25[+]Foxp3[+] T cells,[100–104] transforming growth factor β (TGF-β)-producing T_H3 cells,[100–104] and CD3[+]CD4[−]CD8[−]T cells.[100–104] The so-called natural (n) Tregs (nTregs) are generated in the thymus and are generally anergic to antigenic stimulation but can inhibit proliferation of CD4[+] T_H cells via direct cell contact.[95–108] Thus, the ability to isolate these nTregs holds the promise of immunosuppressive therapy; however, because they constitute only approximately 3% of circulating CD4[+] T cells, their numbers are far too small to be clinically effective. On the other hand, inducible Tregs (iTregs) can be generated in the periphery from nonregulatory CD4[+]CD25[−] T cells, and although they share the phenotype and in vitro suppressive activities of nTreg, they are activated in an antigen-specific fashion.[100–104] In addition, although iTregs can be induced from CD4[+] T cells, it is not known whether these cells function in healthy subjects or whether they could be produced from the peripheral blood of patients with autoimmune diseases. Nonetheless, it is becoming increasingly clear not only that Tregs are the master regulators of immune tolerance mechanisms but also that their deficiency and/or dysregulation may be the critical factor that leads to autoimmunity.[100]

In 2007, 3 reports extended the original observations of Filion and colleagues[81] showing that a breakdown in tolerance induction may be the primary abnormality responsible for ITP induction.[109–111] All 3 reports showed significantly reduced numbers of circulating $CD4^+CD25^+Foxp3^+$ Treg cells in patients with chronic ITP.[109–111] One of them demonstrated that within 4 days after treatment with high-dose dexamethasone (HDDXM), the deficient Treg populations were significantly increased.[110] This increase was correlated with increased platelet counts by 1 week post HDDXM treatment. Their results suggested not only that Treg cells were deficient in patients with chronic ITP but also that therapy may, at least, modulate platelet counts by increasing Treg numbers to perhaps stabilize tolerance mechanisms.

Several noncontrolled trials have demonstrated that rituximab therapy seems efficacious in raising the platelet counts in patients with ITP with an approximate 62% response rate.[112,113] The mechanism of action of rituximab in ITP has been assumed to be due to the selective depletion of $CD20^+$ B cells that subsequently affects auto-antibody development.[114,115] But Stasi and colleagues[114] showed that rituximab actually raised platelet counts in patients with ITP by normalizing faulty T-cell responses resulting from the destruction of the B-cell mass. They further elucidated this surprising finding by demonstrating that the anti-B cell therapy works by specifically restoring defective Tregs in patients with ITP.[115] They suggested that patients with active ITP have a defective Treg compartment that can be significantly modulated by B-cell–targeted therapy. The reasons for these results are not clear but may relate to how B-cell populations may be important in maintaining autoreactive T-cell activation patterns. Alternatively, decreasing the total mass of B cells may cause a collapse of autoreactive T-cell stimulation and normalization of the T-cell repertoire as the B cells begin to return months after the therapy.[115]

Together with Stasi and colleagues' article, 2 other reports were published concurrently that also showed that patients with chronic ITP have reduced numbers of Treg cells and that the Tregs were functionally defective in that they could not suppress T_H-cell activation.[116,117] Olsson and colleagues[116] studied the bone marrow and peripheral blood of patients with chronic ITP and found, particularly in the bone marrow, increased number of infiltrating activated $CD3^+$ T cells with elevated surface expression of VLA-4 and CX3CR1.[116] Compared with healthy controls, the increased T-cell number in the bone marrow was associated with significantly lower number of bone marrow Tregs, suggesting that chronic ITP may be a disease of increased T-cell activation due to a T_{reg} defect within the bone marrow, and this may contribute to suppressed megakaryocyte production in ITP. This latter novel concept is analogous to the studies of MacMillan and colleagues,[118] who demonstrated that autoantibodies from patients with ITP could effectively kill megakaryocytes in vitro. These pathogenic CTL- and autoantibody-mediated mechanisms may be responsible for the notion that bone marrow production of platelets in patients with chronic ITP is faulty or suppressed.

Zhang and colleagues[119] studied whether the defective nTregs from the peripheral blood of patients with ITP could be stimulated in vitro to generate iTregs. They found that platelet Gp-specific iTregs could be generated de novo from nonregulatory $CD4^+CD25^-CD45RA^+$ cells, and these cells could mediate antigen-specific and linked suppression of proliferating $CD4^+$ T_H cells. They found that the iTregs mediated their suppressive effects on T_H cells by modulating the T-cell stimulatory capacity of DCs. A genome-wide assessment of DC changes induced by the antigen-specific iTregs found that TLR Notch and TGF-β signaling pathways were related to the antigen-specific tolerance. These pathways are known to be intimately associated with both pro-and anti-inflammatory responses, and it may be that the balance

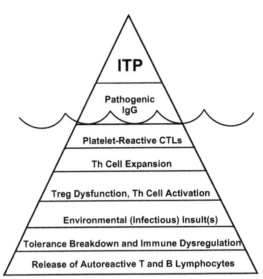

Fig. 2. Underlying immune defects that lead to platelet autoantibody production and ITP. Normally, small numbers of autoreactive T cells are released from the thymus gland and are kept under check by peripheral immune tolerance mechanisms. Abnormal immune dysregulation, either alone or together with an insult (eg, infection), may alter or break tolerance, which results in the abnormal activation of platelet autoreactive T cells. The autoreactive T cells expand to numbers that can potentially activate autoreactive cytotoxic T cells and/or autoantibody production, leading ultimately to enhanced platelet destruction. Thus, targeting the mechanisms of abnormal T-cell activation or tolerance defects are potential ways to significantly alter the autoimmune attack against platelets.

between these DC pathways ultimately control the development of platelet autoimmunity. This study suggests that antigen-specific iTregs may be produced from patients with ITP for antigen-targeted cellular immunotherapy.[119] Taken together, these studies suggest that therapeutically targeting T cells in ITP, even indirectly by the destruction of B cells, is a significant way to effectively reduce platelet destruction and raise platelet counts. It is becoming clear that the presence of antiplatelet antibodies leading to thrombocytopenia may be just the tip of the iceberg in patients with ITP. It now seems that antiplatelet autoantibody production is intimately associated with abnormal T-cell regulation and effector mechanisms that ultimately control the pathogenesis of the disorder (**Fig. 2**).

SUMMARY

The immunopathogenic cause of ITP is not well understood, although there is overwhelming evidence to suggest that a generalized dysfunction of autoreactive T cell is the critical immunopathologic cause of ITP. Disruption of T cells or any of the processes that maintain tolerance of platelet self-antigens are more than likely the potential root cause of the onset of ITP. Superimposed on these abnormal processes are genetic and environmental factors that are also likely to play a significant role in the production of autoantibodies in ITP. More research is warranted to clearly map the underlying immune defects in ITP, and this should lead to the development of more antigen-specific therapies for this bleeding disorder.

REFERENCES

1. Stasi R, Evangelista ML, Stipa E, et al. Idiopathic thrombocytopenic purpura: current concepts in pathophysiology and management. Thromb Haemost 2008;99:4–13.
2. Cines DB, Blanchette VS. Immune thrombocytopenic purpura. N Engl J Med 2002;346:995–1008.
3. Hou M, Stockelberg D, Kutti J, et al. Antibodies against GPIb/IX, GPIIb/IIIa, and other platelet antigens in chronic idiopathic thrombocytopenic purpura. Eur J Haematol 1995;55:307–14.
4. Mehta YS, Pathare AV, Badakere SS, et al. Influence of auto-antibody specificities on the clinical course in patients with chronic and acute ITP. Platelets 2000;11:94–8.
5. Fabris F, Scandellari R, Ruzzon E, et al. Platelet-associated autoantibodies as detected by a solid-phase modified antigen capture ELISA test (MACE) are a useful prognostic factor in idiopathic thrombocytopenic purpura. Blood 2004;103:4562–4.
6. Zhou B, Zhao H, Yang RC, et al. Multi-dysfunctional pathophysiology in ITP. Crit Rev Oncol Hematol 2005;54:107–16.
7. Cines DB, Bussel JB, Liebman HA, et al. The ITP Syndrome: pathogenic and clinical diversity. Blood 2009;113:6511–21.
8. Michel M. Immune thrombocytopenic purpura: epidemiology and implications for patients. Eur J Haematol 2009;82(Suppl 71):3–7.
9. Rodeghiero F, Stasi R, Gernsheimer T, et al. Standardization of terminology, definitions and outcome criteria in immune thrombocytopenic purpura of adults and children: report from an international working group. Blood 2009;113:2386–93.
10. Semple JW, Freedman J. Abnormal cellular immune mechanisms associated with autoimmune thrombocytopenia. Transfus Med Rev 1995;9:327–38.
11. Semple JW. Immunobiology of T helper cells and antigen-presenting cells in autoimmune thrombocytopenic purpura (ITP). Acta Paediatr Suppl 1998;424:41–5.
12. Coopamah M, Garvey MB, Freedman J, et al. Cellular immune mechanisms in autoimmune thrombocytopenic purpura: an update. Transfus Med Rev 2003;17:69–80.
13. Cooper N, Bussel J. The pathogenesis of immune thrombocytopaenic purpura. Br J Haematol 2006;133:364–74.
14. Wright JF, Blanchette V, Wang H, et al. Characterization of platelet-reactive antibodies in children with varicella-associated acute immune thrombocytopenic purpura (ITP). Br J Haematol 1996;95:145–52.
15. Chia WK, Blanchette V, Mody M, et al. Characterization of HIV-1-specific antibodies and HIV-1-crossreactive antibodies to platelets in HIV-1-infected haemophiliac patients. Br J Haematol 1998;103:1014–22.
16. Takahashi T, Yujiri T, Shinohara K, et al. Molecular mimicry by *Helicobacter pylori* CagA protein may be involved in the pathogenesis of *H. pylori*-associated chronic idiopathic thrombocytopenic purpura. Br J Haematol 2004;124:91–6.
17. Nardi M, Tomlinson S, Greco M, et al. Complement-independent, peroxide-induced antibody lysis of platelets in HIV-1-related immune thrombocytopenia. Cell 2000;106:551–61.
18. Nardi M, Feinmark SJ, Hu L, et al. Complement-independent Ab-induced peroxide lysis of platelets requires 12-lipoxygenase and a platelet NADPH oxidase pathway. J Clin Invest 2004;113:973–80.
19. Zhang W, Nardi MA, Borkowsky W, et al. Role of molecular mimicry of HCV protein with platelet GPIIIa in hepatitis C–related immunologic thrombocytopenia. Blood 2009;113:4086–93.

20. Li Z, Nardi MA, Wu J, et al. Platelet fragmentation requires a specific structural conformation of human monoclonal antibody against beta3 integrin. J Biol Chem 2008;283:3224–30.

21. Peterson JA, Nyree CE, Newman PJ, et al. A site involving the "hybrid" and PSI homology domains of GPIIIa (beta 3-integrin subunit) is a common target for antibodies associated with quinine-induced immune thrombocytopenia. Blood 2003;101:937–42.

22. Peterson JA, Nelson TN, Kanack AJ, et al. Fine specificity of drug-dependent antibodies reactive with a restricted domain of platelet GPIIIA. Blood 2008; 111:1234–9.

23. Aster RH. Molecular mimicry and immune thrombocytopenia. Blood 2009;113: 3887–8.

24. Musaji A, Cormont F, Thirion G, et al. Exacerbation of autoantibody-mediated thrombocytopenic purpura by infection with mouse viruses. Blood 2004;104: 2102–6.

25. Gasbarrini A, Fracechi F, Tartaglione R, et al. Regression of autoimmune thrombocytopenia after eradication of *Helicobacter pylori*. Lancet 1998;352:878–9.

26. Jarque I, Andreu R, Llopis I, et al. Absence of platelet response after eradication of *Helicobacter pylori* infection in patients with chronic idiopathic thrombocytopenic purpura. Br J Haematol 2001;115:1002–3.

27. Stasi R, Rossi Z, Stipa E, et al. *Helicobacter pylori* eradication in the management of patients with idiopathic thrombocytopenic purpura. Am J Med 2005;118:420–1.

28. Janeway CA Jr. The immune system evolved to discriminate infectious nonself from noninfectious self. Immunol Today 1992;13:11–6.

29. Medzhitov R, Preston-Hurlburt P, Janeway CA Jr. A human homologue of the Drosophila Toll protein signals activation of adaptive immunity. Nature 1997; 388:394–7.

30. Takeda K, Kaisho T, Akira S. Toll-like receptors. Annu Rev Immunol 2003;21: 335–76.

31. Semple JW, Aslam R, Speck ER, et al. Murine platelets express Toll like receptor 2: a potential regulator of innate and adaptive immunity. Platelets 2004;15:267–8.

32. Shiraki R, Inouea N, Kawasaki S, et al. Expression of Toll-like receptors on human platelets. Thromb Res 2004;113:379–85.

33. Cognasse F, Hamzeh H, Chavarin P, et al. Evidence of Toll-like receptor molecules on human platelets. Immunol Cell Biol 2005;88:196–8.

34. Andonegui G, Kerfoot SM, McNagny K, et al. Platelets express functional Toll-like receptor-4 (TLR4). Blood 2005;106:2417–23.

35. Aslam R, Speck ER, Kim M, et al. Platelet Toll-like receptor expression modulates lipopolysaccharide-induced thrombocytopenia and tumor necrosis factor-production in vivo. Blood 2006;107:637–41.

36. Ståhl A-L, Svensson M, Mörgelin M, et al. Lipopolysaccharide from enterohemorrhagic *Escherichia coli* binds to platelets via TLR4 and CD62 and is detected on circulating platelets in patients with hemolytic uremic syndrome. Blood 2006; 108:167–76.

37. Ward JR, Bingle L, Judge HM, et al. Agonists of toll-like receptor (TLR) 2 and TLR 4 are unable to modulate platelet activation by adenosine diphosphate and platelet activating factor. Thromb Haemost 2005;94:831–8.

38. Patrignani P, Di Febbo C, Tacconelli S, et al. Reduced thromboxane biosynthesis in carriers of Toll-like 4 polymorphisms in vivo. Blood 2006;107:3572–4.

39. Clark SR, Ma AC, Tavener SA, et al. Platelet TLR4 activates neutrophil extracellular traps to ensnare bacteria in septic blood. Nat Med 2007;13:463–9.

40. Kuckleburg CJ, Tiwari R, Czuprynski CJ. Endothelial cell apoptosis induced by bacteria-activated platelets requires caspase-8 and -9 and generation of reactive oxygen species. Thromb Haemost 2008;99:363–72.

41. Semple JW, Aslam R, Kim M, et al. Platelet-bound lipopolysaccharide enhances Fc receptor-mediated phagocytosis of IgG opsonized platelets. Blood 2007; 109:4803–5.

42. Tremblay T, Aubin E, Lemieux R, et al. Picogram doses of lipopolysaccharide exacerbate antibody-mediated thrombocytopenia and reduce the therapeutic efficacy of intravenous immunoglobulin in mice. Br J Haematol 2007;139: 297–302.

43. Asahi A, Nishimoto T, Okazaki Y, et al. *Helicobacter pylori* eradication shifts monocyte Fcγ receptor balance toward inhibitory FcγRIIB in immune thrombocytopenic purpura patients. J Clin Invest 2008;118:2939–49.

44. Sinha AA, Lopez T, McDevitt HO. Autoimmune diseases: the failure of self-tolerance. Science 1990;248:1380–8.

45. Schreuder GM, Tilanus MG, Bontrop RE, et al. HLA-DQ polymorphism associated with resistance to type I diabetes detected with monoclonal antibodies, isoelectric point differences, and restriction fragment length polymorphism. J Exp Med 1986;64:938–43.

46. Karpatkin S. Association of HLA-DRw2 with autoimmune thrombocytopenic purpura. J Clin Invest 1979;63:1085–8.

47. El-Khateeb MS, Awidi AS, Tarawneh MS, et al. HLA antigens, blood groups and immunoglobulin levels in idiopathic thrombocytopenic purpura. Acta Haematol 1986;76:110–4.

48. Goebel KM, Hahn E, Havermann K. HLA matching in autoimmune thrombocytopenic purpura. Br J Haematol 1977;35:341–2.

49. Porges A, Bussel J, Kimberly R, et al. Elevation of platelet associated antibody levels in patients with chronic idiopathic thrombocytopenic purpura expressing the B8 and/or DR3 allotypes. Tissue Antigens 1985;26:132–7.

50. Gratama JW, D'Amaro J, deKoning J, et al. The HLA system in immune thrombocytopenic purpura: its relation to the outcome of therapy. Br J Haematol 1984;56:287–93.

51. Gaiger A, Neumeister A, Heinzl H, et al. HLA class I and II antigens in chronic idiopathic autoimmune thrombocytopenia. Ann Hematol 1994;68:299–302.

52. Nomura S, Matsuzaki T, Ozaki Y, et al. Clinical significance of HLA-DRB1*0410 in Japanese patients with idiopathic thrombocytopenic purpura. Blood 1998;91: 3616–22.

53. Kuwana M, Kaburaki J, Pandey JP, et al. HLA class II alleles in Japanese patients with immune thrombocytopenic purpura. Associations with anti-platelets glycoprotein antibodies and responses to splenectomy. Tissue Antigens 2000;56:337–43.

54. Cao K, Hollenbach J, Shi X, et al. Analysis of the frequencies of HLA-A, B, and C alleles and haplotypes in the five major ethnic groups of the United States reveals high levels of diversity in these loci and contrasting distribution patterns in these populations. Hum Immunol 2001;62:1009–30.

55. Foster CB, Zhu S, Erichsen HC, et al. Polymorphisms in inflammatory cytokines and Fcgamma receptors in childhood chronic immune thrombocytopenic purpura: a pilot study. Br J Haematol 2001;113:596–9.

56. Carcao MD, Blanchette VS, Wakefield CD, et al. Fcgamma receptor IIa and IIIa polymorphisms in childhood immune thrombocytopenic purpura. Br J Haematol 2003;120:135–41.

57. Sood R, Wong W, Jeng M, et al. Gene expression profile of idiopathic thrombo-cytopenic purpura (ITP). Pediatr Blood Cancer 2006;47:675–7.

58. Panzer S. New therapeutic options for adult chronic immune thrombocytopenic purpura: a brief review. Vox Sang 2008;94:1–5.

59. Psaila B, Bussel JB. Refractory immune thrombocytopenic purpura: current strategies for investigation and management. Br J Haematol 2008;143:16–26.

60. Unanue ER. Antigen-presenting function of the macrophage. Annu Rev Immunol 1984;1(Suppl 2):395–429.

61. Lanzavecchia A. Receptor-mediated antigen uptake and its effect on antigen presentation to class II-restricted T lymphocytes. Annu Rev Immunol 1990;8:773–93.

62. Watts C. Capture and processing of exogenous antigens for presentation on MHC molecules. Annu Rev Immunol 1997;15:821–50.

63. Cresswell P. Invariant chain structure and MHC class II function. Cell 1996;84:505–7.

64. Bretscher P, Cohn M. A theory of self-nonself discrimination. Science 1970;169:1042–9.

65. Linsley PS, Clark EA, Ledbetter JA. T-cell antigen CD28 mediates adhesion with B cells by interacting with activation antigen B7/BB-1. Proc Natl Acad Sci U S A 1990;87:5031–6.

66. Liu Y, Linsley PS. Costimulation of T cell growth. Curr Opin Immunol 1992;4:265–70.

67. Lenschow DJ, Walunas TL, Bluestone JA. CD28/B7 system of T cell costimula-tion. Annu Rev Immunol 1996;14:233–58.

68. Fischer Lindahl K, Wilson DB. Histocompatibility antigen-activated cytotoxic T lymphocytes II. Estimates of frequency and specificity of precursors. J Exp Med 1977;145:508–22.

69. The HS, Harley E, Phillips RA, et al. Quantitative studies on the precursors of cytotoxic lymphocytes I. Characteristics of a clonal assay and determination of the size of clones derived from single precursors. J Immunol 1977;118:1049–56.

70. Parker DC. T cell-dependent B cell activation. Annu Rev Immunol 1993;11:331–60.

71. Catani L, Fagioli ME, Tazzari PL, et al. Dendritic cells of immune thrombocyto-penic purpura (ITP) show increased capacity to present apoptotic platelets to T lymphocytes. Exp Hematol 2006;34:879–87.

72. Kissel K, Berbe SR, Nockher A, et al. Human platelets target dendritic cell differ-entiation and production of proinflammatory cytokines. Transfusion 2006;46(5):818–27.

73. Solanilla A, Pasquet JM, Viallard JF, et al. Platelet-associated CD154 in immune thrombocytopenic purpura. Blood 2005;105(1):215–8.

74. Elzey BD, Sprague DL, Ratliff TL. The emerging role of platelets in adaptive immunity. Cell Immunol 2005;238:1–9.

75. Hamzeh-Cognasse H, Cognasse F, Palle S, et al. Direct contact of platelets and their released products exert different effects on human dendritic cell matura-tion. BMC Immunol 2008;9:54–62.

76. Hagihara M, Higuchi A, Tamura N, et al. Platelets, after exposure to a high shear stress, induce IL-10-producing, mature dendritic cells in vitro. J Immunol 2004;172:5297–303.

77. Czapigaa M, Kirk AD, Lekstrom-Himes J. Platelets deliver costimulatory signals to antigen-presenting cells: a potential bridge between injury and immune acti-vation. Exp Hematol 2004;32:135–9.

78. Li N. Platlet-lymphocyte cross-talk. J Leukoc Biol 2008;83:1069–78.
79. Semple JW, Freedman J. Increased antiplatelet T helper lymphocyte reactivity in patients with autoimmune thrombocytopenia. Blood 1991;78:2619–25.
80. Ware RR, Howard TA. Phenotypic and clonal analysis of T lymphocytes in childhood immune thrombocytopenic purpura. Blood 1993;82:2137–42.
81. Filion MC, Bradley AJ, Devine DV, et al. Autoreactive T cells in healthy individuals show tolerance *in vitro* with characteristics similar to but distinct from clonal anergy. Eur J Immunol 1995;25:3123–7.
82. Shimomura T, Fujimura K, Takafuta T, et al. Oligoclonal accumulation of T cells in peripheral blood from patients with idiopathic thrombocytopenic purpura. Br J Haematol 1996;95:732–7.
83. Semple JW, Milev Y, Cosgrave D, et al. Differences in serum cytokine levels in acute and chronic autoimmune thrombocytopenic purpura: relationship to platelet phenotype and antiplatelet T-cell reactivity. Blood 1996;87:4245–54.
84. Guo C, Chu X, Shi Y, et al. Correction of Th1-dominant cytokine profiles by high-dose dexamethasone in patients with chronic idiopathic thrombocytopenic purpura. J Clin Immunol 2007;27:557–62.
85. Wang T, Zhao H, Ren H, et al. Type 1 and type 2 T-cell profiles in idiopathic thrombocytopenic purpura. Haematologica 2005;90:914–23.
86. Liu F, Wu C, Yang X, et al. Polarization and apoptosis of T cell subsets in idiopathic thrombocytopenic purpura. Cell Mol Immunol 2005;25:387–92.
87. Ogawara H, Handa H, Morita K, et al. High Th1/Th2 ratio in patients with chronic idiopathic thrombocytopenic purpura. Eur J Haematol 2003;71:283–8.
88. Mouzaki A, Theodoropoulou M, Gianakopoulos I, et al. Expression patterns of Th1 and Th2 cytokine genes in childhood idiopathic thrombocytopenic purpura (ITP) at presentation and their modulation by intravenous immunoglobulin G (IVIg) treatment: their role in prognosis. Blood 2002;100:1774–9.
89. Kuwana M, Kaburaki J, Ikeda Y. Autoreactive T cells to platelet GPIIb-IIIa in immune thrombocytopenic purpura. Role in production of anti-platelet autoantibody. J Clin Invest 1998;102:1393–402.
90. Kuwana M, Kaburaki J, Kitasato H, et al. Immunodominant epitopes on glycoprotein IIb-IIIa recognized by autoreactive T cells in patients with immune thrombocytopenic purpura. Blood 2001;98:130–9.
91. Sukati H, Watson HG, Urbaniak SJ, et al. Mapping helper T-cell epitopes on platelet membrane glycoprotein IIIa in chronic autoimmune thrombocytopenic purpura. Blood 2007;109:4528–38.
92. Olsson B, Andersson PO, Jacobsson JM, et al. T-cell-mediated cytotoxicity toward platelets in chronic idiopathic thrombocytopenic purpura. Nat Med 2003;9:1123–4.
93. Zhang F, Chu K, Wang L, et al. Cell-mediated lysis of autologous platelets in chronic idiopathic thrombocytopenic purpura. Eur J Haematol 2006;76:427–31.
94. Sabnani I, Tsang P. Therapeutic implications of T-cell clonopathy of unknown significance in chronic immune thrombocytopenic purpura. Platelets 2009;20:135–9.
95. Sakaguchi S. Naturally arising Foxp3-expressing CD25+CD4+ regulatory T cells in immunological tolerance to self and non-self. Nat Immunol 2005;6:345–52.
96. Tang Q, Bluestone JA. The Foxp3+ regulatory T cell: a jack of all trades, master of regulation. Nat Immunol 2008;9:239–44.
97. Hori S, Nomura T, Sakaguchi S. Control of regulatory T cell development by the transcription factor Foxp3. Science 2003;299:1057–61.
98. Fontenot JD, Gavin MA, Rudensky AY. Foxp3 programs the development and function of CD4+CD25+ regulatory Tcells. Nat Immunol 2003;4:330–6.

99. Korn T, Bettelli E, Oukka M, et al. IL-17 and Th17 cells. Annu Rev Immunol 2009; 27:485–517.
100. Bluestone JA, Abbas AK. Natural versus adaptive regulatory T cells. Nat Rev Immunol 2003;3:253–7.
101. Roncarolo MG, Gregori S, Battaglia M, et al. Interleukin-10-secreting type 1 regulatory T cells in rodents and humans. Immunol Rev 2006;212:28–50.
102. Jonuleit H, Schmitt E. The regulatory T cell family: distinct subsets and their inter-relations. J Immunol 2003;171:6323–7.
103. Korn T, Oukka M. Dynamics of antigen-specific regulatory T-cells in the context of autoimmunity. Semin Immunol 2007;19:272–8.
104. Valencia X, Lipsky PE. CD4+CD25+FoxP3+ regulatory T cells in autoimmune diseases. Nat Clin Pract Rheumatol 2007;3:619–26.
105. Crispin JC, Martinez A, Alcocer-Varela J. Quantification of regulatory T cells in patients with systemic lupus erythematosus. J Autoimmun 2003;21:273–6.
106. de Kleer IM, Wedderburn LR, Taams LS, et al. CD4+CD25bright regulatory T cells actively regulate inflammation in the joints of patients with the remitting form of juvenile idiopathic arthritis. J Immunol 2004;172:6435–43.
107. Kukreja A, Cost G, Marker J, et al. Multiple immunoregulatory defects in type-1 diabetes. J Clin Invest 2002;109:131–40.
108. Viglietta V, Baecher-Allan C, Weiner HL, et al. Loss of functional suppression by CD4+CD25+ regulatory T cells in patients with multiple sclerosis. J Exp Med 2004;199:971–9.
109. Sakakura M, Wada H, Tawara I, et al. Reduced Cd4+Cd25+ T cells in patients with idiopathic thrombocytopenic purpura. Thromb Res 2007;120:187–93.
110. Ling Y, Cao X, Yu Z, et al. Circulating dendritic cells subsets and CD4+Foxp3+ regulatory T cells in adult patients with chronic ITP before and after treatment with high-dose dexamethasome. Eur J Haematol 2007;79:310–6.
111. Liu B, Zhao H, Poon MC, et al. Abnormality of CD4(+)CD25(+) regulatory T cells in idiopathic thrombocytopenic purpura. Eur J Haematol 2007;78:139–43.
112. Arnold DM, Dentali F, Crowther MA, et al. Systematic review: efficacy and safety of rituximab for adults with idiopathic thrombocytopenic purpura. Ann Intern Med 2007;146:25–33.
113. Garvey B. Rituximab in the treatment of autoimmune haematological disorders. Brit J Haematol 2008;141:149–69.
114. Stasi R, Del Poeta G, Stipa E, et al. Response to B-cell depleting therapy with rituximab reverts the abnormalities of T cell subsets in patients with idiopathic thrombocytopenic purpura. Blood 2007;110:2924–30.
115. Stasi R, Cooper N, Del Poeta G, et al. Analysis of regulatory T cell changes in patients with idiopathic thrombocytopenic purpura receiving B-cell depleting therapy with rituximab. Blood 2008;112:1147–50.
116. Olsson B, Ridell B, Carlsson L, et al. Recruitment of T cells into bone marrow of ITP patients possibly due to elevated expression of VLA-4 and CX3CR1. Blood 2008;12:1078–84.
117. Yu J, Heck S, Patel V, et al. Defective circulating CD25 regulatory T cells in patients with chronic immune thrombocytopenic purpura. Blood 2008;112:1325–8.
118. McMillan R, Wang L, Tomer A, et al. Suppression of in vitro megakaryocyte production by antiplatelet autoantibodies from adult patients with chronic ITP. Blood 2004;103:1364–9.
119. Zhang X-L, Peng J, Sun J-Z, et al. De novo induction of platelet-specific CD4(+)CD25(+) regulatory T cells from CD4(+)CD25(−) cells in patients with idiopathic thrombocytopenic purpura. Blood 2009;113:2568–77.

Thrombopoietin and Platelet Production in Chronic Immune Thrombocytopenia

David J. Kuter, MD, DPhil[a,b], Terry B. Gernsheimer, MD[c,d],*

KEYWORDS

- ITP • Thrombopoietin • Thrombocytopenia • Platelets • TPO

In 1663 Lazarus de la Rivière (Riverius) recognized that purpura was a manifestation of a systemic bleeding disorder, something he called "thinness of the blood."[1] Although most of his patients probably did not have immune thrombocytopenic purpura (ITP), he stated "But there is one Symptome proper and peculiar to a pestilential Feaver, which doth not happen in other Feavers; viz Purple Specks, or Spots on the whol Body, but especially in the Loyns, the breast and back, like unto Flea-bitings for the most part; which the Italian Physitians name Peticule or Petechio; and these Feavers which have these Symptoms, are commonly named Purpuratae or Petechiales, Purple or Spotted Feavers… wherein the blood boiling, do send forth it's thinner Exhalations to the surface of the Skin."

The first modern description of ITP was probably that of the German physician Paul Gottlieb Werlhof, who in 1775 described a case of "morbus maculosus haemorrhagicus."[2] In 1808 the English dermatologist Robert Willan reported a case of mucosal and cutaneous hemorrhage he called "purpura hemorrhagica."[3] Willan also suggested that "moderate exercise in the open air, a generous diet, and the free use of wine" might be an appropriate treatment. Other reports during the following century clarified the characteristic hemorrhagic features of ITP and ultimately James Homer Wright in his reports of 1902, 1906, and 1910[4–6] related these clinical findings to the lack of platelets. By the beginning of the twentieth century what is now identified as ITP was a known diagnostic entity.[7]

This work was supported by Grants HL82889 (DK), HL072299 (DK) and HL072305 (TG) from the National Institutes of Health.

[a] Harvard Medical School, Boston, MA, USA
[b] Division of Hematology, Yawkey 7940, Massachusetts General Hospital, 55 Fruit Street, Boston, MA 02114, USA
[c] University of Washington, Seattle, WA, USA
[d] Puget Sound Blood Center, 921 Terry Avenue, Seattle, WA 98104, USA
* Corresponding author. Puget Sound Blood Center, 921 Terry Avenue, Seattle, WA 98104.
E-mail address: bldbuddy@u.washington.edu (T.B. Gernsheimer).

Hematol Oncol Clin N Am 23 (2009) 1193–1211
doi:10.1016/j.hoc.2009.09.001
0889-8588/09/$ – see front matter © 2009 Elsevier Inc. All rights reserved.

hemonc.theclinics.com

Theories as to the cause of ITP were developed early in the twentieth century and set the stage for current understanding of ITP. In 1915 the German physician Ernest Frank suggested that ITP was caused by impaired production of platelets from mega-karyocytes.[8] In contrast, in 1916 the Czech medical student Paul Kasnelson specu-lated that ITP was caused by splenic destruction of platelets, as in hemolytic anemia.[9,10] He also succeeded in persuading his supervisor to perform a splenectomy in 1 such patient, with therapeutic success.

The debate as to whether ITP was caused by decreased platelet production or increased platelet destruction was seemingly settled by the experiments of Harrington and Schulman, which suggested a primary role for immune-mediated platelet destruc-tion. In his classic experiment, Harrington infused plasma or whole blood from patients with ITP into himself and his fellows; thrombocytopenia soon ensued (**Fig. 1**).[11] Sternal bone-marrow biopsies performed on these volunteers showed an increase in mega-karyocytes during the thrombocytopenia. Subsequent studies by Shulman showed that the thrombocytopenia induced by ITP plasma infusion was reduced in patients who were splenectomized or pretreated with corticosteroids.[12–14] When combined with the platelet survival and kinetic studies of Harker in 1968, a model emerged that suggested that ITP was caused by immune-mediated platelet destruction accom-panied by a maximal 6-fold compensatory increase in platelet production by the bone marrow.[15–17]

Since 1968, a greater understanding of platelet biology and its regulation by throm-bopoietin (TPO) have emerged. It is now recognized that ITP is a disorder of reduced platelet production and increased platelet destruction. New therapies for ITP with TPO mimetics have emerged that have exploited this new pathophysiologic understanding to the benefit of many patients. This article reviews the biology of TPO, the regulation of its circulating level in ITP, the platelet kinetic data supporting inappropriate platelet production in ITP, and the TPO molecules available to treat ITP. Elsewhere in this

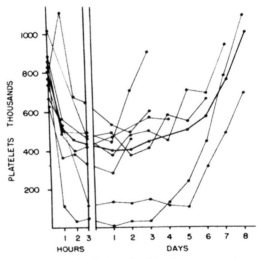

Fig. 1. Infusion of antiplatelet antibody into healthy humans produces thrombocytopenia. Platelet counts after blood or plasma from patients with ITP were infused into health volun-teers. (*From* Harrington WJ, Minnich V, Hollingsworth JW, et al. Demonstration of a throm-bocytopenic factor in the blood of patients with thrombocytopenic purpura. J Lab Clin Med 1951;38:1; with permission.)

issue, the clinical studies in ITP with these TPO mimetics are described in detail (see other articles in this issue).

THROMBOPOIETIN IS THE PRIMARY REGULATOR OF NORMAL PLATELET PRODUCTION

TPO is a 94-kDa protein primarily made in the liver and secreted into the circulation; there is no storage form. Although there is some suggestion of local TPO production in the bone marrow, there is little evidence to show that this is physiologically relevant.[18] Indeed in patients with liver failure, TPO levels are low and patients are thrombocytopenic; on orthotopic liver transplantation, TPO levels increase and the platelet count is restored to normal.[19,20]

There does not seem to be any direct "sensor" of the platelet count and levels are regulated by an efficient, albeit primitive, feedback system (**Fig. 2**).[21] Hepatic TPO production seems to be constant with no transcriptional or posttranscriptional regulation yet identified.[22] Other than liver disease or hepatic resection, no disease or medication is known to affect TPO production. On entering the circulation, TPO is not bound to any specific carrier molecule but does bind with high avidity to TPO receptors on circulating platelets and target bone marrow tissues (megakaryocytes and megakaryocyte precursors).[23] Most of the circulating TPO is cleared by platelets (and possibly megakaryocytes) by binding to the TPO receptor, followed by internalization and catabolism of the bound ligand. Indeed, when platelets were transfused into patients with thrombocytopenia caused by aplastic anemia, the increased TPO levels decreased by 30%.[24] In summary, the circulating TPO level is inversely related to the rate of platelet production: when platelet production is low, less TPO is cleared and levels increase; when platelet production is increased, more TPO is cleared and levels decrease.[25]

When TPO binds to the TPO receptor on platelets there are no major physiologic sequelae other than an increase (at high nonphysiologic concentrations of TPO) in intracellular calcium concentration and an increase in adenosine diphosphate (ADP) in the sensitivity of platelets to weak agonists (half-maximal platelet activation by ADP occurs at half the concentration of ADP usually required for this effect).[26]

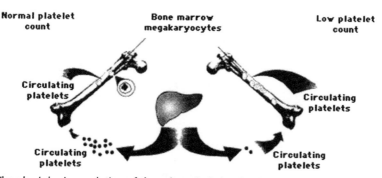

Fig. 2. The physiologic regulation of thrombopoietin levels. The constitutive hepatic production of thrombopoietin (*center*) is cleared by avid thrombopoietin receptors on platelets resulting in normal levels when the platelet production is normal (*left*) and increased levels when the platelet production is reduced (*right*). The bone-marrow megakaryocytes are stimulated to make more platelets as the circulating thrombopoietin concentration rises. (*From* Kuter DJ, Beeler DL, Rosenberg RD. The purification of megapoietin: a physiologic regulator of megakaryocyte growth and platelet production. Proc Natl Acad Sci USA 1994;91:11104; with permission.) Copyright © 1994 National Academy of Sciences U.S.A.

However, on TPO binding to megakaryocytes and megakaryocyte precursors, the TPO receptor is activated and increases megakaryocyte growth, endomitosis, and maturation and reduces the apoptosis rate of these cells.[27] In so doing, megakaryocyte number, ploidy, and viability increase, thereby increasing platelet production (**Fig. 3**).

The importance of TPO for normal platelet production is illustrated by animals in which either TPO or the TPO receptor were "knocked out." In animals homozygous for the absence of TPO or its receptor, the platelet count was reduced by 90% to 95%.[28,29] As expected, the number of megakaryocytes and megakaryocyte precursors were reduced by a similar extent. Myeloid and erythroid precursors were reduced by 70%, but with no effect on the white blood cell (WBC) count or hemoglobin.[30,31] At the time of birth, humans lacking TPO or its receptor have marked thrombocytopenia as a result of the reduced numbers of megakaryocytes and megakaryocyte precursors; however, with time such individuals become pancytopenic.[32–34] Together these data suggest that TPO is necessary for the viability of the pluripotent stem cell and precursors of all lineages, but specifically important for the maturation and development of late megakaryocytes.

TPO LEVELS AND PLATELET PRODUCTION ARE USUALLY NOT INCREASED IN ITP

Seemingly at odds with the long-held understanding that ITP is a disease of antibody-mediated platelet destruction, ITP is also a disorder of inappropriately low platelet production (ie, platelet production remains close to normal and is not increased 6-fold as suggested by Harker).[17] These processes (increased destruction and reduced production) occur simultaneously and probably to a different extent in each patient, hence the widely varying rates of response to many agents. The apparent

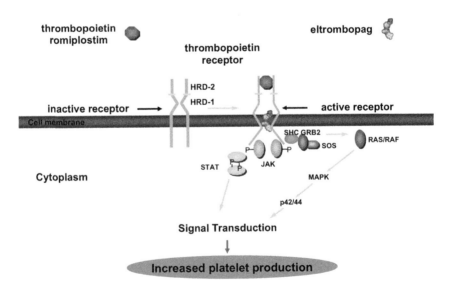

Fig. 3. Activation of the TPO receptor. The TPO receptor has been proposed to exist as an inactive preformed dimer (left receptor dimer) with a proximal (HRD-1) and distal (HRD-2) HRD. On binding of thrombopoietin/romiplostim to the distal HRD-2 or binding of eltrombopag to the transmembrane region, the receptor (right receptor dimer) conformation changes and several signal transduction pathways are activated that increase platelet production.

common mechanism is that the antiplatelet antibody opsonizes platelets, leading to their destruction by the reticuloendothelial (RE) system and inhibits the growth (by accelerated apoptosis) of megakaryocytes and their progenitors (see the article by McMillan in this issue).[35] Two main avenues of investigation support this statement and are reviewed next.

TPO Levels are Not Significantly Elevated in Patients with ITP

As shown in **Fig. 4**, at comparable degrees of thrombocytopenia, TPO levels are increased 10-fold in patients with aplastic anemia (median = 1002 pg/mL, range: 37–161,538 pg/mL) but are virtually normal (median = 64 pg/mL, range: 22–256 pg/mL) in patients with ITP (median = 98 pg/mL, range: 17–313 pg/mL).[25,36] The model described earlier (see **Fig. 2**) helps to explain why.[37] In both patient groups, TPO is being constitutively made by the liver at the same rate. In the aplastic patient, platelet production is reduced below normal, fewer platelets and megakaryocytes are available to bind and clear TPO, and levels increase.[37] In the ITP patient, platelets are still being made at an approximately normal rate (see later discussion) but are being cleared at an increased rate; despite their shortened survival, the platelets can still bind and clear TPO at a normal rate, and TPO levels do not significantly increase.[a]

Platelet Turnover Rates are Not Appreciably Elevated in ITP

Dameshek and Miller[38] attempted to measure platelet production in 1946 by scoring the morphologic appearance of megakaryocytes and platelet budding in the bone

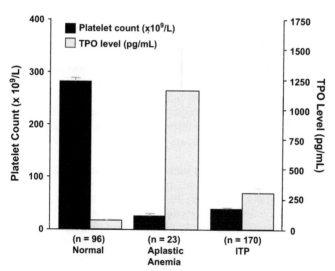

Fig. 4. TPO levels are not increased in patients with ITP. TPO levels ($\pm$ standard deviation [SD]) were measured in thrombocytopenic patients with ITP or aplastic anemia and compared with healthy volunteers.

---

[a] This clearance function is slightly more complex if explored further. There is a log-linear relationship between the TPO level and the rate of platelet production[37]; hence as the rate of platelet production rises in ITP, clearance increases but TPO levels rapidly approach the lower limit of quantitation of the TPO assay. This is the explanation as to why TPO levels become readily increased in disorders of reduced production but usually remain in the broadly normal range when the platelet production rate increases, even if greatly increased.

marrow of patients with chronic and acute ITP, liver disease, and splenomegaly. They found megakaryocytes were present in increased numbers in ITP patients, but noted that these megakaryocytes frequently appeared immature with a "greatly diminished productivity of platelets" and considered the possibility that the spleen exerted "an unusual effect upon the production of platelets from the megakaryocytes."

Taking advantage of the uptake of ^{51}Cr by platelets on in vitro incubation, Aster and Jandl[39] developed a methodology for the measurement of in vivo platelet survival. Radioactivity in serial blood samples collected after transfusion of ^{51}Cr-labeled platelets revealed platelet lifespan in normal patients averaged about 8 days and approximately 30% of the transfused platelets did not circulate and were pooled in the spleen. Platelets were lost from circulation mainly because of senescence with predominantly RE removal in the liver. Najean and colleagues[40] used ^{51}Cr labeling to study platelet survival in 317 patients with ITP on 450 occasions using allogeneic platelets when the patients' platelet counts were less than 80,000/μL and autologous platelets at higher counts. Platelet survivals were always shorter than normal in these patients and directly related to the patients' platelet count whether autologous or allogeneic platelets were used.

Using these same platelet radiolabeling methods Harker and Finch[17] correlated thrombokinetic measurements with studies of megakaryocyte mass (ie, number and volume) to define thrombocytopenic disorders further. They calculated the daily rate of platelet loss from the circulation by the formula:

$$\text{turnover} = \frac{\text{platelet count} \times 10^9 \text{ per liter} \times 90\%}{\text{platelet survival (days)} \times \text{platelet recovery (\%)}}$$

At a steady state, when the peripheral blood platelet count is stable and the number of platelets going into or out of the system is constant, platelet production must equal platelet destruction ("turnover"). At any given platelet count, as platelet survival shortens, the denominator decreases and the resultant production (turnover) rate increases. This makes sense physiologically as the marrow would be expected to increase production in response to thrombocytopenia to reachieve homeostasis, and is consistent with increased numbers of megakaryocytes observed in disorders of increased platelet destruction.

In 15 normal patients studied using autologous radiolabeled platelets, the average platelet count was 250,000 ± 35,000/μL, platelet recovery 65% ± 4, platelet survival 9.9 ± 0.6 days, and platelet production 35,000 ± 4000 platelets/μL/d.[17] Radiolabeled platelet survivals were markedly shortened in 4 patients with ITP, from a mean of 9.9 days in normal patients to 48 to 230 minutes, and calculated production rates in the ITP patients that were 4 to 9 times normal. Platelet kinetic measurements in 7 patients with secondary autoimmune thrombocytopenia were similar to the ITP group. The finding of marked shortening of platelet survival and by implication markedly increased rates of platelet production in ITP was later confirmed by Branehog.[41]

^{111}In was introduced as an alternative radiolabel to ^{51}Cr in 1976.[42] Higher labeling efficiency (64% for ^{111}In and 12% for ^{51}Cr) allowed kinetic measurements with autologous platelets rather than allogeneic platelets in patients with severe thrombocytopenia, and lower levels of erythrocyte binding (1% for ^{111}In and 7.4% for ^{51}Cr) gave more accurate measurements. Higher γ emissions with ^{111}In also permitted investigators to localize platelet uptake reliably using external scanning techniques. Platelet kinetic experiments using ^{111}In-labeled autologous platelets[43,44] avoided potential confounding and adverse effects of homologous (donor) platelets. In dual labeling experiments with [111]In- and ^{51}Cr-labeled autologous and homologous platelets in 13 patients with chronic ITP, autologous platelets survived significantly longer in the circulation than homologous platelets.[43]

A comprehensive evaluation[43] of thrombokinetics using either [51]Cr- or ^{111}In-radiolabeled autologous platelets in 38 patients with ITP (18 patients receiving no treatment, 13 receiving prednisone, and 7 postsplenectomy) found platelet survivals to be less than normal with the exception of 2 postsplenectomy patients in complete remission, and 82% (36 of 44) of platelet survivals were disproportionately less than expected based on the corresponding platelet count.[45] There was a significant relationship between platelet count and autologous platelet survivals only for the splenectomized patients ($r = 0.84$, $P<.001$) and in patients with platelet counts less than 170,000/μL there was no relationship between platelet count and platelet survival ($r = 0.36$, $P>.10$). There was a significant direct correlation between log platelet count and platelet production in all groups ($r = 0.68$, $P<.001$) (**Fig. 5**), suggesting that platelet production rate rather than platelet survival determines platelet counts in ITP patients. Among patients on no treatment, 41% (7 of 17) had decreased platelet production and 53% (9 of 17) were in the normal range. Thus despite normal to increased numbers of marrow megakaryocytes in all ITP patients studied, 94% (16 of 17) of the untreated patients had an inappropriate thrombopoietic response to their low platelet counts. Possible causes of the ineffective thrombopoiesis were postulated to be (1) antibody binding to megakaryocytes interfering with platelet production or release; or (2) antibody-mediated platelet phagocytosis in the bone-marrow RE system preventing their release into circulation.

Improvement in Thrombocytopenia Following Treatment of ITP is Mediated by an Increase in Platelet Production

In contrast to kinetic measurements in untreated ITP patients who characteristically had decreased or normal platelet production rates, 47% (7 of 15) of ITP patients on

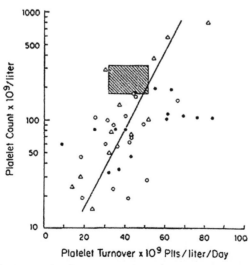

Fig. 5. Relationship between platelet count and platelet turnover. There was a direct relationship between log platelet count and autologous platelet turnover; $r = 0.068$, $P<.001$. Patients were on no treatment (○), prednisone (●), or postsplenectomy (▲). Hatched area represents the normal range.

prednisone were found to have high platelet production.[43] These data suggest that corticosteroid therapy may improve thrombocytopenia in many ITP patients by increasing platelet production. Measurement of platelet kinetics in patients before and after successful treatment with prednisone revealed that an increase in platelet count occurred without a corresponding increase in platelet survival (**Figs. 6** and **7**),[46] supporting the concept that the rate of platelet production is important in determining the circulating platelet count and an increase in platelet count is effected by increasing platelet production or release from the bone marrow. By contrast, successful removal of the spleen in ITP, the primary site of ^{111}In-labeled platelet destruction by γ camera imaging[47] is associated with an increase in platelet survival (**Fig. 8**).[41,46,48]

Li and colleagues[49] observed lower percentages of polyploid and apoptotic mega-karyocytes and decreased in vitro platelet production compared with controls when bone-marrow mononuclear cells and autologous CD8+ T cells from patients with chronic ITP were cocultured, but the addition of dexamethasone to the culture could correct these abnormalities. These studies give further credence to the idea that an improvement in platelet count is mediated by an increase in platelet production and that megakaryocytes can be driven to increase platelet production in ITP.

TPO AND TPO MIMETICS

In the past 15 years several molecules have been developed that bind and activate the TPO receptor.[50] The first generation of TPO molecules were recombinant proteins similar to native TPO but development was halted when antibodies formed against 1 of them. A second generation of TPO molecules was then developed to avoid

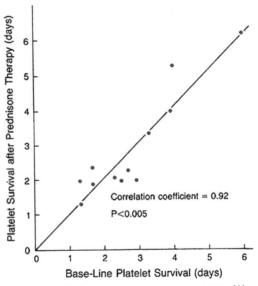

Fig. 6. Platelet survival before and after prednisone treatment. The ^{111}In-labeled autologous platelet survivals of 12 ITP patients were unchanged by prednisone therapy before (base-line) and after therapy with corticosteroids increased their platelet count. The regression line for the data was determined by the equation $y = 0.06 + 1.60$; $r^2 = 0.90$. The correlation coefficient between the platelet survival measurements before and after steroid treatment in the same patient was 0.21 ($P<.005$).

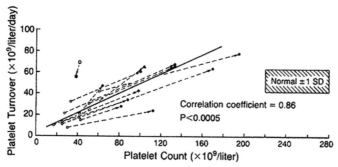

Fig. 7. Platelet turnover and platelet count before and after prednisone treatment. In the 11 patients whose platelet counts improved with treatment there was a direct correlation between the baseline platelet count and platelet turnover rate (○) and between the post-prednisone values (●) (correlation coefficient, 0.86; $P<.0005$). The retreatment and posttreatment data for the 1 patient who had no improvement in the platelet count are denoted by □ and ■, respectively. The regression line for the pretreatment and posttreatment data for the 11 patients who responded to treatment (*solid line*) was predicted by the equation $y = 6.50 + 0.41x$; $r^2 = 0.75$. Individual pretreatment and posttreatment values are connected by dashed lines. The hatched area shows the expected normal relation between platelet count and platelet turnover ± 1 SD.

autoantibody formation and 2 of these are now approved by the US Food and Drug Administration (FDA) for the treatment of ITP. The structure and function of these molecules are discussed next with the detailed results of their clinical studies provided elsewhere in this issue (see article by Bussel).

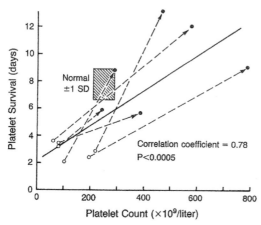

Fig. 8. Platelet survival and platelet count before and after successful splenectomy. The relation between presplenectomy platelet counts and survival data is denoted by (○) and that between postsplenectomy values by (●). The solid regression line for the data was determined by the equation $y = 2.12 + 0.01x$; $r^2 = 0.61$. The correlation coefficient was 0.78 ($P<.0005$). Individual presplenectomy and postsplenectomy values are connected by dashed lines. The hatched area shows the expected normal relation between platelet count and platelet survival ± 1 SD.

First-Generation TPO Molecules

Soon after the discovery of TPO, 2 recombinant TPO molecules entered clinical development. One was a recombinant human TPO (rhTPO) produced in Chinese hamster ovary (CHO) cells, which, except for small differences in its pattern of glycosylation, closely resembled native TPO. The other, pegylated recombinant human megakaryocyte growth and development factor (PEG-rHuMGDF), was composed of the amino-terminal 163 residues of human TPO, was not glycosylated, and had a 30-kDa polyethylene glycol (PEG) moiety attached to keep the molecule stable in the circulation.[50–54]

Preclinical studies in mice and rhesus monkeys showed that both of these recombinant molecules were potent stimulators of megakaryocyte growth and platelet production. These animal studies demonstrated the following important pharmacodynamic aspects of all TPO treatments. After a single dose of TPO, there was a 5-day lag time before the platelet count started to increase (presumably because of TPO stimulation of early, but not late, megakaryocyte progenitors). A platelet count increase followed, peaking on days 12 to 14, which showed a log-linear relationship between the dose of TPO and the peak platelet count.[26] After the platelet peak was reached, the platelet count returned to normal by day 28 with no rebound thrombocytopenia. TPO had no effect on red blood cells or WBC. Prolonged exposure of animals to high doses was well tolerated but did produce reversible marrow fibrosis at these doses.[55–57]

Subsequent human studies in patients who have cancer and who are not receiving chemotherapy showed the same platelet response kinetics: a 5-day lag, peak platelet count at day 12 to 14, and no rebound thrombocytopenia.[58,59] Neither recombinant TPO directly activated human platelets but both reduced by about 50% the threshold for platelet aggregation to weak platelet agonists like ADP.[60]

Between 1995 and 2002 many clinical studies were conducted with both recombinant TPO molecules (for comprehensive reviews see[51,52,61]). In general, both molecules were well tolerated, produced a robust increase in platelets (sometimes to more than several million), were not associated with thrombosis, reduced the extent of thrombocytopenia in nonmyeloablative (but not myeloablative) chemotherapy regimens, and improved the platelet counts in patients with ITP or myelodysplastic syndrome (MDS). In platelet apheresis donors given rhTPO or PEG-rHuMGDF there was a great increase in platelet yields.[62–64] However, subsequent larger safety studies with PEG-rHuMGDF in healthy volunteers demonstrated the appearance of a neutralizing antibody to TPO and development of both first-generation TPO molecules was stopped.[65]

Second-Generation TPO Molecules

The results of the clinical trials with the first-generation TPO molecules were sufficiently encouraging to prompt a search for nonimmunogenic TPO molecules. Two general classes of molecules were developed: TPO peptide mimetics and TPO nonpeptide mimetics. One drug in each class, romiplostim and eltrombopag, has now been approved by the FDA for the treatment of ITP.[50]

Romiplostim (AMG 531, Nplate)

In 1997 a 14-amino acid peptide with no sequence homology with TPO was identified that bound and activated the TPO receptor.[66] Given the requirement of any TPO to bind simultaneously 2 TPO receptor molecules, dimerization of these peptides increased their specific activity about 10,000-fold. The usually short circulatory half-life of peptides often makes them poor pharmacologic agents. Efforts were then directed toward stabilizing the peptide (and yet preserving a dimeric structure) by attaching the peptides to a modified fragment "crystallized" (Fc) receptor.[67]

Initially named Amgen megakaryopoiesis protein-2 (AMP-2), and subsequently developed as AMG-531, romiplostim is a 60-kDa structure composed of 4 of these 14-amino acid peptides attached to a novel IgG heavy chain Fc region (a "peptibody") by glycine bridges (**Fig. 9**).[67,68] To each arm of the Fc region are attached 2 TPO mimetic peptides, again creating a dimeric molecule capable of activating the TPO receptor. The peptides have no sequence homology with endogenous TPO such that if antibodies were to form against romiplostim, they would not cross-react with endogenous TPO. Romiplostim has a circulatory half-life of 120 to 160 hours and is initially removed by the endothelial FcRn receptors, recycled, and eventually cleared by the RE system.[68]

Romiplostim binds to the distal hematopoietic receptor domain (HRD) of the TPO receptor and activates the receptor just like recombinant TPO (see **Fig. 3**). In cultures of bone marrow and TPO-dependent cell lines, romiplostim produces the same effect as recombinant TPO.[69] It does not directly activate platelets, but does lower the threshold for activation by ADP by 50%. Prolonged administration of large doses of romiplostim to mice produced marrow fibrosis that was reversible on stopping the drug.[70]

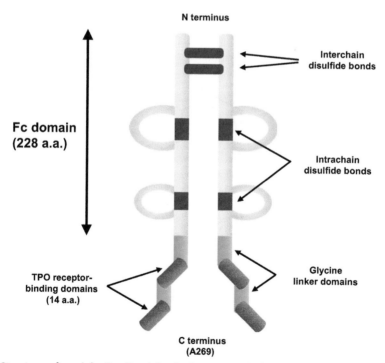

Fig. 9. Structure of romiplostim. Romiplostim is composed of the Fc portion of IgG to which two 14-amino acid TPO peptides (*purple*) are coupled via glycine bridges (*green*) at the carboxy-terminus of each γ heavy chain. Interchain (cysteines C7 and C10) and intrachain (cysteines C42-C102, C148-C206) disulfide bridges are indicated in red. Heavy chain constant domains 2 (CH$_2$) and 3 (CH3) are also shown. Romiplostim has a molecular weight of ~60 kDa.

In healthy human volunteers, single doses of romiplostim produced a dose-dependent increase in platelet count beginning on day 5 and peaking at days 12 to 14.[68] Autoantibody formation did not occur. Romiplostim is now approved by the FDA for the treatment of ITP and is available as a lyophilized powder that is reconstituted with sterile water and injected subcutaneously usually once a week at doses of 1 to 10 µg/kg.[67,68,71,72]

Eltrombopag (SB497115, Promacta)

Screening of libraries of molecules to identify structures that activate the TPO receptor has yielded a large number of "lead compounds."[73,74] Further modification to improve their biologic activity and pharmacologic properties has resulted in several (eltrombopag,[75] AKR-501,[76] LGD-4665,[77] NIP-004,[78] NIP-022,[79] and butyzamide[80,81]) that have undergone clinical development. Only 1, eltrombopag, has completed phase 3 trials and is approved by the FDA for the treatment of ITP.

Although previously known as SB497115, eltrombopag is a small (442 Da) molecule ($C_{25}H_{22}N_4O_4$) with an acidic (COOH) group at 1 end, lipophilic (CH_3) groups at the other end, and a metal chelate group in the center that is a potent, orally available TPO nonpeptide agonist (**Fig. 10**). Single doses have no effect on the platelet count but daily doses for 10 days produce a peak platelet count on day 16.[82]

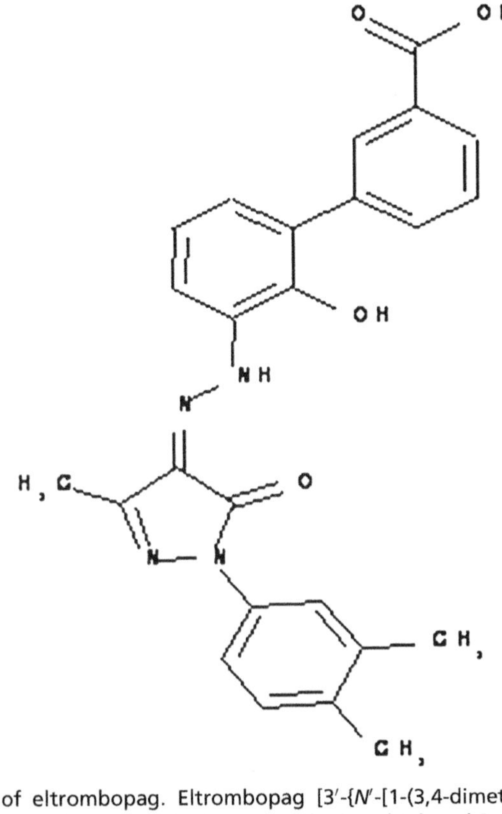

Fig. 10. Structure of eltrombopag. Eltrombopag [3'-{N'-[1-(3,4-dimethyl-phenyl)-3-methyl-5-oxo-1,5-dihydropyrazol-4-ylidene]hydrazino}-2'-hydroxybiphenyl-3-carboxylic acid] is a hydrazone small (442 Da) molecule with an acidic (COOH) group at 1 end, lipophilic (CH_3) groups at the other end, and a metal chelate group in the center.

Eltrombopag has several important features that are representative of this class of molecules:

- It is a small (442 Da) chemical structure that is an orally administered tablet given once a day at a dose of 25 to 75 mg.[83]
- It has specific binding to the TPO receptor and binds only to TPO receptors in humans and chimpanzees.[79,84] This has markedly limited preclinical efficacy studies in small animal models.
- This species specificity is attributed to which amino acid is present at position 499 in the transmembrane region of the TPO receptor: histidine in humans and chimpanzees, leucine in all other species.
- It activates the TPO receptor by binding not to the distal HRD like TPO but to the transmembrane region (see **Fig. 3**).[51,79,81] This makes its biologic effect at least additive to that of TPO.[85]
- It does not directly activate platelets or alter their threshold for activation.[75]
- At maximally tested doses, it increases the platelet count in healthy volunteers 1.5-fold above baseline compared with a 6-fold increase for romiplostim. Whether this difference in potency is of clinical important is unclear.

THE RATIONALE FOR USING TPO IN ITP

Given the new understanding that ITP is a disorder of increased platelet destruction and inappropriately low platelet production, new therapeutic options open up. In addition to using drugs (intravenous immunoglobulin, anti-D) or splenectomy to reduce the rate of platelet destruction, TPO mimetics (the "platelet producers") can now be employed to increase platelet production and thereby ameliorate thrombocytopenia.

Early studies with PEG-rHuMGDF demonstrated that in 3 of 4 Japanese patients with ITP their platelet count increased after administration for 7 days (**Fig. 11**).[86] In

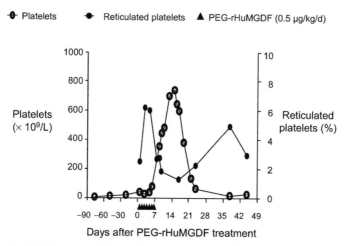

Fig. 11. PEG-rHuMGDF increased the platelet count in a patient with ITP. PEG-rHuMGDF was administered daily for 7 days and the platelet count and reticulated platelets measured daily. The increase in platelet count was preceded by an increase in reticulated platelets. (*Data from* Nomura S, Dan K, Hotta T, et al. Effects of pegylated recombinant human mega-karyocyte growth and development factor in patients with idiopathic thrombocytopenic purpura. Blood 2002;100:728.)

addition, 1 patient with an unusual form of cyclic ITP was maintained on weekly injections of PEG-rHuMGDF for more than 8 years with good control of the platelet count.[87] As presented elsewhere in this issue (see article by Bussel), romiplostim and eltrombopag have been found to be effective in treating patients with ITP.[50]

What has not been thoroughly explored in any of these clinical studies is how TPO mimetics improve the platelet count. Although not directly studied with platelet kinetic approaches, they seem to have little effect on platelet survival in ITP. Indeed, on stopping a TPO mimetic, the platelet count may decrease to life-threatening levels within 5 to 7 days, suggesting (but not formally proving) that platelet survival remains reduced.[72] The simplest explanation for their effect is that TPO mimetics are increasing the number of megakaryocyte precursors, increasing their maturation rate and thereby "overwhelming" the ability of the antiplatelet/megakaryocyte antibody to destroy the increased amount of platelets.

However, studies by Harker[88–90] suggest a more sophisticated mechanism, that is, TPO and TPO mimetics reverse the apoptotic effect of the antiplatelet/megakaryocyte antibody (or local T-cell inhibition) on late megakaryocyte progenitors (probably not on the late megakaryocytes themselves because it takes 5 to 7 days before the platelet count rises in response to a TPO agonist). Harker and colleagues[89] extensively studied 8 patients with human immunodeficiency virus (HIV) thrombocytopenia. Six were given 8 doses of 5 μg/kg PEG-rHuMGDF in a 16-week period and all had their platelet count increase 10-fold within 14 days; 2 patients received placebo and had no increase in platelet count. The megakaryocyte mass before treatment was $69 \pm 37 \times 10^{10}$ fL/kg (normal = 31 ± 5 fL/kg) and remained constant at 76 ± 45 fL/kg during treatment. Because there was no change in platelet survival, antiplatelet antibody or viral load, these results suggested that TPO therapy reduced apoptosis of megakaryocyte progenitors and megakaryocytes and allowed them to produce platelets. Whether this mechanism is true in patients with ITP not infected with HIV awaits further studies; clearly bone-marrow megakaryocytes in patients with ITP not infected with HIV are undergoing accelerated apoptosis.[91]

SUMMARY

Despite normal or increased numbers of megakaryocytes observed in their bone marrow, platelet production seems to be inappropriately low in patients with chronic ITP. Levels of thrombopoietin in the circulation are only moderately increased, if at all, likely because of uptake by platelets targeted for destruction in the RE system. In vitro studies reveal abnormal apoptosis and maturation of megakaryocytes that share antigenic targets with platelets such as glycoprotein IIb/IIIa. Indirect measurements of platelet production using radiolabeled platelet survival measurements are consistent with an abbreviated response in the marrow compartment to the thrombocytopenia. Therapeutic intervention in ITP may increase the platelet count by increasing the numbers of platelets released into the circulation (corticosteroids), or increasing their circulating life span (splenectomy). The findings of inappropriately low levels of thrombopoietin and decreased platelet production by the bone marrow have afforded new opportunities for the therapy for chronic ITP. New agents mimicking the action of thrombopoietin at the megakaryocyte are capable of increasing platelet production and raising the platelet count.

REFERENCES

1. Riverius L. On pestilential feavers. In: Culpepper N, editor. The practice of physick. London: Streator; 1668. p. 618.

2. Werlhof PG. Opera omnia. Hanover, Helwig, 1775, 748. In: Major R, editor. Classical descriptions of disease. 3rd edition. Springfield (IL): CC Thomas; 1965.
3. Willan R. On cutaneous diseases. London: J.G. Barnard; 1808. p. 452.
4. Wright JH. The histogenesis of the blood platelets. J Morphol 1910;21:263.
5. Wright JH. The origin and nature of blood plates. Boston Med Surg J 1906;154:643.
6. Wright JH. A rapid method for the differential staining of blood films and malarial parasites. J Med Res 1902;7:138.
7. Minot G. Studies on a case of idiopathic purpura hemorrhagica. Am J Med Sci 1916;152:48.
8. Frank E. Die essentielle thrombopenie. Berl Klin Wochenschr 1915;52:454 [in German].
9. Kaznelson P. Verschwinden der hamorrhagische diathese bei einem falle von "essentieller thrombopene" (Frank) nach milzexstirpation. Splenogene thrombolytische purpura. Wien Klin Wochenschr 1916;29:1451 [in German].
10. Yoshida Y. Historical review. The light and shadow of Paul Kaznelson: his life and contribution to hematology. Ann Hematol 2008;87:877.
11. Harrington WJ, Minnich V, Hollingsworth JW, et al. Demonstration of a thrombocytopenic factor in the blood of patients with thrombocytopenic purpura. J Lab Clin Med 1951;38:1.
12. Shulman NR, Marder VJ, Weinrach RS. Comparison of immunologic and idiopathic thrombocytopenia. Trans Assoc Am Physicians 1964;77:65.
13. Shulman NR, Marder VJ, Weinrach RS. Similarities between known antiplatelet antibodies and the factor responsible for thrombocytopenia in idiopathic purpura. Physiologic, serologic and isotopic studies. Ann N Y Acad Sci 1965;124:499.
14. Shulman NR, Weinrach RS, Libre EP, et al. The role of the reticuloendothelial system in the pathogenesis of idiopathic thrombocytopenic purpura. Trans Assoc Am Physicians 1965;78:374.
15. Harker LA. Kinetics of thrombopoiesis. J Clin Invest 1968;47:458.
16. Harker LA. Regulation of thrombopoiesis. Am J Phys 1970;218:1376.
17. Harker LA, Finch CA. Thrombokinetics in man. J Clin Invest 1969;48:963.
18. McIntosh B, Kaushansky K. Transcriptional regulation of bone marrow thrombopoietin by platelet proteins. Exp Hematol 2008;36:799.
19. Peck-Radosavljevic M, Wichlas M, Zacherl J, et al. Thrombopoietin induces rapid resolution of thrombocytopenia after orthotopic liver transplantation through increased platelet production. Blood 2000;95:795.
20. Peck-Radosavljevic M, Zacherl J, Meng YG, et al. Is inadequate thrombopoietin production a major cause of thrombocytopenia in cirrhosis of the liver? J Hepatol 1997;27:127.
21. Kuter DJ, Beeler DL, Rosenberg RD. The purification of megapoietin: a physiological regulator of megakaryocyte growth and platelet production. Proc Natl Acad Sci U S A 1994;91:11104.
22. Yang C, Li J, Kuter DJ. The physiological response of thrombopoietin (c-Mpl ligand) to thrombocytopenia in the rat. Br J Haematol 1999;105:478.
23. Li J, Xia Y, Kuter DJ. Interaction of thrombopoietin with the platelet c-mpl receptor in plasma: binding, internalization, stability and pharmacokinetics. Br J Haematol 1999;106:345.
24. Scheding S, Bergmann M, Shimosaka A, et al. Human plasma thrombopoietin levels are regulated by binding to platelet thrombopoietin receptors in vivo. Transfusion 2002;42:321.
25. Emmons RV, Reid DM, Cohen RL, et al. Human thrombopoietin levels are high when thrombocytopenia is due to megakaryocyte deficiency and low when due to increased platelet destruction. Blood 1996;87:4068.

26. Harker LA, Marzec UM, Hunt P, et al. Dose-response effects of pegylated human megakaryocyte growth and development factor on platelet production and function in nonhuman primates. Blood 1996;88:511.

27. Kaushansky K. Lineage-specific hematopoietic growth factors. N Engl J Med 2006;354:2034.

28. de Sauvage FJ, Carver-Moore K, Luoh SM, et al. Physiological regulation of early and late stages of megakaryocytopoiesis by thrombopoietin. J Exp Med 1996; 183:651.

29. de Sauvage FJ, Villeval JL, Shivdasani RA. Regulation of megakaryocytopoiesis and platelet production: lessons from animal models. J Lab Clin Med 1998;131: 496.

30. Alexander WS, Roberts AW, Nicola NA, et al. Deficiencies in progenitor cells of multiple hematopoietic lineages and defective megakaryocytopoiesis in mice lacking the thrombopoietic receptor c-Mpl. Blood 1996;87:2162.

31. Carver-Moore K, Broxmeyer HE, Luoh SM, et al. Low levels of erythroid and myeloid progenitors in thrombopoietin- and c-mpl-deficient mice. Blood 1996; 88:803.

32. Ballmaier M, Germeshausen M, Schulze H, et al. c-mpl mutations are the cause of congenital amegakaryocytic thrombocytopenia. Blood 2001;97:139.

33. Ihara K, Ishii E, Eguchi M, et al. Identification of mutations in the c-mpl gene in congenital amegakaryocytic thrombocytopenia. Proc Natl Acad Sci U S A 1999;96:3132.

34. van den Oudenrijn S, Bruin M, Folman CC, et al. Mutations in the thrombopoietin receptor, Mpl, in children with congenital amegakaryocytic thrombocytopenia. Br J Haematol 2000;110:441.

35. McMillan R, Wang L, Tomer A, et al. Suppression of in vitro megakaryocyte production by antiplatelet autoantibodies from adult patients with chronic ITP. Blood 2004;103:1364.

36. Nichol JL. Thrombopoietin levels after chemotherapy and in naturally occurring human diseases. Curr Opin Hematol 1998;5:203.

37. Kuter DJ. The physiology of platelet production. Stem Cells 1996;14:88.

38. Dameshek W, Miller E. The megakaryocytes in idiopathic thrombocytopenic purpura, a form of hypersplenism. Blood 1946;1:27.

39. Aster RH, Jandl JH. Platelet sequestration in man. I. Methods. J Clin Invest 1964; 43:843.

40. Najean Y, Ardaillou N, Dresch C, et al. The platelet destruction site in thrombocytopenic purpuras. Br J Haematol 1967;13:409.

41. Branehog I, Kutti J, Weinfeld A. Platelet survival and platelet production in idiopathic thrombocytopenic purpura (ITP). Br J Haematol 1974;27:127.

42. Thakur ML, Welch MJ, Joist JH, et al. Indium-LLL labeled platelets: studies on preparation and evaluation of in vitro and in vivo functions. Thromb Res 1976;9:345.

43. Ballem PJ, Segal GM, Stratton JR, et al. Mechanisms of thrombocytopenia in chronic autoimmune thrombocytopenic purpura. Evidence of both impaired platelet production and increased platelet clearance. J Clin Invest 1987;80:33.

44. Heyns Adu P, Badenhorst PN, Lotter MG, et al. Platelet turnover and kinetics in immune thrombocytopenic purpura: results with autologous ^{111}In-labeled platelets and homologous ^{51}Cr-labeled platelets differ. Blood 1986;67:86.

45. Hanson SR, Slichter SJ. Platelet kinetics in patients with bone marrow hypoplasia: evidence for a fixed platelet requirement. Blood 1985;66:1105.

46. Gernsheimer T, Stratton J, Ballem PJ, et al. Mechanisms of response to treatment in autoimmune thrombocytopenic purpura. N Engl J Med 1989;320:974.

47. Stratton JR, Ballem PJ, Gernsheimer T, et al. Platelet destruction in autoimmune thrombocytopenic purpura: kinetics and clearance of indium-111-labeled autologous platelets. J Nucl Med 1989;30:629.
48. Louwes H, Vellenga E, Houwerzijl EJ, et al. Effects of prednisone and splenectomy in patients with idiopathic thrombocytopenic purpura: only splenectomy induces a complete remission. Ann Hematol 2001;80:728.
49. Li S, Wang L, Zhao C, et al. CD8+ T cells suppress autologous megakaryocyte apoptosis in idiopathic thrombocytopenic purpura. Br J Haematol 2007;139:605.
50. Kuter DJ. Thrombopoietin and thrombopoietin mimetics in the treatment of thrombocytopenia. Annu Rev Med 2009;60:193.
51. Kuter DJ. New drugs for familiar therapeutic targets: thrombopoietin receptor agonists and immune thrombocytopenic purpura. Eur J Haematol Suppl 2008;69:9.
52. Kuter DJ. New thrombopoietic growth factors. Blood 2007;109:4607.
53. Kuter DJ. Thrombopoietin: biology, clinical applications, role in the donor setting. J Clin Apheresis 1996;11:149.
54. Kuter DJ. Thrombopoietins and thrombopoiesis: a clinical perspective. Vox Sang 1998;74:75.
55. Frey BM, Rafii S, Teterson M, et al. Adenovector-mediated expression of human thrombopoietin cDNA in immune- compromised mice: insights into the pathophysiology of osteomyelofibrosis. J Immunol 1998;160:691.
56. Villeval JL, Cohen-Solal K, Tulliez M, et al. High thrombopoietin production by hematopoietic cells induces a fatal myeloproliferative syndrome in mice. Blood 1997;90:4369.
57. Yan XQ, Lacey D, Hill D, et al. A model of myelofibrosis and osteosclerosis in mice induced by overexpressing thrombopoietin (mpl ligand): reversal of disease by bone marrow transplantation. Blood 1996;88:402.
58. Basser RL, Rasko JE, Clarke K, et al. Thrombopoietic effects of pegylated recombinant human megakaryocyte growth and development factor (PEG-rHuMGDF) in patients with advanced cancer. Lancet 1996;348:1279.
59. Fanucchi M, Glaspy J, Crawford J, et al. Effects of polyethylene glycol-conjugated recombinant human megakaryocyte growth and development factor on platelet counts after chemotherapy for lung cancer. N Engl J Med 1997;336:404.
60. Harker LA, Hunt P, Marzec UM, et al. Regulation of platelet production and function by megakaryocyte growth and development factor in nonhuman primates. Blood 1833;87:1996.
61. Kuter DJ, Begley CG. Recombinant human thrombopoietin: basic biology and evaluation of clinical studies. Blood 2002;100:3457.
62. Goodnough LT, Kuter DJ, McCullough J, et al. Prophylactic platelet transfusions from healthy apheresis platelet donors undergoing treatment with thrombopoietin. Blood 2001;98:1346.
63. Kuter DJ, Goodnough LT, Romo J, et al. Thrombopoietin therapy increases platelet yields in healthy platelet donors. Blood 2001;98:1339.
64. Vadhan-Raj S, Kavanagh JJ, Freedman RS, et al. Safety and efficacy of transfusions of autologous cryopreserved platelets derived from recombinant human thrombopoietin to support chemotherapy-associated severe thrombocytopenia: a randomised cross-over study. Lancet 2002;359:2145.
65. Li J, Yang C, Xia Y, et al. Thrombocytopenia caused by the development of antibodies to thrombopoietin. Blood 2001;98:3241.
66. Cwirla SE, Balasubramanian P, Duffin DJ, et al. Peptide agonist of the thrombopoietin receptor as potent as the natural cytokine. Science 1997;276:1696.

67. Bussel JB, Kuter DJ, George JN, et al. AMG 531, a thrombopoiesis-stimulating protein, for chronic ITP. N Engl J Med 2006;355:1672.

68. Wang B, Nichol JL, Sullivan JT. Pharmacodynamics and pharmacokinetics of AMG 531, a novel thrombopoietin receptor ligand. Clin Pharmacol Ther 2004; 76:628.

69. Broudy VC, Lin NL. AMG531 stimulates megakaryopoiesis in vitro by binding to Mpl. Cytokines 2004;25:52.

70. Kuter DJ, Mufti G, Bain B, et al. Evaluation of bone marrow reticulin formation in romiplostim-treated adult patients with chronic ITP. Blood 2008;112:1171a.

71. ODAC meeting briefing document. Available at:http://www.fda.gov/ohrms/dockets/ac/08/briefing/2008-4345b1-02-AMGEN.pdf. Accessed November 5, 2008.

72. Kuter DJ, Bussel JB, Lyons RM, et al. Efficacy of romiplostim in patients with chronic immune thrombocytopenic purpura: a double-blind randomised controlled trial. Lancet 2008;371:395.

73. Duffy KJ, Darcy MG, Delorme E, et al. Hydrazinonaphthalene and azonaphthalene thrombopoietin mimics are nonpeptidyl promoters of megakaryocytopoiesis. J Med Chem 2001;44:3730.

74. Duffy KJ, Price AT, Delorme E, et al. Identification of a pharmacophore for thrombopoietic activity of small, non-peptidyl molecules. 2. Rational design of naphtho[1,2-d]imidazole thrombopoietin mimics. J Med Chem 2002;45:3576.

75. Jenkins JM, Williams D, Deng Y, et al. Phase 1 clinical study of eltrombopag, an oral, nonpeptide thrombopoietin receptor agonist. Blood 2007;109:4739.

76. Desjardins RE, Tempel DL, Lucek R, et al. Single and multiple oral doses of AKR-501 (TM477) increase the platelet count in healthy volunteers. Blood 2006;108:145a.

77. Dziewanowska ZE, Matsumoto RM, Zhang JK, et al. Single and multiple oral doses of LGD-4665, a small molecule thrombopoietin receptor agonist, increase platelet counts in healthy male subjects. Blood 2007;110:1298.

78. Nakamura T, Miyakawa Y, Miyamura A, et al. A novel nonpeptidyl human c-Mpl activator stimulates human megakaryopoiesis and thrombopoiesis. Blood 2006; 107:4300.

79. Nogami W, Yoshida H, Koizumi K, et al. The effect of a novel, small non-peptidyl molecule butyzamide on human thrombopoietin receptor and megakaryopoiesis. Haematologica 2008;93:1495.

80. Yamane N, Takahashi K, Tanaka Y, et al. Discovery of novel non-peptide thrombopoietin mimetic compounds that induce megakaryocytopoiesis. Biosci Rep 2008; 28:275.

81. Yamane N, Tanaka Y, Ohyabu N, et al. Characterization of novel non-peptide thrombopoietin mimetics, their species specificity and the activation mechanism of the thrombopoietin receptor. Eur J Pharmacol 2008;586:44.

82. Jenkins J, Nicholl R, Williams D, et al. An oral, non-peptide, small molecule thrombopoietin receptor agonist increases platelet counts in healthy subjects. Blood 2004;104:797a.

83. Bussel JB, Cheng G, Saleh MN, et al. Eltrombopag for the treatment of chronic idiopathic thrombocytopenic purpura. N Engl J Med 2007;357:2237.

84. Erickson-Miller C, Delorme E, Iskander M, et al. Species specificity and receptor domain interaction of a small molecule TPO receptor agonist. Blood 2004;104: 795a.

85. Fukushima-Shintani M, Suzuki K, Iwatsuki Y, et al. AKR-501 (YM477) in combination with thrombopoietin enhances human megakaryocytopoiesis. Exp Hematol 2008;36:1337.

86. Nomura S, Dan K, Hotta T, et al. Effects of pegylated recombinant human megakaryocyte growth and development factor in patients with idiopathic thrombocytopenic purpura. Blood 2002;100:728.
87. Rice L, Nichol JL, McMillan R, et al. Cyclic immune thrombocytopenia responsive to thrombopoietic growth factor therapy. Am J Hematol 2001;68:210.
88. Cole JL, Marzec UM, Gunthel CJ, et al. Ineffective platelet production in thrombocytopenic human immunodeficiency virus-infected patients. Blood 1998;91:3239.
89. Harker LA, Carter RA, Marzec UM, et al. Correction of thrombocytopenia and ineffective platelet production in patients infected with human immunodeficiency virus (HIV) by PEG-rHuMGDF therapy. Blood 1998;92:707a.
90. Harker LA, Marzec UM, Novembre F, et al. Treatment of thrombocytopenia in chimpanzees infected with human immunodeficiency virus by pegylated recombinant human megakaryocyte growth and development factor. Blood 1998;91:4427.
91. Houwerzijl EJ, Blom NR, van der Want JJ, et al. Ultrastructural study shows morphologic features of apoptosis and para-apoptosis in megakaryocytes from patients with idiopathic thrombocytopenic purpura. Blood 2004;103:500.

Chronic Immune Thrombocytopenia in Adults: Epidemiology and Clinical Presentation

Patrick F. Fogarty, MD

KEYWORDS

• Chronic ITP • Bleeding • Natural history • Epidemiology

EPIDEMIOLOGY OF CHRONIC IMMUNE THROMBOCYTOPENIA

Data regarding the incidence and prevalence of immune thrombocytopenia (ITP) are scant, and derive mostly from European and North American population-based analyses. Whereas the *incidence* of newly diagnosed ITP ranges from 1.6 to 3.9 per 100,000 persons per year,[1–3] analyses of *prevalence* indicate a higher frequency among affected adults, due to the propensity of the disorder to become chronic and the resulting accumulation of cases in the population. Recent studies concerning the epidemiology of ITP in adults are summarized in **Table 1**; for comparison, studies defining both incidence (which indicates cases of new-onset ITP) and prevalence (which identifies persistent or chronic cases) of ITP in adults are included.

An analysis of the available epidemiologic data concerning chronic ITP requires a careful consideration of definitions. Until very recently, "chronic" ITP required persistence of thrombocytopenia for at least 6 months following diagnosis.[7,8] A clarification of terminology now requires that the disorder be present for at least 12 months in order for the disease to be called "chronic;" in contrast, ITP characterized by low platelet counts for at least 3 but fewer than 12 months after diagnosis is referred to as "persistent" ITP.[9] Thus, according to the current definition, older studies may consider shorter time periods of observation when designating cases as having "chronic" ITP.

Incidence is defined as the number of new cases of a disease in a population over a specified period of time, and, accordingly, studies describing incidence rates of ITP

Financial disclosure: P.F.F. has received research support and honoraria from GSK, and research support and honoraria from Amgen.

Division of Hematology/Oncology, Department of Medicine, University of California, San Francisco, 505 Parnassus Avenue, Room M-1286, San Francisco, CA 94143-1270, USA

E-mail address: pfogarty@medicine.ucsf.edu

Hematol Oncol Clin N Am 23 (2009) 1213–1221
doi:10.1016/j.hoc.2009.08.004
0889-8588/09/$ – see front matter © 2009 Elsevier Inc. All rights reserved.

Table 1
Epidemiology of new-onset or chronic immune thrombocytopenic purpura in adults

Study	N	Design	Incidence/Prevalence (per 100,000 Persons)[a]	Female: Male Ratio	Comments
Frederiksen and Schmidt, 1999[1]	221	Retrospective (Denmark)	Incidence = 2.25/y[b] Doubling of incidence with age >60 y	1.7	Cases defined by clinical criteria[c]
Neylon et al, 2003[3]	245	Prospective (UK)	Incidence = 1.6/y Incidence highest among age >60 y	1.2[d]	Cases defined by clinical criteria[e]
Abrahamson et al, 2009[2]	840	Retrospective (UK)	Incidence = 3.9/y	1.4[f]	Cases defined by administrative data[g]
Segal and Powe, 2006[4]	454	Retrospective (Maryland, USA)	Period prevalence = 5.6–16[h] Prevalence increases with age	>1.9[i]	Cases defined by administrative data[j]
Landgren et al, 2006[5]	7196	Retrospective (US Veterans hospital system)	Period prevalence = 189 (black) Period prevalence = 176 (white)	n/a	Cases defined by administrative data[k]
Feudjo-Tepie et al, 2008[6]	4943	Retrospective (USA)	Period prevalence = 20.0 Peak prevalence in middle-adult years	1.8	Cases defined by administrative data[l]

[a] Age-adjusted.

[b] Incidence = 2.68/y if platelets $<100 \times 10^9$/L considered.

[c] Patients with presenting platelet count $<100 \times 10^9$/L included; alternative causes of thrombocytopenia (eg, myelodysplasia, disseminated intravascular coagulation), cancer, infectious thrombocytopenia excluded.

[d] Female predominance in age 45–59 years only.

[e] Patients with presenting platelet count $<50 \times 10^9$/L included; bone marrow examination required; proven causes of thrombocytopenia (eg, gestational, drug-related) excluded; infectious thrombocytopenia not excluded.

[f] Incidence in women higher than men only until age 70 years.

[g] Patients aged ≥ 18 years included; one continuous year of observation required to exclude prevalent cases.

[h] Period prevalence decreases to 4.5 per 100,000 when a duration of disease of at least 180 days is considered.

[i] Data include children.

[j] Age ≥ 65 years and cases with concurrent human immunodeficiency virus infection, bone marrow failure, and leukemia/lymphoma excluded; cases from a single calendar year only included; at least 2 diagnosis codes separated by ≥ 30 days required.

[k] Males and hospitalized cases only considered; follow-up for ≥ 1 year required; variance in diagnosis codes over 30-year study period leading to inclusion of non-ITP thrombocytopenia possible.

[l] Age-unrestricted inclusion criteria; cases with concurrent human immunodeficiency virus infection, bone marrow failure, and leukemia/lymphoma excluded; cases across calendar years permitted; at least 2 diagnosis codes separated by ≥ 6 months required.

among adults reflect new-onset ITP, and are mostly European (see **Table 1**). Estimates of the frequency of persistent or chronic ITP, conversely, derive from analyses of *prevalence* (defined as the number of established cases among a defined population), and most of the recent work in this regard has been performed in the United States (see **Table 1**).

In one retrospective United States study, administrative data from the state of Maryland during one calendar year (2002) was used to estimate the period prevalence of chronic ITP.[4] Two diagnoses codes separated by at least 30 days were required, in an effort to eliminate transient cases from the analysis. The age-adjusted prevalence was 9.5 per 100,000 persons, increasing from 4.1 per 100,000 among 19- to 24-year-olds to 16 per 100,000 among 55- to 64-year-olds. That the *prevalence* of ITP increased with age was consistent with prior studies reporting an increased *incidence* of ITP (ie, new cases) with advancing age.[1,3] Importantly, however the age-adjusted period prevalence decreased to 4.5 per 100,000 persons when 2 diagnosis codes separated by at least 180 days were required. Using the current definitions,[9] this figure more closely approximates the prevalence of persistent ITP and may overestimate the prevalence of chronic ITP (at least 12 months of disease). In this study, the female-to-male ratio among cases was 1.9, with most of the female predominance occurring in middle age.

In a similar, larger analysis of administrative data derived from a claims database among United States persons diagnosed with ITP lasting for at least 6 months, a higher period prevalence of 20.0 per 100,000 was reported, potentially as a result of an expanded consideration of cases (see **Table 1**).[6] An increasing prevalence with age and a higher prevalence among women also were observed.

Although some data has suggested a lower prevalence of ITP among black as compared with white Americans,[10] a retrospective population-based analysis showed a comparable prevalence of ITP among black and white military veterans, suggesting no ethnic variation (see **Table 1**).[5]

CLINICAL PRESENTATION AND NATURAL HISTORY OF CHRONIC IMMUNE THROMBOCYTOPENIA
Clinical Presentation

By definition, individuals with chronic ITP have carried the diagnosis for at least 12 months,[9] and either exhibit a reduced platelet count or require ongoing treatment to maintain a normal platelet count. Due to the well-recognized propensity of the disorder to become chronic in adults, it has long been held that most nonpediatric patients who are diagnosed with symptomatic, new-onset ITP will retain the diagnosis at 1 year and require therapy.[7,8,11] This assumption, however, has been challenged in some recent series.[3,12–14]

Although symptomatic bleeding is expected to be related to the baseline platelet count,[7,8,11,15] data regarding the distribution of severity thrombocytopenia (ie, mild, moderate, or severe) among patients beyond the initial phase of the disease are limited. Because the available series of adult patients with ITP either specify platelet thresholds *a priori*[13] or lack consistency in terms of timing of follow-up assessments,[3,16,17] data regarding the severity of thrombocytopenia at the onset of the persistent or chronic phase of the disease are not as available in adults as they are in children, in whom prospective registrations with adequate long-term follow-up have been performed.[18]

The manifestations of disease (if any) may vary considerably among patients with chronic ITP, and besides the platelet count may be influenced by additional factors including the age of the patient.[19] Patients with mild or moderate thrombocytopenia may manifest almost no bleeding symptoms, whereas severe thrombocytopenia (platelets, <20–30 × 10^9/L) is commonly associated with spontaneous mucocutaneous bleeding including petechiae, purpura, epistaxis, and gingival bleeding.[7,8,15] The most feared complication of severe thrombocytopenia is intracranial hemorrhage, although other types of severe internal bleeding (such as gastrointestinal) also are possible.

When first evaluating a patient who carries a diagnosis of chronic ITP, assurance of exclusion of other causes of chronic thrombocytopenia is critical. These causes include infectious-related (human immunodeficiency virus or hepatitis C virus infections),[20] lymphoproliferative disease-related (such as chronic lymphocytic leukemia or lymphoma)[21] and, rarely, congenital (commoner in younger patients or those with a compelling family history).[22,23] Suspicion for an alternative cause of chronic thrombocytopenia may be heightened if the platelet count never has responded to standard immunomodulatory treatments. In older patients, myelodysplasia (including chronic myelomonocytic leukemia) should be considered and excluded; according to current guidelines,[7,8] bone marrow aspiration in patients older than 60 years is appropriate.

Natural History of Chronic Immune Thrombocytopenia and Clinical Outcomes

Although the majority of patients with ITP are symptomatic at diagnosis,[1,3,11] studies addressing disease manifestations in patients who continue to be affected at 12 months after diagnosis are relatively few. In addition, because adults with new-onset ITP typically receive treatment, fewer true natural history data are available for adults than for children with ITP. Instead, series of patients with new-onset disease with follow-up beyond the initial phase of the disorder, or of patients who are identified as having persistent or chronic disease, provide insight into clinical outcomes for adults with longer-lasting disease (**Table 2**).

In a European population-based study, 245 adult patients with new-onset ITP (confirmed by bone marrow examination) identified over a 7-year period were followed prospectively for a median of 60 months.[3] At 6 months post diagnosis, fewer than 25% of patients who had presented with platelet counts of less than 20 × 10^9/L were reported to have chronic ITP (defined as a platelet count <50 × 10^9/L) that required ongoing treatment. Of the 27 deaths that occurred during the study period, only 3 were interpreted as being directly caused by ITP. Further, 5 of 45 patients who did not receive treatment spontaneously remitted. These observations led the investigators to infer a better prognosis of adult ITP than previously thought. Data on outcomes beyond 6 months in all patients, however, were not presented, and relapses beyond the study period could not be excluded. In addition, patients with platelet counts of 50 × 10^9/L or more at presentation, in whom disease progression could have occurred, were not included in the study population.

In a study of 178 elderly individuals (mean age, 72 years) presenting to a single Italian institution with ITP of varying clinical severity over a 17-year period, 13.4% of 90 patients who never received treatment had platelet counts of less than 50 × 10^9/L at 6 months' or longer follow-up.[12] Of the 49 patients who were designated as having experienced a complete or partial response at 1 month following initial treatment, 28.6% experienced a relapse (defined as platelet count <50 × 10^9/L) at a mean of 13 months. Of 28 patients who experienced no response at 1 month following initial treatment, 43% were reported as achieving a late response at a median of 65 months post diagnosis and 57% remained nonresponders. Of note, spontaneous remission (defined as platelets $\geq$150 × 10^9/L) occurred in 5.5% of the 90 patients who never received treatment at a median follow-up of 43 months. That 87% of untreated patients either achieved or maintained a platelet count of 50 × 10^9/L or more without bleeding, however, may have been the result of inclusion of very mild cases (up to platelet counts of 139 × 10^9/L), predisposing the study population to more favorable outcomes. Response duration was not reported in this study.

In an Italian, single-center, retrospective evaluation over a 20-year period of 94 adults with "chronic" ITP (defined as platelet count <50 × 10^9/L at ≥6 months post diagnosis) who underwent splenectomy, 11% still had a platelet count of less than 50 × 10^9/L at 12 months post splenectomy, increasing to 16% at a median 84 months' follow-up.[25] Whereas 2 patients died of sepsis at 85 and 96 months post splenectomy, no patient (including nonresponders) died of hemorrhage. In a similar, prospective study at a single institution in France, 183 ITP patients with "chronic" ITP (defined as platelet count <50 × 10^9/L at ≥6 months post diagnosis) underwent splenectomy, and 71% had responded at 3 years' follow-up.[16] Of the 47 ITP patients who had failed to respond durably to splenectomy (defined as platelet counts <100 × 10^9/L at 3 months post procedure; 7 children inclusive in this subpopulation), at a median follow-up of 90 months, 10.6% remained severely thrombocytopenic (platelets, <20 × 10^9/L) and fatal bleeding occurred in 6%.

The long-term outcome of a combined series of 310 children and adults (median age, 40 years; age range, 8–87 years) with chronic ITP (defined as persistence of platelets <150 × 10^9/L for at least 6 months following diagnosis) was assessed in a single-center, Italian study.[17] At a median follow-up of 121 months, 34 patients had platelet counts of less than 30 × 10^9/L and the majority (56%) of this cohort were not receiving treatment. Major bleeding (requiring hospitalization or leading to a decline in hemoglobin of 2 g/dL) was observed in 9 patients, and one death due to intracranial hemorrhage occurred. Of note, 7 of 9 episodes of major bleeding occurred in patients younger than 60 years.

A United States–based, retrospective study of 114 adults with chronic ITP who had failed to respond durably to splenectomy (defined as platelet count after splenectomy ≤30 × 10^9/L) demonstrated that 28.6% of evaluable patients remained severely thrombocytopenic (platelet count, ≤30 × 10^9/L) at a median follow-up of 110 months post splenectomy, whereas the majority achieved a complete or stable partial remission at a median of 46 months.[13] Thirty-two deaths occurred during the study period, due to bleeding (10.2% of the evaluable study population) or complications of therapy (5.6%).

In a single-institution, retrospective Dutch study of 152 adults with ITP accrued over a 20-year period, an 85% response rate (defined as a platelet count >30 × 10^9/L while on no ITP-specific medications 2 years post diagnosis) was observed among evaluable patients.[14] Although the current terminology indicates that some individuals in this cohort actually would have had chronic ITP,[9] the mortality rate was similar to that of the non-ITP population. In contrast, in the 9% of patients with severe thrombocytopenia (platelets ≤30 × 10^9/L) at 2 years' follow-up the mortality rate was fourfold that of the general population, with a comparable causation of infectious complications and bleeding. Among individuals who required immunomodulatory medications to maintain a platelet count of greater than 30 × 10^9/L at 2 years' follow-up (6% of the evaluable patients), the mortality rate was only slightly increased and ITP-related hospital admissions occurred frequently, pointing to augmented morbidity of the (then) available therapies among patients with chronic ITP.

To better define the risk of bleeding among adults with severe, chronic ITP (defined as platelet count <30 × 10^9/L at least 1 year following diagnosis), a pooled analysis of clinical series comprising more than 1800 patients identified an annual incidence of fatal hemorrhage of 1.6 to 3.9 cases per 100 patient-years (0.4% and 13% per year in patients younger than 40 and older than 60 years, respectively), confirming an

Table 2
Clinical outcomes in persistent and chronic ITP[a] in adults

Study	Population	N	Platelet Count (×10⁹/L)	Median Age, Range (y)	Follow-up (Median) (Mo)	Bleeding	Deaths	No. of Spontaneous Remissions (%)
Stasi et al, 1995[24]	New-onset ITP	208	$\leq$120	51 (19–86)	92	—	5 deaths due to ICH	8 (3.8%)[b]
Portielje et al, 2001[14]	New-onset ITP[c]	152	<100	39[d] (15–86)	113	—	4-fold increase in mortality in 9% of patients with platelets $\leq$30 × 10⁹/L at 2 y follow-up	—
Neylon et al, 2003[3]	New-onset ITP[e]	245	<50	56 (16–91)	60	—	2 deaths "attributable to ITP…later in the course of…disease" and 1 septic death following splenectomy	5 (2%)[f]
Bizzoni et al, 2006[12]	New-onset ITP, elderly	178	1–139 (median 49)	70 (65–87)	43	Bleeding score not found to correlate with age $\geq$ or <75 years	1 death (ICH) at 48 mo follow-up	5 (2.8%)[g]
Vianelli et al, 2001[17]	Persistent/chronic ITP[h]	310	<150	40 (8–87)	121	9 major bleeding events	1 death (ICH)	0 (0%)[i]
Mazzucconi et al, 1999[25]	Persistent/chronic ITP;[j] post splenectomy	94	<50	31 (15–57)	84	—	No hemorrhagic deaths[k]	—

Bourgeois et al, 2003[16]	Persistent/chronic ITP,[j] refractory to splenectomy	40[l]	<30	41 (16–74)	7.5	3 hospitalizations due to bleeding[m]	2 deaths (ICH and gastrointestinal bleeding) at 5 and 0 mo post splenectomy, respectively	—
McMillan and Durette, 2004[13]	Chronic ITP,[n] refractory to splenectomy	114	<30	n/a[o]	110	—	Death due to bleeding in 10.2% or complications of therapy in 5.6% of 105 evaluable patients	—
Cohen et al, 2000[19]	Chronic ITP[p] (pooled analysis)	1817	<30	n/a[q]	n/a[r]	Fatal and nonfatal hemorrhage: 0.4%–14%/y and 3%–71%, respectively[s]	5-y mortality: 2.2% (<40 y old), 47.8% (>60 y old)	—

Abbreviation: ICH, intracranial hemorrhage.

a Designation of duration of disease is per current terminology[9] and may differ from the original designation.

b Defined as platelets ≥ 120 × 10^9/L; frequency of spontaneous remission increases to 9.2% if only patients who did not receive treatment (n = 87) are considered.

c At 2 years' follow-up, 6% of evaluable patients required immunomodulatory medications to maintain platelets >30 × 10^9/L.

d Mean age.

e At a median 60 months' follow-up, fewer than 25% of the initial study population of 245 patients had platelets ≤50 × 10^9/L for at least 6 months post diagnosis.

f Defined as platelets ≥ 100 × 10^9/L; frequency of spontaneous remission increases to 11% if only patients who did not receive treatment (n = 45) are considered.

g Defined as platelets ≥ 150 × 10^9/L; frequency of spontaneous remission increases to 5.5% if only patients who did not receive treatment (n = 90) are considered.

h Defined as platelets ≤ 150 × 10^9/L for ≥ 6 months post diagnosis.

i Defined as platelets ≥ 150 × 10^9/L.

j Defined as platelet count < 50 × 10^9/L at ≥ 6 months post diagnosis.

k Two deaths due to sepsis at 85 and 96 months post splenectomy, respectively, occurred.

l Initial study population included 183 patients, and 7 of the 47 patients who failed splenectomy were children.

m Could include cases of bleeding in children.

n Defined as platelet count <30 × 10^9/L despite splenectomy.

o Median age at diagnosis = 37 years.

p Defined as platelets <30 × 10^9/L at ≥1 year post diagnosis.

q Pooled analysis yielded 9 of 17 studies reporting age distribution of cohorts.

r Pooled analysis identified 1258 to 3023 patient-years at risk.

s Lower estimate is for cases <40 years and higher estimate is for cases >60 years old.

increasing risk of fatal bleeding with advancing age.[19] By comparison, the rate of nonfatal hemorrhage was estimated to be 3% and 71% per year in patients younger than 40 and older than 60 years, respectively. In this analysis, the predicted 5-year mortality rates ranged from 2.2% among those younger than 40 to 47.8% among those older than 60 years, suggesting a worse prognosis among older individuals with severe thrombocytopenia than younger patients or those with milder disease.

SUMMARY

Data concerning the prevalence of chronic ITP among adults are limited, and are confounded by lack of concordance of definitions of stage of disease. In the largest series of outpatients, prevalence has been estimated to range from 5.6 to 20 per 100,000 population and increases with advancing age. A female predominance is most pronounced among middle-aged patients, and no racial variation is apparent. Adult patients with chronic ITP may have a better prognosis than previously thought, although bleeding risk increases dramatically in association with severe thrombocytopenia and older age; a small minority of patients may recover spontaneously. More systematic analyses, with standardized definitions of cases and adequate duration of follow-up, are needed.

REFERENCES

1. Frederiksen H, Schmidt K. The incidence of idiopathic thrombocytopenic purpura in adults increases with age. Blood 1999;94(3):909–13.
2. Abrahamson PE, Hall SA, Feudjo-Tepie M, et al. The Incidence of idiopathic thrombocytopenic purpura (ITP) among adults: a population-based study and literature review. Eur J Haematol 2009;83:83–9.
3. Neylon AJ, Saunders PW, Howard MR, et al. Clinically significant newly presenting autoimmune thrombocytopenic purpura in adults: a prospective study of a population-based cohort of 245 patients. Br J Haematol 2003;122(6):966–74.
4. Segal JB, Powe NR. Prevalence of immune thrombocytopenia: analyses of administrative data. J Thromb Haemost 2006;4(11):2377–83.
5. Landgren O, Gridley G, Fears TR, et al. Immune thrombocytopenic purpura does not exhibit a disparity in prevalence between African American and White veterans. Blood 2006;108(3):1111–2.
6. Feudjo-Tepie MA, Robinson NJ, Bennett D. Prevalence of diagnosed chronic immune thrombocytopenic purpura in the US: analysis of a large claim database. J Thromb Haemost 2008;6(4):711–2.
7. British Committee for Standards in Haematology General Haematology Task Force. Guidelines for the investigation and management of idiopathic thrombocytopenic purpura in adults, children and in pregnancy. Br J Haematol 2003;120(4): 574–96.
8. George JN, Woolf SH, Raskob GE, et al. Idiopathic thrombocytopenic purpura: a practice guideline developed by explicit methods for the American Society of Hematology. Blood 1996;88(1):3–40.
9. Rodeghiero F, Stasi R, Gernsheimer T, et al. Standardization of terminology, definitions and outcome criteria in immune thrombocytopenic purpura of adults and children: report from an international working group. Blood 2009;113(11): 2386–93.
10. Teeling JL, Jansen-Hendriks T, Kuijpers TW, et al. Therapeutic efficacy of intravenous immunoglobulin preparations depends on the immunoglobulin G dimers: studies in experimental immune thrombocytopenia. Blood 2001;98(4):1095–9.

11. Cines DB, McMillan R. Management of adult idiopathic thrombocytopenic purpura. Annu Rev Med 2005;56:425–42.
12. Bizzoni L, Mazzucconi MG, Gentile M, et al. Idiopathic thrombocytopenic purpura (ITP) in the elderly: clinical course in 178 patients. Eur J Haematol 2006;76(3):210–6.
13. McMillan R, Durette C. Long-term outcomes in adults with chronic ITP after splenectomy failure. Blood 2004;104(4):956–60.
14. Portielje JE, Westendorp RG, Kluin-Nelemans HC, et al. Morbidity and mortality in adults with idiopathic thrombocytopenic purpura. Blood 2001;97(9):2549–54.
15. Cines DB, Blanchette VS. Immune thrombocytopenic purpura. N Engl J Med 2002;346(13):995–1008.
16. Bourgeois E, Caulier MT, Delarozee C, et al. Long-term follow-up of chronic auto-immune thrombocytopenic purpura refractory to splenectomy: a prospective analysis. Br J Haematol 2003;120(6):1079–88.
17. Vianelli N, Valdre L, Fiacchini M, et al. Long-term follow-up of idiopathic thrombo-cytopenic purpura in 310 patients. Haematologica 2001;86(5):504–9.
18. Imbach P, Kuhne T, Muller D, et al. Childhood ITP: 12 months follow-up data from the prospective registry I of the Intercontinental Childhood ITP Study Group (ICIS). Pediatr Blood Cancer 2006;46(3):351–6.
19. Cohen YC, Djulbegovic B, Shamai-Lubovitz O, et al. The bleeding risk and natural history of idiopathic thrombocytopenic purpura in patients with persistent low platelet counts. Arch Intern Med 2000;160(11):1630–8.
20. Liebman HA. Viral-associated immune thrombocytopenic purpura. Hematology Am Soc Hematol Educ Program 2008;2008:212–8.
21. Liebman HA. Recognizing and treating secondary immune thrombocytopenic purpura associated with lymphoproliferative disorders. Semin Hematol 2009;46(1 suppl 2):S33–6.
22. De Boeck K, Degreef H, Verwilghen R, et al. Thrombocytopenia: first symptom in a patient with dyskeratosis congenita. Pediatrics 1981;67(6):898–903.
23. Fogarty PF, Yamaguchi H, Wiestner A, et al. Late presentation of dyskeratosis congenita as apparently acquired aplastic anaemia due to mutations in telome-rase RNA. Lancet 2003;362(9396):1628–30.
24. Stasi R, Stipa E, Masi M, et al. Long-term observation of 208 adults with chronic idiopathic thrombocytopenic purpura. Am J Med 1995;98(5):436–42.
25. Mazzucconi MG, Arista MC, Peraino M, et al. Long-term follow-up of autoimmune thrombocytopenic purpura (ATP) patients submitted to splenectomy. Eur J Haematol 1999;62(4):219–22.

Chronic Immune Thrombocytopenia in Children: Epidemiology and Clinical Presentation

Carolyn M. Bennett, MD, MSc[a],*, Michael Tarantino, MD[b]

KEYWORDS

- Chronic childhood immune thrombocytopenic purpura • ITP
- Bleeding • Splenectomy • Intracranial hemorrhage

Immune thrombocytopenic purpura (ITP) is one of the most common acquired bleeding disorders in children. The natural history of ITP in the pediatric population differs significantly from that in adults. Most adults will have chronic ITP, persistent thrombocytopenia beyond 6 months from diagnosis, and many will require some form of ongoing therapy. In contrast, most children with ITP will have the acute form of disease, self-limited thrombocytopenia that resolves completely within weeks or months, with or without therapy. Twenty percent to 30% of children with acute ITP will go on to have persistent thrombocytopenia, but nearly a quarter of these children will have disease resolution by 12.[1] Only a small subset of children with ITP has clinically significant disease with severe thrombocytopenia and/or bleeding that requires intervention. Treatment for these children is an ongoing clinical challenge, as few therapies offer long-term remission, and all have significant side effects and toxicities. Treatment-related toxicity is not trivial and should weigh in the decision to intervene, or not, with drug therapy. More effective therapies that have minimal toxicity are sorely needed.

This article focuses on the management of chronic ITP in the pediatric population.

PATHOPHYSIOLOGY

Until the past 10 to 20 years, the pathophysiology of ITP has largely been attributed to platelet autoantibody production and resultant platelet destruction by macrophages in

[a] Aflac Cancer Center and Blood Disorders Service, Emory University School of Medicine and Children's Healthcare of Atlanta, 5455 Meridian Mark Road, Suite 400, Atlanta, GA 30342, USA
[b] University of Illinois College of Medicine-Peoria, 1 Illini Drive, Peoria, IL 61656-1649, USA
* Corresponding author.
E-mail address: carolyn.bennett@choa.org (C.M. Bennett).

Hematol Oncol Clin N Am 23 (2009) 1223–1238
doi:10.1016/j.hoc.2009.08.002
0889-8588/09/$ – see front matter © 2009 Elsevier Inc. All rights reserved.

hemonc.theclinics.com

the reticuloendothelial system.[2] Although autoantibody-mediated destruction of platelets is a critical part of the disease, recent evidence suggests a more multifactorial and complex pathogenesis involving both cellular and humoral immunity. Studies investigating the interaction between cellular and humoral immune responses have identified unrecognized mechanisms of platelet autoimmune destruction in ITP and potential targets for future therapy.[3] New treatment strategies targeted at specific immune mechanisms may prove to be more effective in managing ITP in both children and adults.

The earliest informative studies of ITP were done by Harrington and colleagues,[4] in the 1950s. These studies showed that ITP involved an "antiplatelet factor" in plasma of affected patients and later confirmed that this factor was immunoglobulin. Later studies showed that ITP resulted from Fc-receptor–mediated autoimmune destruction of antibody-coated platelets by macrophages in the reticuloendothelial system.[5] The autoantibody in most patients with ITP is of the IgG subclass and is reactive to multiple platelet antigens, most commonly glycoproteins IIb/IIa and Ib/IX.[6] Anti-GP IIb/IIIa antibodies can be detected in a high percentage of children with both acute and chronic ITP.[7] However, in some patients with ITP, both adults and children with acute and chronic disease, no antibodies can be detected even with highly sensitive direct platelet-bound antibody identification methods.[8] Although antibodies clearly play a crucial role in the development of thrombocytopenia in ITP, other mechanisms of platelet destruction are important for disease pathogenesis.

Recent evidence has shown that cellular immunity plays a critical role in the development of ITP. T-cell abnormalities have been demonstrated in patients with ITP and CD4+, T helper cell activation appears to be an important trigger for platelet autoantibody production.[9] Imbalances in cytokine secretion have been measured in children and adults with ITP indicating altered cellular immunity. T cell clones from the peripheral blood of children and adults with chronic ITP secrete increased levels of interleukin (IL)-2 when incubated with platelets in vitro.[10,11] Increased serum levels of inflammatory cytokines, IL-10, IL-2, and interferon (IFN)-γ, have been measured in children and adults with chronic ITP.[12,13] Cytokine gene expression by peripheral blood mononuclear cells from chronic ITP patients was measured ex vivo and after in vitro activation by mitogens and also showed increases in both IL-2 and IFN-γ.[14] More recent studies have shown that cytotoxic CD3+ T cells from chronic ITP patients have increased expression of genes involved in cell-mediated cytotoxicity and that these cytotoxic T cells can destroy platelets with a high effector cell to target ratio.[15,16]

Clearly, increased platelet destruction is an important part of the pathogenesis of ITP, but decreased platelet production also plays a critical role, particularly in adults.[17] Increased megakaryocyte numbers in the bone marrow of patients is a hallmark of ITP, but in up to 40% of adults, this increase may be inappropriate for the degree of platelet destruction.[18] Antibodies may inhibit megakaryocyte maturation, induce apoptosis, impair platelet release, or megakaryocyte destruction may occur within the bone marrow.[17,19] In many ITP patients, circulating thrombopoietin (TPO) levels are either normal or only slightly increased indicating that ineffective megakaryopoiesis may be responsible for severe thrombocytopenia in some patients.[20] New thrombopoietin mimetics have shown good efficacy in the treatment of ITP in adults with the disease and studies in children are under way.[21,22]

Ongoing research has shown that ITP results from a complex interplay between cellular and humoral immunity, which leads to a loss of self-tolerance and the autoimmune destruction of platelets and decreased megakaryopoiesis.[23] Targeted treatment strategies are being developed and used for clinical management of the disease and may prove as or more effective than previous therapeutic strategies.

CLINICAL FEATURES OF IMMUNE THROMBOCYTOPENIC PURPURA IN CHILDHOOD

ITP may present at any age including infancy, but the peak age of diagnosis in children is between 5 and 6 years, with 70% presenting between 1 and 10 years.[24] Often the onset of symptoms is preceded by a presumed viral illness or by immunization with a live virus vaccine.[24] Approximately two-thirds of children with ITP will experience a preceding febrile illness and numerous viruses have been associated with immune thrombocytopenia, including rubella, varicella, mumps, rubeola, cytomegalovirus, Epstein-Barr virus, and hepatitis, among others.[23] The risk of ITP is increased in children after immunization with measles, mumps, and rubella (MMR) vaccine.[25,26] In the vast majority of children with ITP, no specific infection can be documented.

ITP is a diagnosis of exclusion and other causes of thrombocytopenia must be considered before making the diagnosis.[27] In most cases, the diagnosis can be made based on careful history, physical examination, and review of peripheral blood smear.[27] Children with ITP typically present acutely with the sudden onset of mucocutaneous bleeding and isolated thrombocytopenia with surprisingly few other signs or symptoms.[28–30] Skin findings of bruising and petechiae can be extensive, but many children with ITP have only minimal evidence of bleeding despite profound thrombocytopenia.[31,32] Typical bleeding manifestations include purpura, petechiae, epistaxis, hematuria, and menorrhagia (in teenage girls).[29–31,33] The physical examination is usually normal otherwise. Findings such as fever, malaise, other constitutional symptoms, pain, limp, lymphadenopathy, and splenomegaly are atypical and warrant further investigation.[28,34] Complete blood count reveals profound thrombocytopenia with large platelets, but is otherwise normal. Most children have severe thrombocytopenia at presentation with platelets under 20×10^9/L, but serious or life-threatening bleeding is unusual.[32] Mild anemia may be present because of bleeding, but other blood cell abnormalities are not typical and should be investigated further if present.[34] Bone marrow evaluation is unnecessary for the diagnosis in most typical cases, but is indicated in the presence of atypical physical or laboratory findings. Testing for the presence of antiplatelet antibodies is not useful diagnostically or prognostically, as neither the antigenic specificity nor the serum titer of antiplatelet antibodies correlates with severity of the thrombocytopenia or predicts disease course.[7,8,35,36]

In most children with ITP, the thrombocytopenia resolves spontaneously within weeks irrespective of treatment.[37–41] About 20% to 30% of children will have chronic ITP, defined as persistence of thrombocytopenia beyond 6 months from diagnosis.[27] In a prospective study of 2540 patients with acute ITP by the Intercontinental ITP Study (ICIS) group, about two-thirds of children had resolution of disease by 6 months.[24] Another 25% had resolution of disease by 12 months.[1] There is a high rate of long-term spontaneous remission and in most patients with chronic ITP, the outcome is favorable.[1,38–41] Only about 5% to 10% of children with ITP will have clinically significant, chronic ITP 2 years after diagnoses.[42,43]

Certain clinical and laboratory features have been associated with the subsequent development of chronic ITP including an insidious onset of symptoms, female gender, older age, and higher platelet count at presentation.[39–41,44,45] Unfortunately, although these findings are interesting and may provide clues to the pathophysiology of ITP, in general these characteristics are not useful for clinical management or for prognosis. Chronic ITP affects children of all ages including infants, but it is more common in children older than 10 years. Children of both sexes can be affected but most studies report higher incidence in teenage girls. In general, children who develop chronic ITP have higher platelet counts at presentation than children who have acute disease. In a recent review of the Canadian experience with 198 children age 1 to 19 years with chronic ITP, the median platelet count at diagnosis was 40×10^9/L with a range of 1 to 136×10^9/L, which is consistent with other published reports.[1,39,41,45] Most children with chronic ITP have either no bleeding symptoms or mild intermittent bleeding episodes that may not require treatment. A small but significant minority of children has severe, clinically symptomatic thrombocytopenia requiring therapy.

The prevention of serious and life-threatening bleeding, particularly intracranial hemorrhage, is the major motivation for treatment in children with ITP. Fortunately, the risk in children with chronic ITP is low, but predicting severe bleeding in individual patients is exceedingly difficult. The incidence of intracranial hemorrhage (ICH) in patients with newly diagnosed ITP has been estimated at 0.1% to 0.5% of cases. Most studies reporting incidence of ICH in ITP include patients with acute disease, so the true incidence in chronic ITP is not known with accuracy. Because the overall risk of hemorrhage is proportional to the severity of the thrombocytopenia and its duration, the risk in chronic ITP is presumed to be somewhat higher, but it is still an uncommon event. In the Canadian study of children with chronic ITP, none of the 198 patients with chronic ITP had ICH or other life-threatening bleeding complications. Other retrospective reviews of children confirm the low incidence of ICH in chronic ITP.[37,40] Few, if any, long-term longitudinal studies include enough patients and observation time to accurately assess the true risk of ICH in children with chronic ITP. Unfortunately, there are no reliable predictors of ICH in children with ITP. The rarity of ICH and other severe bleeding makes the identification of risk factors very difficult. Platelet count alone is an insufficient measure of bleeding risk. However, the overwhelming majority of patients who experience ICH have platelet counts less than 10×10^9/L near or at the time of the bleeding event.[46] Nevertheless, many patients have severely low platelet count and little if any symptomatic bleeding. Therefore, management decisions must be individualized and based on bleeding symptoms, platelet counts, and individual child and family needs and concerns.

IMMUNE THROMBOCYTOPENIC PURPURA WITH ATYPICAL FEATURES

Children with atypical clinical or laboratory findings or children whose disease is refractory to treatment should be evaluated for other causes of thrombocytopenia.

Bone marrow failure and myelodysplastic syndrome can present with thrombocytopenia as a presenting feature. Other clinical and laboratory findings are usually present, but anemia, lymphadenopathy, or splenomegaly may be mild at first and may not cause concern on initial examination. Children with bone marrow failure or myelodysplasia are unlikely to respond to standard first-line ITP therapy. Bone marrow aspiration and biopsy should be performed in patients who have refractory disease or who have persistent or progressive clinical or laboratory abnormalities.[47]

Immune thrombocytopenia is a common feature of autoimmune rheumatologic disease and develops in about 5% of patients with systemic lupus erythematosus (SLE).[23,48,49] The thrombocytopenia is usually mild, but in rare cases can be severe and refractory and can be accompanied by other cytopenias.[50] Careful physical and laboratory evaluation including antinuclear antibody, double-stranded DNA, serum complement (C3 and C4) and antineutrophil cytoplasmic antibodies (ANCA) should performed in patients with rheumatologic features or combined cytopenias.[51]

Children with common variable immunodeficiency (CVID) or other immunodeficiency syndromes can present with thrombocytopenia.[23,52-54] CVID is a rare disorder characterized by defects in B-cell development; clinical manifestations include recurrent infections, allergic symptoms, and autoimmune disease.[23] Laboratory findings include immune cytopenias, including ITP, autoimmune hemolytic anemia (AIHA) and neutropenia, low serum immunoglobulin, and insufficient antibody response to protein and polysaccharide antigens. Children with ITP with other immune cytopenias or with recurrent infections should be evaluated for CVID.

Evans syndrome is defined as the combination of ITP with direct antibody positive AIHA.[55] About half of patients with Evans syndrome develop autoimmune neutropenia and up to 10% have all three cell lines affected.[56,57] Patients with Evans syndrome may have evidence of other autoimmune disease such as autoimmune lymphoprolifer- ative syndrome (ALPS, see the following paragraph).[58,59] Chronic and refractory disease is more common in Evans syndrome and splenectomy may be ineffective.[55] Rituximab therapy has been used successfully to treat the cytopenias of Evans syndrome and may be beneficial in severe and refractory cases.[60]

Immune thrombocytopenia is a common feature of ALPS, a rare inherited autoim- mune disorder of defective B- and T-cell apoptosis. Mutations in the Fas receptor, Fax ligand, and caspase gene are present in most patients with ALPS.[61] Patients typi- cally present with profound lymphadenopathy and hepatosplenomegaly and flow cy- tometry testing reveals a polyclonal population of T cells that are double negative, ie, do not express CD4 or CD8, but express the α/β T-cell receptor.[62] Children who present with ITP in combination with other immune cytopenias, hepatosplenomegaly, and lymphadenopathy should be evaluated for ALPS.[63] Mycophenolate mofetil (MMF) and sirolimus have been used effectively as steroid- and splenectomy-sparing treat- ments for the cytopenias of ALPS.[64,65] Splenectomy should be avoided in patients with ALPS because of the increased risk of postsplenectomy sepsis.[61]

Myosin heavy chain 9 (MYH9)–related platelet disorders are inherited thrombocyto- penias that can be mistaken for ITP. Patients with MYH9 disorders usually present with mild bleeding symptoms and have mild to moderate thrombocytopenia with large platelets on peripheral smear.[66] Several mutations in the MYH9 gene lead to prema- ture release of platelets from the bone marrow, macrothrombocytopenia, and cyto- plasmic inclusion bodies within leukocytes.[66] Four overlapping syndromes, known as May-Hegglin anomaly, Epstein syndrome, Fechtner syndrome, and Sebastian platelet syndrome, describe different clinical manifestations of MYH9 gene mutations. Macrothrombocytopenia is present in all affected individuals. Sebastian syndrome and the May-Hegglin anomaly predominately affect platelet size and are uncommonly associated with serious bleeding. Patients with Epstein syndrome and Fechtner syndrome may have otologic and/or renal abnormalities.

TREATMENT

The goal of treatment for children with ITP is to maintain a hemostatically safe platelet count while avoiding potential severe side effects of therapy.[36,67] Many children with chronic ITP have mild to moderate thrombocytopenia and few signs or symptoms of bleeding. These children may not require treatment other than close observation. A relapsing form of ITP is common in children with chronic ITP who may have prolonged periods of normal to near normal platelet counts followed by acute episodes of severe thrombocytopenia and overt bleeding requiring therapy.[42] These episodes may be preceded by viral or bacterial infection, but often have no clear inciting event. Patients following this clinical pattern may be managed with close observation until the episode resolves or may be given intermittent treatment with courses of corticosteroids, intra- venous immune globulin, or anti-D immune globulin (in patients who are Rhesus posi- tive and have intact spleens). A small but significant minority of children have severe disease with platelets chronically under $20 \times 10^9/L$ and symptomatic bleeding.

Clinically significant chronic ITP presents a difficult therapeutic challenge, particularly in active children.

There is no current standard of care for children with symptomatic, chronic ITP and therefore treatment choice is largely based on patient needs, age and activity level, practitioner experience, anecdotal evidence, case reports, and expert opinion. An individual approach must be used when managing children and adolescents with chronic ITP. The benefits and risks of each treatment must be considered carefully before initiation of therapy. Many therapies are available, but none offers high efficacy and all have significant real and potential toxicities. Quality of life issues are extremely important for children and families and should not be overlooked when considering a management plan.

"STANDARD" THERAPY

Many children with chronic ITP can be managed intermittently as needed for severe thrombocytopenia or bleeding with "standard" therapies: corticosteroids, intravenous immunoglobulin (IVIG), and anti-D immune globulin.[67,68] There is extensive experience with these medications for the treatment of acute and chronic ITP in children and adults, but there are few randomized controlled trials comparing treatments in children with chronic ITP. All three treatments are effective in the sense that most children will respond with increased platelet counts and reduced bleeding symptoms. Approximately three-quarters of patients will respond to any of these treatments[69]; however, responses are typically temporary and none induces long-term remission or cure. There is no evidence to suggest that any of these treatments alters the natural history of the disease. Nonetheless, corticosteroids, IVIG, and anti-D are useful in the management of children with symptomatic ITP.[67,68]

Corticosteroids

Various doses and regimens of corticosteroids have been used successfully to treat chronic ITP in children. Short-course, relatively high-dose corticosteroids without a taper are effective in increasing the platelet count rapidly (within 24–48 hours) with mild side effects and can be used intermittently to treat symptomatic ITP.[34,70] Many other steroid treatments, oral and IV, have been used effectively in the treatment of chronic, childhood ITP. Low-dose prednisone at 0.1 to 0.2 mg/kg/day orally can be useful in some patients without serious side effects.[47] High-dose and/or prolonged courses of corticosteroid therapy are associated with increased, potentially irreversible, adverse side effects, so long-term therapy is not recommended. Advantages of corticosteroids include availability of an oral route and low cost. Short-term side effects are mild and include irritability and behavioral disturbances, hyperglycemia, hypertension and headache. Long-term therapy is not recommended because of the well-known risks of immunosuppression, hirtsutism, weight gain, growth delay, osteoporosis, and cataracts.

Intravenous Immunoglobulin

IVIG is effective in rapidly raising the platelet counts in children with ITP.[69,71–73] Various regimens have been used over the years with success, but doses of 0.8 to 1.0 g/kg are effective in increasing the platelet count quickly and effectively in most patients.[34,69] Higher doses do not improve response and are associated with more adverse effects, particularly headache, and are not recommended.[74] Repeated infusions may be given as needed every 2 to 6 weeks for symptomatic thrombocytopenia.[47] IVIG is expensive and must be given as a slow IV infusion. Infusion-related side effects such as flushing, fever, and (sometimes severe) headache are common and usually mild, but more serious allergic reactions and aseptic meningitis can occur. IVIG is a blood product derived from pooled donor plasma and there is the potential risk of pathogen transmission, but stringent donor screening and pathogen inactivation steps have substantially reduced these risks.

Anti-D Immune Globulin

Anti-D immunoglobulin is effective in increasing platelet counts in children with ITP who are Rhesus positive and have intact spleens.[75] A study comparing the efficacy of high- and low-dose anti-D showed the superiority of the 75 μg/kg dose.[76] The side effects are usually mild and consist of infusion-related headache, chills, and fatigue. Mild anemia resulting from alloantibody-induced extravascular hemolysis is common; with an average drop in hemoglobin of 0.8 to 1.4 g/dL reported.[75] Severe hemolytic anemia with disseminated vascular coagulation and acute renal failure is a rare (approximately 1 in 20,000–30,000 infusions) but significant side effect.[77] Anti-D must be given via short IV infusion, although reports of efficacy with subcutaneous administration have been reported.[78] Like IVIG, it is a blood product and carries the potential risk of pathogen transmission, but screening and pathogen inactivation treatment have lowered this risk considerably.

SECOND-LINE THERAPY
Splenectomy

Although early splenectomy is a standard treatment for most adults with chronic ITP, splenectomy is performed much less often in the pediatric population particularly before 12 months disease duration. Splenectomy is effective in this population, but is less commonly performed because of the high rate of spontaneous remission in this age group, the surgical and anesthesia risks in young children, and the small but significant risk for fatal postsplenectomy sepsis.

There is a wealth of evidence and successful clinical practice to support the effectiveness of splenectomy children with ITP. The practice guidelines developed by the American Society of Hematology (ASH) reported a 72% overall complete remission rate after splenectomy in 271 children with ITP in 16 case series published over 40 years.[27] In a more recent prospective study from the ICIS group, 134 children underwent splenectomy for ITP and 83.6% achieved complete response (platelets over 150 $\times$ 10^9/L).[79] Eighty percent of complete responders in this study maintained this response at 1 year. Factors that were weakly associated with a higher probability to achieve complete remission in the ICIS study were older age, longer duration of ITP, and male gender.[79] Other case series of splenectomy in children with chronic ITP have shown similar response rates ranging from 67% to 81%.[80–84] Splenectomy patients typically have significantly lower mean platelet counts at diagnosis of chronic ITP, are older, and have longer duration of severe disease than nonsplenectomy patients.[39]

The disinclination to perform splenectomy in children with ITP stems from the increased risk of fatal infection with encapsulated organisms. Very few long-term follow-up studies of children with chronic ITP who have undergone splenectomy have been performed and late failure rates and rates of infection are not known with any accuracy. Patient numbers are very small and clinical practice has changed over the past 20 years, so any information must be used with care in patient management. In the ICIS study, a prospective study with relatively short follow-up, there were no fatal infections, but there were seven episodes of nonfatal sepsis.[79] Other retrospective reviews have reported similar efficacy rates, and sepsis-related mortality appears to be quite low.[80,82,84] The availability of vaccines against *Streptococcus pneumoniae*, *Neisseria meningitides*, and *Haemophilus influenzae* type b may have reduced the risk of sepsis substantially in recent years. Laparoscopic technique has significantly lowered the surgical risks associated with splenectomy and reduced the recovery time.

Guidelines for splenectomy in children who have ITP are conservative. The panel from the ASH group recommended consideration for elective splenectomy in children with chronic ITP only under certain circumstances: persistence of disease for at least at 12 months, bleeding symptoms with severe thrombocytopenia, or thrombocytopenia that is refractory to first-line therapy with corticosteroid, IVIG, or anti D.[27] A similar group from the United Kingdom supported the consideration of splenectomy in the setting of severe lifestyle restrictions and/or severe bleeding or life-threatening bleeding.[85] However, there were insufficient data to make evidence-based recommendations for specific indications and timing for splenectomy.

In summary, splenectomy is effective for the treatment of chronic ITP in childhood and is one of the only options that offer potential long-term disease remission. However, splenectomy is not without serious potential morbidity and mortality and the risk of fatal sepsis remains a concern. Splenectomy should not be considered a standard, first-line treatment for children with chronic ITP. Splenectomy should be delayed for as long as possible and should be reserved for children with severe disease that has failed other conservative management. If splenectomy is performed, the laparoscopic technique is preferable. Before elective splenectomy, immunization against *N meningitides*, *S pneumonia*, and *H influenza* type b should be performed. Preoperative treatment with corticosteroids, IVIG, or anti-D is usually necessary to bring the platelets to a hemostatically safe range ($\sim$ 50–75 $\times$ 10^9/L) for surgery. Children who achieve remission with splenectomy must be followed closely for the remainder of their lives to prevent infection. Children younger than 5 years should receive daily prophylaxis with penicillin or equivalent antibiotic when penicillin allergic. The optimal duration of prophylactic penicillin treatment is debatable. All febrile episodes should be evaluated and treatment with parenteral antibiotics should be considered to prevent life-threatening bacterial sepsis. When ineffective, patients must be followed similarly and must cope with this lifelong risk without any benefit.

Other Therapies

Numerous therapies have been tried with varying degrees of success to treat patients with symptomatic ITP including rituximab, azathioprine and 6-mercatopurine (6-MP), MMF, cyclosporin, sirolimus, dapsone, vincristine, and cyclophosphamide. Evidence supporting the efficacy and safety in children with severe chronic ITP is unsatisfactory. To date, no third-line therapy offers proven long-term efficacy; all have serious potential and real side effects. Usually the decision regarding such therapy is based on physician experience, patient needs, and family preference. Randomized controlled trials measuring response to therapy based on platelet count, bleeding symptoms, quality of life, and safety are desperately needed.

Rituximab

Rituximab is a human murine chimeric monoclonal antibody directed against the CD 20 antigen expressed on pre-B and mature B lymphocytes. Rituximab eliminates circulating B cells with recovery in 6 to 12 months from treatment. Rituximab is approved by the Food and Drug Administration (FDA) for the treatment of B-cell lymphomas in adults, but has been used to treat a variety of antibody-mediated auto-immune disease with some success. Studies in adults with chronic ITP have shown a response rate of about 50%.[86–88] In a recent systematic review of 313 adult patients from 19 studies, 62.5% of patients achieved a platelet count of 50×10^9/L or greater.[89] Studies in children have shown similar response rates.[60,90] In a prospective study of 36 pediatric patients with severe and/or refractory ITP, the response rate, defined as a platelet count of 50×10^9/L or greater during 4 consecutive weeks starting in weeks 9 to 12, after 4 weekly doses of rituximab (375 mg/m^2/dose) was 31%.[60] In a 1-year follow-up study, 8 of the 11 initial responders maintained a platelet count over 150×10^9/L for the duration of the study (72.7%).[91]

Severe short- and medium-term adverse effects associated with rituximab treatment in children with ITP are rare.[89] Common side effects of therapy include infusion-related headache, fever, chills, and transient hypotension. Therapy-related serum sickness was more common in the pediatric age group (5%).[60,90] Severe adverse events, such as bacterial infections and reactivation of preexisting chronic infection and serious bacterial infections, particularly hepatitis B, have been reported in adults but are unusual in children with ITP.[89,92] Two patients with SLE treated with rituximab developed fatal progressive multifocal leukoencephalopathy after rituximab.[93] These reports raise concern for using this drug as a treatment in children with chronic ITP. To date, there have been no reports of hepatitis infection or leukoencephalopathy in children with chronic ITP treated with rituximab.

Rituximab is attractive because it is one of the few treatment options for children with ITP that offers potential long-term remission. However, it is effective in only half of treated patients and long-term safety has not been established. Randomized controlled trials to define the role of rituximab as a treatment for chronic ITP are greatly needed.

6-MP/Azathioprine

Azathioprine and 6-MP are thiopurine antimetabolites, cytotoxic immunosuppressive agents that have been used for many years to treat leukemia and autoimmune disease. Azathioprine is slowly but completely metabolized to 6-MP, which is then metabolized to 6-thioguanine nucleotide. Experience using these drugs in patients with chronic ITP is limited, but early reports suggested favorable outcome.[94,95] A recent retrospective review of 6-MP in childhood cytopenias, including autoimmune thrombocytopenia and ITP, showed surprising results: an overall response rate of 83% and a response rate in chronic ITP of 85%. Side effects included reversible increases in aspartate aminotransferase and alanine aminotransferase and neutropenia. This study was retrospective and had small numbers of patients so the results should be considered carefully before initiation of therapy.

Thiopurine drugs are metabolized by thiopurine S-methyltransferase (TPMT). An inherited deficiency of TPMT activity increases the risk of adverse events, particularly myelosuppression and hepatotoxicity.[96] Testing for TPMT genotype and enzyme activity are available and should be considered at the onset of therapy.

Mycophenolate Mofetil

MMF is an immunosuppressive agent that has been used to reduce rejection in solid organ transplant. It has been used successfully as a single agent in small case series involving primarily adults with severe and refractory chronic ITP.[97–100] Response rates ranged from 39% to 80%, but patient numbers in each study were small. No serious side effects were reported. Experience in children with chronic ITP is limited.

Vincristine

Low-dose weekly vincristine has been used as a single agent and in combination therapy to treat adults and children with ITP.[101,102] Two studies from the 1970s report favorable overall response rates in 27 children with chronic ITP.[101] Vincristine has well documented side effects including neurotoxicity, constipation, and jaw pain, which limit long-term use.

Other Agents

Cyclosporin, cyclophosphamide, dapsone, and numerous other agents have been used to treat severe chronic ITP.[103,104] There are few clinical trials using these drugs in children and lack of documented efficacy and well-described toxicities limit widespread use in children. These agents should be tried in only the most severe and refractory cases, if at all.

New Agents

Decreased platelet production is a contributing factor in the pathogenesis of ITP and recent studies have focused on the development and use of agents that increase platelet count via the stimulation of megakaryopoiesis.[105] Thrombopoietin is the primary growth factor responsible for platelet production and two agents, romiplostim and eltrombopag, thrombopoietin mimetics, are currently approved for the treatment of chronic ITP in adults with chronic ITP. Romiplostim is a thrombopoietic peptibody that is administered as weekly subcutaneous injections.[21] Eltrombopag is an oral nonpeptide molecule given as a daily oral dose.[106] Both agents have shown robust platelet responses in adults with chronic ITP.[106,107] Other than reversible bone marrow fibrosis in a few adult patients treated with romiplostim, drug-specific side effects are tolerable, but long-term studies have not been completed. Trials using these drugs in the pediatric population are under way and their place in the management of childhood ITP remains to be determined.

FUTURE DIRECTIONS

Clinically significant chronic ITP in childhood remains a difficult clinical challenge. Treatment decisions are based largely on small trials, personal experience, or anecdotal evidence. Available treatments have low efficacy or significant toxicities or both. The optimal treatment for children with severe disease is the subject of ongoing debate. Because the outcome of ITP in childhood is generally favorable, management practices that preserve quality of life and limit toxicities are important. Ongoing research into new therapies and prospective trials comparing agents are necessary.

REFERENCES

1. Imbach P, Kuhne T, Muller D, et al. Childhood ITP: 12 months follow-up data from the prospective registry I of the Intercontinental Childhood ITP Study Group (ICIS). Pediatr Blood Cancer 2006;46(3):351–6.
2. Cines DB, McMillan R. Pathogenesis of chronic immune thrombocytopenic purpura. Curr Opin Hematol 2007;14(5):511–4.
3. Gernsheimer T. Epidemiology and pathophysiology of immune thrombocytopenic purpura. Eur J Haematol Suppl 2008;69:3–8.
4. Harrington WJ, Minnich V, Hollingsworth JW, et al. Demonstration of a thrombocytopenic factor in the blood of patients with thrombocytopenic purpura. J Lab Clin Med 1951;38(1):1–10.

5. Cines DB, Blanchette VS. Immune thrombocytopenic purpura. N Engl J Med 2002;346(13):995–1008.

6. Berchtold P, Wenger M. Autoantibodies against platelet glycoproteins in autoimmune thrombocytopenic purpura: their clinical significance and response to treatment. Blood 1993;81(5):1246–50.

7. Taub JW, Warrier I, Holtkamp C, et al. Characterization of autoantibodies against the platelet glycoprotein antigens IIb/IIIa in childhood idiopathic thrombocytopenia purpura. Am J Hematol 1995;48(2):104–7.

8. Berchtold P, Muller D, Beardsley D, et al. International study to compare antigen-specific methods used for the measurement of antiplatelet autoantibodies. Br J Haematol 1997;96(3):477–83.

9. Semple JW. Immune pathophysiology of autoimmune thrombocytopenic purpura. Blood Rev 2002;16(1):9–12.

10. Semple JW, Freedman J. Increased antiplatelet T helper lymphocyte reactivity in patients with autoimmune thrombocytopenia. Blood 1991;78(10):2619–25.

11. Ware RE, Howard TA. Phenotypic and clonal analysis of T lymphocytes in childhood immune thrombocytopenic purpura. Blood 1993;82(7):2137–42.

12. Garcia-Suarez J, Prieto A, Reyes E, et al. Abnormal gamma IFN and alpha TNF secretion in purified CD2+ cells from autoimmune thrombocytopenic purpura (ATP) patients: their implication in the clinical course of the disease. Am J Hematol 1995;49(4):271–6.

13. Semple J, Milev Y, Cosgrave D, et al. Differences in serum cytokine levels in acute and chronic autoimmune thrombocytopenic purpura: relationship to platelet phenotype and antiplatelet T-cell reactivity. Blood 1996;87(10):4245–54.

14. Panitsas FP, Theodoropoulou M, Kouraklis A, et al. Adult chronic idiopathic thrombocytopenic purpura (ITP) is the manifestation of a type-1 polarized immune response. Blood 2004;103(7):2645–7.

15. Andersson J. Cytokines in idiopathic thrombocytopenic purpura (ITP). Acta Paediatr Suppl 1998;424:61–4.

16. Olsson B, Andersson PO, Jernas M, et al. T-cell-mediated cytotoxicity toward platelets in chronic idiopathic thrombocytopenic purpura. Nat Med 2003;9(9): 1123–4.

17. Ballem PJ, Segal GM, Stratton JR, et al. Mechanisms of thrombocytopenia in chronic autoimmune thrombocytopenic purpura—evidence of both impaired platelet production and increased platelet clearance. J Clin Invest 1987;80(1): 33–40.

18. Louwes H, Zeinali Lathori OA, Vellenga E, et al. Platelet kinetic studies in patients with idiopathic thrombocytopenic purpura. Am J Med 1999;106(4):430–4.

19. Houwerzijl EJ, Blom NR, van der Want JJ, et al. Ultrastructural study shows morphologic features of apoptosis and para-apoptosis in megakaryocytes from patients with idiopathic thrombocytopenic purpura. Blood 2004;103(2): 500–6.

20. Aledort LM, Hayward CP, Chen MG, et al. Prospective screening of 205 patients with ITP, including diagnosis, serological markers, and the relationship between platelet counts, endogenous thrombopoietin, and circulating antithrombopoietin antibodies. Am J Hematol 2004;76(3):205–13.

21. Kuter DJ, Bussel JB, Lyons RM, et al. Efficacy of romiplostim in patients with chronic immune thrombocytopenic purpura: a double-blind randomised controlled trial. Lancet 2008;371(9610):395–403.

22. Bussel JB, Cheng G, Saleh MN, et al. Eltrombopag for the treatment of chronic idiopathic thrombocytopenic purpura. N Engl J Med 2007;357(22):2237–47.

23. Cines DB, Bussel JB, Liebman HA, et al. The ITP syndrome: pathogenic and clinical diversity. Blood 2009;113(26):6511–21.

24. Kuhne T, Buchanan GR, Zimmerman S, et al. A prospective comparative study of 2540 infants and children with newly diagnosed idiopathic thrombocytopenic purpura (ITP) from the Intercontinental Childhood ITP Study Group. J Pediatr 2003;143(5):605–8.

25. Rajantie J, Zeller B, Treutiger I, et al. Vaccination associated thrombocytopenic purpura in children. Vaccine 2007;25(10):1838–40.

26. Black C, Kaye JA, Jick H. MMR vaccine and idiopathic thrombocytopaenic purpura. Br J Clin Pharmacol 2003;55(1):107–11.

27. George JN, Woolf SH, Raskob GE, et al. Idiopathic thrombocytopenic purpura: a practice guideline developed by explicit methods for the American Society of Hematology. Blood 1996;88(1):3–40.

28. Lusher JM, Iyer R. Idiopathic thrombocytopenic purpura in children. Semin Thromb Hemost 1977;3(3):175–99.

29. Lusher JM, Zuelzer WW. Idiopathic thrombocytopenic purpura in childhood. J Pediatr 1966;68(6):971–9.

30. Choi SI, McClure PD. Idiopathic thrombocytopenic purpura in childhood. Can Med Assoc J 1967;97(11):562–8.

31. Bolton-Maggs PH, Moon I. Assessment of UK practice for management of acute childhood idiopathic thrombocytopenic purpura against published guidelines. Lancet 1997;350(9078):620–3.

32. Neunert CE, Buchanan GR, Imbach P, et al. Severe hemorrhage in children with newly diagnosed immune thrombocytopenic purpura. Blood 2008;112(10): 4003–8.

33. Blanchette VS, Carcao M. Childhood acute immune thrombocytopenic purpura: 20 years later. Semin Thromb Hemost 2003;29(6):605–17.

34. Blanchette V, Bolton-Maggs P. Childhood immune thrombocytopenic purpura: diagnosis and management. Pediatr Clin North Am 2008;55(2):393–420 ix.

35. Stasi R, Stipa E, Masi M, et al. Long-term observation of 208 adults with chronic idiopathic thrombocytopenic purpura. Am J Med 1995;98(5):436–42.

36. George JN, Raskob GE. Idiopathic thrombocytopenic purpura: a concise summary of the pathophysiology and diagnosis in children and adults. Semin Hematol 1998;35(1 Suppl 1):5–8.

37. Glanz J, France E, Xu S, et al. A population-based, multisite cohort study of the predictors of chronic idiopathic thrombocytopenic purpura in children. Pediatrics 2008;121(3):e506–12.

38. Jayabose S, Levendoglu-Tugal O, Ozkaynkak MF, et al. Long-term outcome of chronic idiopathic thrombocytopenic purpura in children. J Pediatr Hematol Oncol 2004;26(11):724–6.

39. Belletrutti M, Ali K, Barnard D, et al. Chronic immune thrombocytopenic-purpura in children—a survey of the Canadian experience. J Pediatr Hematol Oncol 2007;29(2):95–100.

40. Donato H, Picon A, Martinez M, et al. Demographic data, natural history, and prognostic factors of idiopathic thrombocytopenic purpura in children: a multicentered study from Argentina. Pediatr Blood Cancer 2009;52(4):491–6.

41. Watts RG. Idiopathic thrombocytopenic purpura: a 10-year natural history study at the Children's Hospital of Alabama. Clin Pediatr (Phila) 2004;43(8): 691–702.

42. Lilleyman JS. Chronic childhood idiopathic thrombocytopenic purpura. Baillieres Best Pract Res Clin Haematol 2000;13(3):469–83.

43. Imbach P, Akatsuka J, Blanchette V, et al. Immunothrombocytopenic purpura as a model for pathogenesis and treatment of autoimmunity. Eur J Pediatr 1995; 154(9 Suppl 4):S60–4.

44. Kuhne T. Investigation and management of newly diagnosed childhood idiopathic thrombocytopenic purpura: problems and proposed solutions. J Pediatr Hematol Oncol 2003;25(Suppl 1):S24–7.

45. Zeller B, Rajantie J, Hedlund-Treutiger I, et al. Childhood idiopathic thrombocytopenic purpura in the Nordic countries: epidemiology and predictors of chronic disease. Acta Paediatr 2005;94(2):178–84.

46. Butros LJ, Bussel JB. Intracranial hemorrhage in immune thrombocytopenic purpura: a retrospective analysis. J Pediatr Hematol Oncol 2003;25(8):660–4.

47. Kalpatthi R, Bussel JB. Diagnosis, pathophysiology and management of children with refractory immune thrombocytopenic purpura. Curr Opin Pediatr 2008;20(1):8–16.

48. Ziakas PD, Giannouli S, Zintzaras E, et al. Lupus thrombocytopenia: clinical implications and prognostic significance. Ann Rheum Dis 2005;64(9): 1366–9.

49. Hazzan R, Mukamel M, Yacobovich J, et al. Risk factors for future development of systemic lupus erythematosus in children with idiopathic thrombocytopenic purpura. Pediatr Blood Cancer 2006;47(Suppl 5):657–9.

50. Arnal C, Piette JC, Leone J, et al. Treatment of severe immune thrombocytopenia associated with systemic lupus erythematosus: 59 cases. J Rheumatol 2002; 29(1):75–83.

51. Liebman HA, Stasi R. Secondary immune thrombocytopenic purpura. Curr Opin Hematol 2007;14(5):557–73.

52. Heeney MM, Zimmerman SA, Ware RE. Childhood autoimmune cytopenia secondary to unsuspected common variable immunodeficiency. J Pediatr 2003;143(5):662–5.

53. Michel M, Chanet V, Galicier L, et al. Autoimmune thrombocytopenic purpura and common variable immunodeficiency: analysis of 21 cases and review of the literature. Medicine (Baltimore) 2004;83(4):254–63.

54. Wang J, Cunningham-Rundles C. Treatment and outcome of autoimmune hematologic disease in common variable immunodeficiency (CVID). J Autoimmun 2005;25(1):57–62.

55. Blouin P, Landman-Parker J, Thuret I, et al. Evans syndrome: a retrospective study from the SHIP (French Society of Pediatric Hematology and Immunology). Blood 2002;100(11):3810.

56. Norton A, Roberts I. Management of Evans syndrome. Br J Haematol 2006; 132(2):125–37.

57. Wang WC. Evans syndrome in childhood: pathophysiology, clinical course, and treatment. Am J Pediatr Hematol Oncol 1988;10(4):330–8.

58. Cines DB, Liebman H, Stasi R. Pathobiology of secondary immune thrombocytopenia. Semin Hematol 2009;46(1):S2–14.

59. Teachey DT, Manno CS, Axsom KM, et al. Unmasking Evans syndrome: T cell phenotype and apoptotic response reveal autoimmune lymphoproliferative syndrome (ALPS). Blood 2005;105(6):2443–8.

60. Bennett CM, Rogers ZR, Kinnamon DD, et al. Prospective phase 1/2 study of rituximab in childhood and adolescent chronic immune thrombocytopenic purpura. Blood 2006;107(7):2639–42.

61. Rao VK, Straus SE. Causes and consequences of the autoimmune lymphoproliferative syndrome. Hematology 2006;11(1):15–23.

62. Holzelova E, Vonarbourg C, Stolzenberg MC, et al. Autoimmune lymphoproliferative syndrome with somatic Fas mutations. N Engl J Med 2004;351(14): 1409–18.

63. Hundt M, Posovszky C, Schmidt RE. A new disorder of lymphocyte apoptosis: combination of autoimmunity, infectious lymphadenopathy, double negative T cells, and impaired activation-induced cell death. Immunobiology 2002;206(5): 514–8.

64. Rao VK, Dugan F, Dale JK, et al. Use of mycophenolate mofetil for chronic, refractory immune cytopenias in children with autoimmune lymphoproliferative syndrome. Br J Haematol 2005;129(4):534–8.

65. Teachey DT, Greiner R, Seif A, et al. Treatment with sirolimus results in complete responses in patients with autoimmune lymphoproliferative syndrome. Br J Haematol 2009;145(1):101–6.

66. Althaus K, Greinacher A. MYH9-related platelet disorders. Semin Thromb Hemost 2009;35(2):189–203.

67. Provan D, Newland A, Norfolk D, et al. Guidelines for the investigation and management of idiopathic thrombocytopenic purpura in adults, children and in pregnancy. Br J Haematol 2003;120(4):574–96.

68. George JN, Woolf SH, Raskob GE. Idiopathic thrombocytopenic purpura: a guideline for diagnosis and management of children and adults. American Society of Hematology. Ann Med 1998;30(1):38–44.

69. Blanchette V, Imbach P, Andrew M, et al. Randomised trial of intravenous immunoglobulin G, intravenous anti-D, and oral prednisone in childhood acute immune thrombocytopenic purpura. Lancet 1994;344(8924):703–7.

70. Jayabose S, Patel P, Inamdar S, et al. Use of intravenous methylprednisolone in acute idiopathic thrombocytopenic purpura. Am J Pediatr Hematol Oncol 1987; 9(2):133–5.

71. Imbach P, d'Apuzzo V, Hirt A, et al. High dose intravenous gammaglobulin for idiopathic thrombocytopenic purpura in childhood. Lancet 1981;317(8232): 1228–31.

72. Bussel JB. The use of intravenous gamma-globulin in idiopathic thrombocytopenic purpura. Clin Immunol Immunopathol 1989;53(2):S147–55.

73. Beck CE, Nathan PC, Parkin PC, et al. Corticosteroids versus intravenous immune globulin for the treatment of acute immune thrombocytopenic purpura in children: a systematic review and meta-analysis of randomized controlled trials. J Pediatr 2005;147(4):521–7.

74. Blanchette VS, Luke B, Andrew M, et al. A prospective, randomized trial of high-dose intravenous immune globulin G therapy, oral prednisone therapy, and no therapy in childhood acute immune thrombocytopenic purpura. J Pediatr 1993;123(6):989–95.

75. Scaradavou A, Woo B, Woloski BM, et al. Intravenous anti-D treatment of immune thrombocytopenic purpura: experience in 272 patients. Blood 1997; 89(8):2689–700.

76. Tarantino MD, Young G, Bertolone SJ, et al. Single dose of anti-D immune globulin at 75 microg/kg is as effective as intravenous immune globulin at rapidly raising the platelet count in newly diagnosed immune thrombocytopenic purpura in children. J Pediatr 2006;148(4):489–94.

77. Gaines AR. Disseminated intravascular coagulation associated with acute hemoglobinemia or hemoglobinuria following Rho(D) immune globulin intravenous administration for immune thrombocytopenic purpura. Blood 2005;106(5): 1532–7.

78. Meyer O, Kiesewetter H, Hermsen M, et al. Efficacy and safety of anti-D given by subcutaneous injection to patients with autoimmune thrombocytopenia. Eur J Haematol 2004;73(1):71–2.

79. Kuhne T, Blanchette V, Buchanan GR, et al. Splenectomy in children with idiopathic thrombocytopenic purpura: a prospective study of 134 children from the Intercontinental Childhood ITP Study Group. Pediatr Blood Cancer 2007; 49(6):829–34.

80. Aronis S, Platokouki H, Avgeri M, et al. Retrospective evaluation of long-term efficacy and safety of splenectomy in chronic idiopathic thrombocytopenic purpura in children. Acta Paediatr 2004;93(5):638–42.

81. El-Alfy MS, El-Tawil MM, Shahein N. 5-to 16-year follow-up following splenectomy in chronic immune thrombocytopenic purpura in children. Acta Haematol 2003;110(1):20–4.

82. Mantadakis E, Buchanan GR. Elective splenectomy in children with idiopathic thrombocytopenic purpura. J Pediatr Hematol Oncol 2000;22(2):148–53.

83. Milen M. Critical issues concerning splenectomy for chronic idiopathic thrombocytopenic purpura in childhood. Pediatr Blood Cancer 2006;47(Suppl 5):734–6.

84. Ramenghi U, Amendola G, Farinasso L, et al. Splenectomy in children with chronic ITP: long-term efficacy and relation between its outcome and responses to previous treatments. Pediatr Blood Cancer 2006;47(Suppl 5):742–5.

85. Eden OB, Lilleyman JS. Guidelines for management of idiopathic thrombocytopenic purpura. Arch Dis Child 1992;67(8):1056–8.

86. Stasi R, Pagano A, Stipa E, et al. Rituximab chimeric anti-CD20 monoclonal antibody treatment for adults with chronic idiopathic thrombocytopenic purpura. Blood 2001;98(4):952–7.

87. Giagounidis AA, Anhuf J, Schneider P, et al. Treatment of relapsed idiopathic thrombocytopenic purpura with the anti-CD20 monoclonal antibody rituximab: a pilot study. Eur J Haematol 2002;69(2):95–100.

88. Zaja F, Iacona I, Masolini P, et al. B-cell depletion with rituximab as treatment for immune hemolytic anemia and chronic thrombocytopenia. Haematologica 2002; 87(2):189–95.

89. Arnold DM, Dentali F, Crowther MA, et al. Systematic review: efficacy and safety of rituximab for adults with idiopathic thrombocytopenic purpura. Ann Intern Med 2007;146(1):25–33.

90. Wang J, Wiley JM, Luddy R, et al. Chronic immune thrombocytopenic purpura in children: assessment of rituximab treatment. J Pediatr 2005;146(2):217–21.

91. Mueller BU, Bennett CM, Feldman HA, et al. One year follow-up of children and adolescents with chronic immune thrombocytopenic purpura (ITP) treated with rituximab. Pediatr Blood Cancer 2009;52(2):259–62.

92. Ram R, Ben-Bassat I, Shpilberg O, et al. The late adverse events of rituximab therapy—rare but there!. Leuk Lymphoma 2009;50(7):1083–95.

93. Carson KR, Evens AM, Richey EA, et al. Progressive multifocal leukoencephalopathy after rituximab therapy in HIV-negative patients: a report of 57 cases from the Research on Adverse Drug Events and Reports project. Blood 2009; 113(20):4834–40.

94. Hilgartner MW, Lanzkowsky P, Smith CH. The use of azathioprine in refractory idiopathic thrombocytopenic purpura in children. Acta Paediatr Scand 1970; 59(4):409–15.

95. Quiquandon I, Fenaux P, Caulier MT, et al. Re-evaluation of the role of azathioprine in the treatment of adult chronic idiopathic thrombocytopenic purpura: a report on 53 cases. Br J Haematol 1990;74(2):223–8.

96. Gurwitz D, Rodriguez-Antona C, Payne K, et al. Improving pharmacovigilance in Europe: TPMT genotyping and phenotyping in the UK and Spain. Eur J Hum Genet 2009;17(8):991–8.
97. Hou M, Peng J, Shi Y, et al. Mycophenolate mofetil (MMF) for the treatment of steroid-resistant idiopathic thrombocytopenic purpura. Eur J Haematol 2003; 70(6):353–7.
98. Kotb R, Pinganaud C, Trichet C, et al. Efficacy of mycophenolate mofetil in adult refractory auto-immune cytopenias: a single center preliminary study. Eur J Haematol 2005;75(1):60–4.
99. Provan D, Moss AJ, Newland AC, et al. Efficacy of mycophenolate mofetil as single-agent therapy for refractory immune thrombocytopenic purpura. Am J Hematol 2006;81(1):19–25.
100. Zhang WG, Ji L, Cao XM, et al. Mycophenolate mofetil as a treatment for refractory idiopathic thrombocytopenic purpura. Acta Pharmacol Sin 2005;26(5): 598–602.
101. Hicsonmez G, Ozsoylu S. Vincristine for treatment of chronic thrombocytopenia in children. N Engl J Med 1977;296(8):454–5.
102. Williams JA, Boxer LA. Combination therapy for refractory idiopathic thrombocytopenic purpura in adolescents. J Pediatr Hematol Oncol 2003;25(3):232–5.
103. Zver S, Zupan IP, Cernelc P. Cyclosporin A as an immunosuppressive treatment modality for patients with refractory autoimmune thrombocytopenic purpura after splenectomy failure. Int J Hematol 2006;83(3):238–42.
104. Damodar S, Viswabandya A, George B, et al. Dapsone for chronic idiopathic thrombocytopenic purpura in children and adults—a report on 90 patients. Eur J Haematol 2005;75(4):328–31.
105. Nurden AT, Viallard JF, Nurden P. New-generation drugs that stimulate platelet production in chronic immune thrombocytopenic purpura. Lancet 2009; 373(9674):1562–9.
106. Bussel JB, Provan D, Shamsi T, et al. Effect of eltrombopag on platelet counts and bleeding during treatment of chronic idiopathic thrombocytopenic purpura: a randomised, double-blind, placebo-controlled trial. Lancet 2009;373(9664): 641–8.
107. Bussel JB, Kuter DJ, Pullarkat V, et al. Safety and efficacy of long-term treatment with romiplostim in thrombocytopenic patients with chronic ITP. Blood 2009; 113(10):2161–71.

Immune Thrombocytopenia in Patients with Connective Tissue Disorders and the Antiphospholipid Antibody Syndrome

Daniel G. Arkfeld, MD[a],*, Ilene C. Weitz, MD[b]

KEYWORDS

- Thrombocytopenia • Lupus • Sjögren syndrome
- Rheumatoid arthritis • Still disease
- Antiphospholipid antibody syndrome

Autoimmunity involving the adaptive immune system with T- and B-cell mediated effects plays a central role in the complex pathophysiology of connective tissue disorders, and is fundamental to the development and progression of many rheumatic diseases and immune thrombocytopenia (ITP).[1] Many rheumatologic conditions have been associated with thrombocytopenia, most often due to antibody-mediated platelet destruction, but also intravascular consumption and decreased platelet production. Comorbid factors such as infections, medications, and vaccinations can also confuse the physician's attempt for prompt and appropriate therapy.

Systemic lupus erythematosus (SLE) and antiphospholipid syndrome (APL) are 2 of the most recognizable connective tissue disorders associated with ITP. Although laboratory evidence of autoimmunity, such as a positive antinuclear antibody, is common in ITP,[2] only a few patients are likely to develop SLE or other conditions if they do not present with additional symptoms or signs of a connective tissue disorder.[3] The pathophysiology of ITP in connective tissue disorders is similar to that of primary ITP and is mediated by antiplatelet autoantibodies.[4] Fc-γ receptors

---

[a] Division of Rheumatology and Immunology, University of Southern California–Keck School of Medicine, HMR 711, 2011 Zonal Avenue, Los Angeles, CA 90033, USA
[b] Division of Hematology, University of Southern California–Keck School of Medicine, HMR 711, 2011 Zonal Avenue, Los Angeles, CA 90033, USA
* Corresponding author.
E-mail address: arkfeld@usc.edu (D.G. Arkfeld).

Hematol Oncol Clin N Am 23 (2009) 1239–1249
doi:10.1016/j.hoc.2009.08.010
0889-8588/09/$ – see front matter © 2009 Elsevier Inc. All rights reserved.

play a central role in platelet phagocytosis,[5] and modulation of these receptors can induce improvements in the platelet count.[6] Decreased platelet production, as in primary ITP, may also be involved in the pathogenesis of ITP in patients with the secondary form of the disorder.[5] Platelet autoantibodies and antithrombopoietin receptor (Mpl) antibodies can induce both peripheral platelet destruction and decreased platelet production.[7,8]

SYSTEMIC LUPUS ERYTHEMATOSIS

SLE is a systemic inflammatory disease that can affect any organ system in the body, including the hematological system, which is 1 of 11 criteria for the diagnosis of the disease.[9] Hematological manifestations include leukopenia, hemolytic anemia, and thrombocytopenia, all of which can be present at the onset of disease. However, given its varied clinical presentations, SLE can be difficult to diagnose.[10] Twenty percent to 25% of patients with SLE have platelet counts of less than 100×10^9/L, although it is rarely severe, with less than 10% with platelet counts of less than 30×10^9/L.[10,11] A recent Chinese study reported an incidence of 24.2%.[12] In patients with SLE, thrombocytopenia with platelet counts less than 100×10^9/L is more prevalent in patients with high-titer anticardiolipin antibodies.[13] It was once speculated that splenectomy for refractory ITP triggered SLE. It was subsequently shown that these patients would have eventually developed SLE, and that hematological manifestations were a presenting symptom and harbinger of the disorder. Splenectomy, although it may result in an improvement in the platelet count, may place patients with SLE at greater risk of infection, particularly if they need additional immunosuppression.[14] Splenectomy should therefore be avoided if possible.

Platelet destruction in SLE can be multifactorial. Potential mechanisms for the pathogenesis of thrombocytopenia in patients with lupus include antibody mediated destruction by antiplatelet glycoprotein (GP) IIb/IIIa and GP Ib/IX antibodies or, possibly, antiphospholipid antibodies. Autoantibodies to platelet glycoproteins and the c-Mpl receptor[7,8] may induce megakaryocyte apoptosis and other bone marrow alterations, not classically characteristic of ITP, and may result in decreased platelet production.[5,12,15] Lupus vasculitis, thrombotic microangiopathy, and hemophagocytosis are immunopathologic disorders in which platelets are destroyed secondary to a microvascular inflammatory process. Thrombocytopenia in these disorders reverses with correction of the primary process. There are no studies of plasma thrombopoietin levels in patients with SLE and thrombocytopenia, but it can be assumed that they are similar to that reported in patients with ITP.[15]

A low platelet count in SLE can also result from several other mechanisms including drug-induced thrombocytopenia, infections, or pregnancy. Antimalarial agents have been reported to frequently induce thrombocytopenia.[16] Infections including *Helicobacter pylori*, hepatitis C virus (HCV), human immunodeficiency virus (HIV), and other viral illnesses can further contribute to the risk of developing thrombocytopenia.[5,17,18] Two disorders associated with thrombocytopenia, Evans syndrome and Graves disease, are both reported to have an increased frequency in patients with SLE.[5,17] Thrombocytopenia in pregnant patients with SLE can result from the HELLP (Hemolysis, Elevated Liver enzymes, Low Platelets) syndrome, and in the postpartum period SLE flares can make the diagnosis of ITP difficult in these patients.[19]

Treatment of SLE can be either systemic or organ directed. However, when patients with SLE have associated ITP, therapy is predominately systemic. Available therapies for SLE include antimalarial agents such as hydroxychloroquine, which are used predominantly for treatment of cutaneous, musculoskeletal manifestations, and symptoms of fatigue.[20] However, there are no data to demonstrate the efficacy of this drug in patients with SLE and ITP. In patients with SLE alone, corticosteroids can provide rapid relief of an SLE flare and can be used in short-term bridging therapy to other immunosuppressant agents. In patients with SLE and ITP, corticosteroids remain the primary treatment modality, although every effort should be made to switch to a steroid-sparing therapy. All efforts are directed to minimize the long-term use of corticosteroids. Immunosuppressant agents such as methotrexate, azathioprine, leflunomide, dapsone, cyclosporine, mycophenolate mofetil, and cyclophosphamide are often used as disease-modifying and steroid-sparing agents in SLE.[20] Each of these agents has reported responses in patients with chronic ITP.[2] Several case series on the use of B-lymphocyte depletion with rituximab, an agent with documented responses in refractory ITP, have also reported clinical benefit in refractory SLE patients.[21] Newer potential therapies including both T- and B-cell directed therapies can also be used in SLE and ITP, although they did not meet their end point in recent lupus studies.[20] Future development of immune system modulators targeting such as double-stranded DNA, modulating Fc-γ receptors, inhibiting interleukin-6 expression, and anti-BLyS and other B-cell receptor antibodies, as well as immune therapy with T-regulatory lymphocytes, are some of the potential new therapeutic agents for SLE that could also benefit patients with ITP.

SJÖGREN SYNDROME

Sjögren syndrome, which is also called autoimmune exocrinopathy, is the second most common autoimmune disorder, with a community prevalence of the primary form ranging from 0.1% to 0.6%, the majority of whom are female (> 90% of cases).[22] In this disorder, patients suffer from dry mouth and dry eyes often in association with systemic inflammation. Autoantibodies, including those to the extractable nuclear antigens of Ro and La that attack the salivary and ocular glands, are believed to lead to sicca symptoms.[23] Another name for the anti-Ro and anti-La antibodies is anti-SSA and anti-SSB, respectively. HIV infection can also present with a sicca complex, but is pathophysiologically different due to a predominance of CD8+ lymphocytes and not memory CD4+ T cells or B cells on lip or parotid biopsy.[22] HCV infection has also been implicated in the development of Sjögren syndrome, as has H pylori.[24] These infectious causes should be considered in the differential diagnosis of patients presenting with sicca,[22] and are also associated with the development of immune thrombocytopenia.[16,25]

ITP has been reported in patients with Sjögren syndrome, but its overall incidence is unknown.[26,27] Many of the cases reported also demonstrate other autoimmune manifestations that may reflect a broader defect in immune regulation.[26,27] However, most patients seem to respond to standard ITP therapy. Adding to this complexity is an increased risk of lymphoma with primary Sjögren syndrome that needs to be considered during patient evaluation, which should include a careful examination for lymphadenopathy. Evolution to a high-grade lymphoma can occur after transformation from a mucosa-associated lymphoid tissue (MALT) lymphoma, which is believed to result from the ongoing inflammatory lymphoepithelial sialadenitis.[22]

RHEUMATOID ARTHRITIS

Rheumatoid arthritis (RA) is systemic inflammatory disorder leading to painful, destructive arthritis. The disease results from aberrant T- and B-lymphocyte regulation, leading to the abnormal expression of inflammatory cytokines. Case reports of ITP in patients with RA are rare, and frequently include patients with multiorgan system involvement.[28] The majority of case reports of thrombocytopenia developing in patients with RA seem to be the direct result of disease treatment. Treatment of RA with sulfasalazine, gold salts, hydroxychloroquine, and most recently anti-tumor necrosis factor (TNF) agents, have all been associated with the development of thrombocytopenia.[29–32] In patients with RA and thrombocytopenia, drug-induced thrombocytopenia should first be excluded before a diagnosis of ITP is made. In RA patients with the additional diagnosis of ITP, many of the therapeutic agents for RA, especially corticosteroids and B-cell directed therapy with rituximab, have documented efficacy in immune thrombocytopenia.

VASCULITIC SYNDROMES

The vasculitic syndromes are a heterogeneous collection of autoimmune inflammatory disorders, resulting in arterial vascular injury. These syndromes can be associated with mild to moderate thrombocytopenia. However, in most cases thrombocytopenia does not result from immune-mediated platelet destruction. Leukocytoclastic vasculitis skin lesions need to be differentiated from thrombocytopenic purpura, although the presence of palpable purpura suggests vasculitis, and biopsy should be used for confirmation. The vasculitic disorders can affect any artery and are broadly separated into those with involvement of small, medium, or large vessels. The majority of case reports of ITP associated with vasculitis has been in patients with medium vessel vasculitis.[32–35] Cryoglobulins, which are immune complexes characterized by their ability to precipitate from serum in cold conditions, are associated with small vessel vasculitis and have also been associated with ITP[5]; this is particularly true when the cryoglobulins result from HCV infection.[5] Kawasaki syndrome, a vasculitis associated with coronary artery involvement, has been associated with ITP.[32,33] Wegener granulomatosis, a vasculitis associated with antinuclear cytoplasmic antibodies (ANCA),[35,36] can be associated with either thrombocytosis or thrombocytopenia. An early study suggesting that thrombocytopenia in this disorder was associated with antiphospholipid antibodies was not confirmed in a larger study.[35] In ANCA-associated vasculitis with thrombocytopenia, it can be difficult to differentiate between immune and nonimmune mechanisms for the thrombocytopenia, and response to immunosuppressive treatment alone may not help to differentiate between immune or nonimmune platelet destruction. Although ITP associated with large vessel vasculitis, such as giant cell arteritis or Takayasu vasculitis, is rarely reported,[34] thrombocytopenia may complicate treatment, because aspirin therapy or anticoagulation may be indicated to prevent vascular thrombosis.[34]

STILL DISEASE

Still disease is a systemic inflammatory disorder found in both juvenile and adult forms.[37] Still disease patients may present with ITP and atypical bone marrow changes.[38] Thrombotic thrombocytopenic purpura and hemophagocytic syndromes have also been reported in Still disease patients, supporting the need for a careful review of the peripheral smear in these patients and possibly a bone marrow examination.[39–41] For patients with ITP and Still disease, treatment should be directed toward treating the Still disease. Treatment of adult-onset Still disease (AOSD) with ITP would include corticosteroids and other disease-modifying agents. Recent use of biologic agents, including anti-TNF inhibitory drugs anakinra, rituximab, and tocilizumab, have been reported with success,[38] but except for rituximab none of these have demonstrated efficacy in patients with ITP. Autologous bone marrow transplantation has been used for treating refractory Still disease patients.[42]

OTHER RHEUMATOLOGIC DISORDERS

Mixed connective tissue disease (MCTD) can present with overlapping features of SLE, RA, and polymyositis, with varying degrees of organ involvement.[43] MCTD patients typically have a very high serum ribonucleoprotein, which is helpful in the diagnosis. A case report of ITP in MCTD related the 2 disorders in etiology.[44] Because there is a close relationship of MCTD with lupus, finding autoimmune thrombocytopenia would not be unexpected.

Polymyositis, dermatomyositis, and inclusion body myositis are the most common members of a group of inflammatory myopathies.[45] ITP has been reported in association with myositis in a few case studies.[46–49] In patients older than 35 years, dermatomyositis may develop as a manifestation of an underlying malignancy.[45] Differentiating a primary autoimmune myositis from one associated with a malignancy with hematological involvement can be difficult due to similar clinical presentations. In addition, ITP in patients with autoimmune myositis frequently present with additional autoimmune manifestations suggestive of a more generalized defect in immune regulation.[46–49] Treatment of ITP in these patients may be complicated by the severity of the patient's clinical presentation. Because a muscle biopsy may be necessary for definitive diagnosis, initial therapy with intravenous immunoglobulin to increase the platelet count allows for a safe procedure. Case reports have also shown an association between ITP and seronegative spondylarthropathies, including ankylosing spondylitis.[50,51]

The increasing use of targeted therapies in the treatment of rheumatologic disorders by disrupting the organ-specific inflammatory response may result in the evolution of new autoimmune manifestations in these patients. An example is a recent report of a patient with psoriasis treated with an anti-TNF agent who subsequently developed ITP.[52] There are currently 5 Food and Drug Administration approved anti-TNF agents (etanercept, infliximab, adalimumab, golimumab, and certolizumab), 3 of which have been reported to be associated with the development of thrombocytopenia.[28,29]

ANTIPHOSPHOLIPID SYNDROME AND IMMUNE THROMBOCYTOPENIA

The antiphospholipid syndrome (APS) is a complex disorder characterized by recurrent fetal loss and recurrent thromboembolic events. This section reviews the association between APS and thrombocytopenia, the incidence of antiphospholipid antibodies (APLA) in ITP, and the pathophysiology and relationship of these antibodies to thrombosis and other complications of the antiphospholipid syndrome.

The APS is a disorder defined by recurrent fetal loss as well as recurrent venous or arterial thromboembolic events. In the most severe form, catastrophic antiphospholipid syndrome (CAPS), multiple organ dysfunction may occur, involving the central nervous system, liver, kidney, bone marrow necrosis, nonbacterial endocarditis, and skin.[53] Although frequently associated with SLE, over half of the patients with APS do not have clinical evidence of SLE.[54,55]

Thrombocytopenia in association with APS is more common in patients with SLE than in primary APS (PAPS), although well described in both.[56] The incidence of thrombocytopenia reported in various studies is between 22% and 42%.[57] Thrombocytopenia in APS tends to be less severe than that seen with ITP, usually ranging from 70 to 120 × 10^9 platelets/L, and does not usually require intervention.[55] As a result, it is less commonly associated with bleeding manifestations than ITP. APS may present with isolated thrombocytopenia without other signs and symptoms. The presence of thrombocytopenia does not seem to have an effect on the thromboembolic complication of the disorder, as rates of thrombosis were similar with and without thrombocytopenia.[54] Whereas the findings of cardiac valvular vegetations and myocardial infarction did not have any association with thrombocytopenia, valvular leaflet thickening showed a strong statistical correlation with thrombocytopenia.[54] Chorea, arthritis, and livido reticularis similarly were associated with the presence of thrombocytopenia.[54]

The pathogenesis of thrombocytopenia in APS is still uncertain. The incidence of the lupus anticoagulant (LA), a defining characteristic of the disorder, is higher in APS than in ITP. Antibodies to β2-glycoprotein 1b are also high and, like the lupus anticoagulant, are associated with an increased risk of thrombosis.[58] Anticardiolipin IgM antibodies were also more frequent in patients with APS than in patients with ITP.[59] Antibodies to specific glycoprotein receptors such as GP 1b/IX and IIbIIIa were detected in 40% of patients with APLA.[58,60] Giannakopoulos and colleagues[61] noted that in 11 of 15 (73%) patients with APS and platelet counts of less than 50 × 10^9/L, antiplatelet antibodies to specific platelet glycoproteins could be identified. It has been proposed that binding of antibodies to β2-glycoprotein 1b induces dimerization of the receptor, stimulating phosphorylation of the abetalipoprotein E receptor. This process results in activation of mitogen-activated protein kinase, generating thromboxane A2 as well as phosphatidylinositol-3-kinase and Akt through glycoprotein IIIa, inducing platelet activation and sensitization to other agonists.[5,62] Antiphospholipid antibodies bind to anionic phospholipids on the inner platelet membrane, which suggests that platelet activation or aggregation may be required for membrane exposure of these phospholipids to the antibodies.[63,64] In patients with both SLE and PAPS, antiplatelet antibodies were found much more frequently in patients with thrombocytopenia compared with their counterparts without thrombocytopenia. In addition, there was a strong association between PAPS with thrombocytopenia and anticardiolipin (ACL) antibodies, LA, and specific platelet glycoprotein antibodies.[65] Antiphospholipid antibodies inducing endothelial cell activation are present in a significant number of patients with APS, both with and without thrombocytopenia. β2-Glycoprotein 1 has been demonstrated to bind to endothelial cells as well as trophoblasts, and to induce endothelial cell activation. This activation results in increased cytokine and adhesion molecule expression.[66] However, the prevalence of the LA was higher in the groups with PAPS and thrombocytopenia than with ITP. In contrast, endothelial cell activation was noted in ITP patients only when antiphospholipid antibodies were present. It has been postulated that endothelial cell activation by APLA leads to overexpression of leukocyte adhesion molecules as well as increasing the risk of thrombosis, even in patients with severe thrombocytopenia.[67,68] Polymorphism in Toll-like receptors may enhance the endothelial binding and activation by the antibodies.[69]

In patients presenting with ITP, 66% of patients may have antiphospholipid antibodies.[70] IgG against pure phospholipid is frequent.[58] In an analysis of 146 patients with ITP by Stasi,[70] 46% of patients had evidence of LA activity or ACL antibodies, but no correlation was found between LA ratios and the titers of ACL IgG or IgM with age, sex, degree of thrombocytopenia, or hemorrhage. There was similarly no correlation with APLA. However, in the 52% of patients with platelet counts of less than 50 × 10^9/L, high levels of APLA were seen in one-half of the patients. The presence of APLA was not predictive of response to treatment. In 2 recent analyses, APLA were found in 26% and 38% of ITP patients.[71–73] As in the earlier study, the presence of APLA was not predictive of response to steroids or splenectomy. However, thrombosis did correlate with the detection of an LA with APLA in patients with ITP. This result may identify a unique subset of patients at increased the risk of thromboembolic complications, particularly after therapy-induced platelet recovery.[60,68] There is scant literature on the role of prophylactic anticoagulation in the absence of thrombosis in this subset of patients.

Thrombocytopenia in APS rarely requires treatment unless the platelet count is less than 30×10^9/L. In addition to prednisone, there are some case reports indicating response to rituximab with improvement in the platelet count, as well as reduction or disappearance of anticardiolipin antibodies.[74,75]

SUMMARY

It has been theorized that ITP is a syndrome characterized by various defects in immune regulation, resulting in a common phenotype, decreased blood platelets, and symptoms of mucocutaneous bleeding. Most often, successful treatment of the underlying connective tissue disorder with corticosteroids or other disease-modifying agents can simultaneously improve concurrent thrombocytopenia. The best evidence to date would support the targeting of treatment to the connective tissue disorder, expecting a simultaneous improvement in the platelet count. Due to the frequent relapses associated with many of the connective tissue disorders and the frequent use of immunosuppressant agents, splenectomy should be undertaken only in highly refractory patients.

Differentiating the varying immunopathic etiologies that contribute to development of connective tissue disorders may lead to a better understanding of the mechanisms of thrombocytopenia in a subset of these patients. The use of target therapies to treat connective tissue disorders has the potential of reducing the risk of the development of ITP or, conversely, inducing the development of immune thrombocytopenia.

REFERENCES

1. Arkfeld DG. The potential utility of B cell-directed biologic therapy in autoimmune diseases. Rheumatol Int 2008;28:205–15.
2. McMillan R. Therapy for adults with refractory chronic immune thrombocytopenic purpura. Ann Intern Med 1997;126:307–14.
3. Altintas A, Ozel A, Okur N, et al. Prevalence and clinical significance of elevated antinuclear antibody test in children and adult patients with idiopathic thrombocytopenic purpura. J Thromb Thrombolysis 2007;24:163–8.
4. Karpatkin S, Lackner HL. Association of antiplatelet antibody with functional platelet disorders. Autoimmune thrombocytopenic purpura, systemic lupus erythematosus and thrombopathia. Am J Med 1975;59:599–604.
5. Cines DB, Bussel JB, Liebman HA, et al. The ITP syndrome: a diverse set of disorders with different immune mechanisms. Blood 2009;113:6511–21.
6. Asahi A, Nishimoto T, Okazaki Y, et al. *Helicobacter pylori* eradication shifts monocyte Fcγ receptor balance toward inhibitory FcγRIIB in immune thrombocytopenic purpura patients. J Clin Invest 2008;118:2939–49.
7. McMillan R, Wang L, Tomer A, et al. Suppression of in vitro megakaryocyte production by antiplatelet autoantibodies from adult patients with chronic ITP. Blood 2004;103:1364–9.
8. Katsumata Y, Suzuki T, Kuwana M, et al. Autoantibody to c-Mpl (thrombopoietin receptor) in systemic lupus erythematosus: relationship to thrombocytopenia with megakaryocytic hypoplasia. Arthritis Rheum 2002;46:2148–59.
9. Rahman A, Isenberg DA. Systemic lupus erythematosus. N Engl J Med 2008;358:929–39.
10. Ziakas PD, Routsias JG, Giannouli S, et al. Suspects in the tale of lupus-associated thrombocytopenia. Clin Exp Immunol 2006;145:71–80.

11. Ziakas PD, Poulou LS, Giannouli S, et al. Thrombocytopenia in lupus: baseline C3 as an independent risk factor for relapse. Ann Rheum Dis 2007;66:130–1.

12. Chen JL, Huang XM, Zeng XJ, et al. Hematological abnormalities in systemic lupus erythematosus and clinical significance there of: comparative analysis of 236 cases. Zhonghua Yi Xue Za Zhi 2007;87(19):1330–3.

13. Nojima J, Suehisa E, Kuratsune H, et al. High prevalence of thrombocytopenia in SLE patients with a high level of anticardiolipin antibodies combined with lupus anticoagulant. Am J Hematol 1998;58:55–60.

14. Arnal C, Piette JC, Léone J, et al. Treatment of severe immune thrombocytopenia associated with systemic lupus erythematosus: 59 cases. J Rheumatol 2002; 29(1):75–83.

15. Gernsheimer T. Chronic idiopathic thrombocytopenic purpura: mechanisms of pathogenesis. Oncologist 2009;14(1):12–21.

16. George JN, Raskob GE, Shah SR, et al. Drug-induced thrombocytopenia: a systematic review of published case reports. Ann Intern Med 1998;129:886–90.

17. Cines DB, Liebman H, Stasi R. Pathobiology of secondary immune thrombocytopenia. Semin Hematol 2009;46(Suppl 2):S2–14.

18. Zandman-Goddard G, Shoenfeld Y. HIV and autoimmunity. Autoimmun Rev 2002; 1:329–37.

19. Tincani A, Bazzani C, Zingarelli S, et al. Lupus and the antiphospholipid syndrome in pregnancy and obstetrics: clinical characteristics, diagnosis, pathogenesis, and treatment. Semin Thromb Hemost 2008;34(3):267–73.

20. Manzi S, Kao AH. Systemic lupus erythematosus C. Treatment and assessment. In: Stone JH, Klippel JH, Crofford LJ, et al, editors. The primer on rheumatic diseases. 13th edition. New York: Springer; 2008. p. 327–38.

21. Ramos-Casals M, Soto M, Cuadrado M, et al. Rituximab in systemic lupus erythematosus. A systematic review of off-label use in 188 cases. Lupus 2009;18: 767–76.

22. Wada M, Kamimoto H, Park SY, et al. Autoimmune hepatitis concomitant with hypergammaglobulinemic purpura, immune thrombocytopenia, and Sjögren's syndrome. Intern Med 2001;40(4):308–11.

23. Daniels T. Sjögren's syndrome. In: Stone JH, Klippel JH, Crofford LJ, White PH, editors. The primer on rheumatic diseases. 13th edition. New York: Springer; 2008. p. 389–97.

24. Delaleu N, Immervoll H, Cornelius J, et al. Biomarker profiles in serum and saliva of experimental Sjögren's syndrome: associations with specific autoimmune manifestations. Arthritis Res Ther 2008;10(1):R22.

25. Ramos-Casals M, Loustaud-Ratti V, De Vita S, et al. Sjögren syndrome associated with hepatitis C virus: a multicenter analysis of 137 cases. Medicine (Baltimore) 2005;84(2):81–9.

26. Watanabe M, Fujimoto T, Iwano M, et al. Report of a patient of primary Sjögren syndrome, IgA nephropathy and chronic idiopathic thrombocytopenic purpura. Nihon Rinsho Meneki Gakkai Kaishi 2002;25:191–8.

27. Yamada Y, Kuroe K. A case of rheumatoid arthritis complicated with idiopathic thrombocytopenic purpura and Hashimoto's disease. Ryumachi 1991;31:413–9.

28. Pathare SK, Heycock C, Hamilton J. TNF alpha blocker-induced thrombocytopenia. Rheumatology (Oxford) 2006;45:1313–4.

29. Vidal F, Fontova R, Richart C. Severe neutropenia and thrombocytopenia associated with infliximab. Ann Intern Med 2003;139:W–W63.

30. Cantarini L, Tinazzi I, Biasi D, et al. Sulfasalazine-induced immune thrombocytopenia. Postgrad Med J 2007;83(980):e1.

31. Levin MD, van t Veer MB, de Veld JC, et al. Two patients with acute thrombocytopenia following gold administration and five-year follow-up. Neth J Med 2003; 61:223–5.
32. Hara T, Mizuno Y, Akeda H, et al. Thrombocytopenia: a complication of Kawasaki disease. Eur J Pediatr 1988;147:51–3.
33. Asano T, Sudoh M, Watanabe M, et al. Transient thrombocytopenia with large platelets in Kawasaki disease. Pediatr Hematol Oncol 2007;24:551–4.
34. Matsuzaki K, Shiiya N, Kubota S, et al. A case of an ascending aortic aneurysm due to mesoaortitis complicated with idiopathic thrombocytopenic purpura. Ann Thorac Cardiovasc Surg 2001;7:315–8.
35. Meyer MF, Schnabel A, Schatz H, et al. Lack of association between antiphospholipid antibodies and thrombocytopenia in patients with Wegener's granulomatosis. Semin Arthritis Rheum 2001;31:4–11.
36. Wiik A. Autoantibodies in vasculitis. Arthritis Res Ther 2003;5(3):147–52.
37. Lin SJ, Jaing TH. Thrombocytopenia in systemic-onset juvenile chronic arthritis: report of two cases with unusual bone marrow features. Clin Rheumatol 1999;18(3):241–3.
38. Fautrel B. Adult-onset Still disease. Best Pract Res Clin Rheumatol 2008;22(5): 773–92.
39. Gopal M, Cohn CD, McEntire MR, et al. Thrombotic thrombocytopenic purpura and adult onset Still's disease. Am J Med Sci 2009;337:373–6.
40. Sayarlioglu M, Sayarlioglu H, Ozkaya M, et al. Thrombotic thrombocytopenic purpura-hemolytic uremic syndrome and adult onset Still's disease: case report and review of the literature. Mod Rheumatol 2008;18:403–6.
41. Yoshizaki A, Kawakami A, Aramaki T, et al. Preferential recovery by an intensive initial therapy from hemophagocytic syndrome complicated with adult onset Still's disease presenting as agranulocytosis and hypercytokinemia. Clin Exp Rheumatol 2008;26:383.
42. Passweg J, Tyndall A. Autologous stem cell transplantation in autoimmune diseases. Semin Hematol 2007;44(4):278–85.
43. Pope JE. Other manifestations of mixed connective tissue disease. Rheum Dis Clin North Am 2005;31(3):519–33, vii.
44. Richart C, Pujol-Borrell R. Autoimmune hemolytic anemia and idiopathic thrombocytopenic purpura preceding a mixed connective tissue disease. Med Clin (Barc) 1983;81(8):370.
45. Christopher-Stine L, Plotz PH. Myositis: an update on pathogenesis. Curr Opin Rheumatol 2004;16:700–6.
46. Chang DK, Yoo DH, Kim TH, et al. Induction of remission with intravenous immunoglobulin and cyclophosphamide in steroid-resistant Evans' syndrome associated with dermatomyositis. Clin Rheumatol 2001;20:63–6.
47. Takaku T, Kuriyama Y, Shoji N, et al. Simultaneous development of factor V inhibitor and autoimmune thrombocytopenia in a patient with dermatomyositis. Rinsho Ketsueki 2002;43:1050–4.
48. Kaneoka H, Sasatomi Y, Miyagi K, et al. A rare case of dermatomyositis associated with immune-complex type glomerulonephritis, idiopathic thrombopenic purpura, pulmonary fibrosis and lung cancer. Clin Exp Rheumatol 2003;21:801–2.
49. Williams SF, Mincey BA, Calamia KT. Inclusion body myositis associated with celiac sprue and idiopathic thrombocytopenic purpura. South Med J 2003;96: 721–3.
50. Tsai CY, Yu CL, Tsai YY, et al. Osteochondroma in a patient with juvenile ankylosing spondylitis associated with idiopathic thrombocytopenic purpura and alpha thalassemia. Scand J Rheumatol 1996;25:61–2.

51. Uozumi K, Makino T, Shimotakahara S, et al. Cyclic thrombocytopenia with chronic thyroiditis and ankylosing spondylitis. Rinsho Ketsueki 1992;33:1215–20.

52. Brunasso AM, Massone C. Thrombocytopenia associated with the use of anti-tumor necrosis factor-alpha agents for psoriasis. J Am Acad Dermatol 2009;60: 781–5.

53. Miyakis S, Lockshin MD, Atsumi T, et al. International consensus statement on an update of the classification criteria for definite antiphospholipid syndrome. J Thromb Haemost 2006;4:295–306.

54. Krause I, Blank M, Fraser A, et al. The association of thrombocytopenia with systemic manifestations in the antiphospholipid syndrome. Immunobiology 2005;210:749–54.

55. Chong BH, Brighton TC, Chesterman CN. Antiphospholipid antibodies and platelets. Semin Thromb Hemost 1995;21:76–84.

56. Galli M, Finazzi G, Barbui T. Thrombocytopenia in the antiphospholipid syndrome. Br J Haematol 1996;93:1–5.

57. Uthman I, Godeau B, Tahaer A, et al. The hematologic manifestations of the antiphospholipid syndrome. Blood Rev 2008;22:187–94.

58. Bidot CJ, Jy W, Horstman LL, et al. Antiphospholipid antibodies (APLA) in immune thrombocytopenic purpura (ITP) and antiphospholipid syndrome (APS). Am J Hematol 2006;81:391–6.

59. Godeau B, Piette JC, Fromont P, et al. Specific antiplatelet glycoprotein autoantibodies are associated with the thrombocytopenia of primary antiphospholipid syndrome. Br J Haematol 1997;98(4):873–9.

60. Galli M, Luciani D, Bertoli G, et al. Anti beta-2-glycoprotein I, antiprothrombin antibodies, and the risk of thrombosis in the antiphospholipid syndrome. Blood 2003; 102:2717–23.

61. Giannakopoulos B, Passam F, Rahgozar S, et al. Current concepts on the pathogenesis of the antiphospholipid syndrome. Blood 2007;109(2):422–30.

62. Vega-Ostertag ME, Pierangeli SS. Mechanisms of aPL-thrombosis: effect of aPL on endothelium and platelets. Curr Rheumatol Rep 2007;9:190–7.

63. Nojima J, Suehisa E, Akita N, et al. Risk of arterial thrombosis in patients with anticardiolipin antibodies and lupus anticoagulant. Br J Haematol 1997;96:447–50.

64. Macchi L, Rispal P, Clofent-Sanchez G, et al. Anti-platelet antibodies in patients with SLE and the primary anitphospholipid antibody syndrome: their relationship with the observed thrombocytopenia. Br J Haematol 1997;98:336–41.

65. Meroni PL, Rashchi E, Camera M, et al. Endothelial activation by aPL: a potential pathogenetic mechanism for the clinical manifestations of the syndrome. J Autoimmun 2000;15:237–40.

66. Dunoyer-Geindre S, Boehlen F, Favier R, et al. Endothelial cell activation by immunoglobulins from patients with immune thrombocytopenic purpura or with antiphospholipid syndrome. Haematologica 2008;93(4):635–6.

67. Atsumi T, Furukawa S, Amengual O, et al. Antiphospholipid antibody associated with thrombocytopenia and the paradoxical risk of thrombosis. Lupus 2005;14: 499–504.

68. Pierangeli SS, Vega-Ostertag ME, Raschi E, et al. Toll-like receptor and antiphospholipid mediated thrombosis: in vivo studies. Ann Rheum Dis 2007;66:1327–33.

69. Harris EN, Gharavi AE, Hegde U, et al. Anticardiolipin antibodies in autoimmune thrombocytopenic purpura. Br J Haematol 1985;59:231–4.

70. Stasi R. Prevalence and clinical significance of elevated antiphospholipid antibodies in patients with idiopathic thrombocytopenic pupura. Blood 1990;84: 4203–8.

71. Despujol CPD, Michel M, Khellaf, et al. Antiphospholipid antibodies in adults with immune thrombocytopenic purpura. Br J Haematol 2008;142:638–43.
72. Diz-Kucukkaya R, Hachihanefioglu A, Yenerel M. Antiphospholipid antibodies and antiphospholipid syndrome in patients presenting with the immune thrombocytopenic purpura: a prospective cohort study. Blood 2001;98:1760–4.
73. Kravitz MS, Shoenfeld Y. Thrombocytopenic conditions- autoimmunity and hypercoagulability: commonalities and differences in ITP, TTP, HIT, and APS. Am J Hematol 2005;80(3):232–42.
74. Trapp R, Loew A, Thuss-Patience P. Successful treatment of thrombocytopenia in primary antiphospholipid antibody syndrome with the anti-CD20 antibody rituximab—monitoring of antiphospholipid and anti GP antibodies: a case report. Ann Hematol 2006;85:134–5.
75. Ruckert A, Glimm H, Lubbert M, et al. Successful treatment of life threatening Evans' syndrome due to antiphospholipid antibody syndrome by rituximab-based regimen: a case with long-term follow up. Lupus 2008;17:757.

Thyroid Disease in Patients with Immune Thrombocytopenia

Eric Cheung, MD, Howard A. Liebman, MD*

KEYWORDS

- Immune thrombocytopenia • Thyroid diseases
- Hyperthyroidism • Graves disease

The first patient case report of hyperthyroidism and thrombocytopenia was published in 1931.[1] Since then, more than 160 cases of hyperthyroidism associated with immune thrombocytopenic purpura (ITP) have been reported.[2] Similar reports of ITP and immune-mediated hypothyroidism (Hashimoto thyroiditis) would suggest that there is more than casual relationship between autoimmune thyroid disease and ITP. Although this association between thyroid disease and ITP is well documented, many questions remain regarding true prevalence and whether the presence of thyroid disease in patients with ITP defines a different subset of patients that may impact its management. This is due to the medical literature regarding thyroid disease and ITP being composed mostly of case reports and small retrospective studies.

A strong association between other systemic autoimmune diseases and autoimmune thyroid diseases is also well documented.[3–5] Therefore, the combination of autoimmune thyroid disease and ITP could reflect a more significant defect in the immune self-tolerance of these patients compared with those who have primary ITP alone.[6] Such defects may characterize an ITP patient population as more refractory to standard ITP therapy.[6]

THE THYROID GLAND AND AUTOIMMUNE THYROID DISEASE

The thyroid gland is anatomically composed of loose follicles responsible for the regulated secretion of the 2 biologically active thyroid hormones, thyroxine (T4) and 3,5,3'-triiodothyronine (T3). Thyroid hormones are essential for the development of the brain in infants and for metabolic activity in adults. Thyroid hormone balance is regulated by the extrathyroidal conversion of T4 to T3; by nutritional, hormonal, and illness-related factors; and by thyrotropin (thyroid-stimulating hormone [TSH]).

University of Southern California-Keck School of Medicine, Jane Anne Nohl Division of Hematology, Norris Comprehensive Cancer Center, Room 3466, 1441 Eastlake Avenue, Los Angeles, CA 90033-0800, USA
* Corresponding author.
E-mail address: liebman@usc.edu (H.A. Liebman).

Hematol Oncol Clin N Am 23 (2009) 1251–1260
doi:10.1016/j.hoc.2009.08.003
0889-8588/09/$ – see front matter © 2009 Elsevier Inc. All rights reserved.

Thyrotropin, in turn, is regulated by thyrotropin-releasing hormone, a glycoprotein synthesized and secreted by the anterior pituitary gland.

Different disorders can cause hyperthyroidism. The etiologic difference of these disorders can be distinguished via 24-hour I^{131} radioiodine uptake. A high radioiodine uptake indicates increased de novo synthesis of the thyroid hormones and is observed in Graves disease,[7] autoimmune (Hashimoto) thyrotoxicosis,[8] toxic adenomas, and multi-nodular goiters. Low radioiodine uptake in the presence of hyperthyroidism indicates excessive unregulated thyroid hormone release due to inflammatory or infection-related destruction of thyroid tissue, with the release of preformed hormone (thyroiditis) or an extrathyroidal source of hormone (ectopic hyperthyroidism).

Graves disease is the most common cause of hyperthyroidism and is an autoimmune disorder resulting from thyrotropin-receptor–stimulating antibodies. Graves disease is part of a systemic syndrome consisting of hyperthyroidism, goiter, and ophthalmopathy.[7] Several immune mechanisms have been implicated in the pathogenesis of Graves hyperthyroidism, including molecular mimicry, thyroid-cell expression of human leukocyte antigens (HLA), and bystander activation. The clinical manifestations of Graves disease, such as ophthalmopathy,[9] may be present even in the absence of hyperthyroidism, suggesting that it is only one manifestation of this systemic disease.

Subclinical hyperthyroidism is defined by normal serum thyroxine and triiodothyronine concentrations and a low serum TSH concentration. The causes of subclinical hyperthyroidism are the same as those for overt hyperthyroidism. Treatment of patients with subclinical hyperthyroidism is often recommended because of decreased bone density and the presence of atrial fibrillation in elderly patients.

Hypothyroidism can result from a defect anywhere along the hypothalamic-pituitary-thyroid axis. Hypothyroidism may be transient when secondary to thyroiditis or pregnancy, may be drug-induced, or it may result from hypothalamic or pituitary disease. Most often, hypothyroidism results from progressive thyroid disease (primary hypothyroidism) caused by autoimmune destruction of the thyroid gland.[8] Hypothyroidism may develop in the later stages of Graves disease or Hashimoto thyroiditis, either as the result of progressive immune gland destruction or from ablative treatment of hyperthyroidism.

Subclinical hypothyroidism is defined as a normal serum-free thyroxine concentration and an elevated serum thyrotropin concentration. The causes of subclinical hypothyroidism are the same as those of overt hypothyroidism. Although the American College of Physicians Guidelines[10] questions the sufficiency of data with regard to treatment recommendations, many investigators recommend hormone replacement for correction of abnormal serum lipids and to prevent progression to overt hypothyroidism.

ITP AND THYROID DISEASE: A DISTINCT SYNDROME?

Multiple case reports and retrospective studies have documented the concurrence of ITP and autoimmune disease. Although the recent standardization of terminology for ITP[11] has designated these patients as having secondary ITP, specific terms such as thyroid disease-associated ITP may not reliably characterize patients with a history of ITP and thyroid disease.[11] The separation of primary from secondary ITP was developed with the view that patients with secondary forms of the disease may require a different approach to management.[6] However, this distinction is not clear with regard to the association between ITP and autoimmune thyroid diseases.

Autoimmune thyroid disorders, such as hypothyroidism resulting from Hashimoto thyroiditis[12–17] or hyperthyroidism, from Graves disease,[2,16,18–26] have been repeatedly reported in patients with ITP. However, the clinical course of thyroid disease and ITP may be widely separated in time of onset and clinical expression. Also, the clinical course of ITP in patients with overt symptomatic thyroid disease may also be different from that of patients with subclinical thyroid disease. In many of the case reports of ITP and thyroid disease, patients present with other autoimmune disorders such as myasthenia gravis,[12] Guillain-Barré syndrome[17] systemic lupus erythematosus,[24] and scleroderma-dermatomyositis.[25] The management of these disorders may take precedence over the management of the thrombocytopenia or, at least, complicate the treatment of the ITP. These patients, in particular, may have an even more significant defect in immune self-tolerance.[6]

This defect in immune self-tolerance is again reflected in multiple cases of Graves disease reported in patients with Evan syndrome, the combination of ITP and autoimmune hemolytic anemia.[27–32] In addition, many of these case reports are found in the Japanese and Asian medical literature, suggesting a possible genetic propensity for both disorders in these populations.

Thyroid disease associated with ITP has occasionally been reported in the pediatric literature.[33] A familial presentation of both diseases has also been reported.[34] Bizzaro[34] reported the coexistence of ITP and Graves disease in several members of the same family. Four related women developed autoimmune thrombocytopenia, of which, 2 also presented with hyperthyroidism. The HLA phenotype for these women was determined and B8 and DR3 antigens, previously reported in high frequencies in Graves Disease, were present.[35] The 2 women with hyperthyroidism were found to have high titers of antiplatelet and thyroid-stimulating immunoglobulins.[34]

TIMING OF ONSET OF DISORDERS

The time between the onset of clinically overt thyroid disease and immune ITP can be variable. Reports of simultaneous presentations of ITP and autoimmune thyroid disease are often seen, as are case reports of patients who develop thyroid disease or ITP during the treatment of one or the other disorder.[2,19,20,22,26,33] Jacobs and colleagues[22] reported on 6 patients with hyperthyroidism and ITP. In 5 patients, the diseases occurred simultaneously. In 1 patient, thyrotoxicosis developed after successful treatment of the thrombocytopenia. Kamei and colleagues[25] reported on a 35-year-old Japanese woman with a combination of scleroderma-dermatomyositis overlap syndrome and Graves disease who developed ITP during therapy for the Graves disease with antithyroid drugs and steroids.

Other cases of ITP may present earlier or at a significantly different time to the diagnosis of thyroid disorders. Timing between the diagnosis of ITP and thyroid disease can vary from months[33] to years.[15,17,21,31,36] Kohli and colleagues[17] reported a 21-year-old Caucasian woman with a past history of Hashimoto thyroiditis who later presented with symptoms due to Guillain-Barré syndrome and a simultaneous platelet count of 6000/L, 1 week after an upper respiratory infection.[17]

Bowles and colleagues[15] reported on a 52-year-old woman with chronic severe refractory thrombocytopenia present for 3 years before the discovery of hypothyroidism. A 31-year-old black women diagnosed with Graves' disease had been successfully treated for ITP with splenectomy at 12 years of age.[21] The development of hyperthyroidism was not associated with a relapse in her ITP. In contrast, a 39-year-old Japanese woman with a 10-year history of Graves disease, treated with methimazole for 2 years, presented with severe thrombocytopenia on relapse of her hyperthyroidism.[36]

In the largest published studies on thyroid disease and thrombocytopenia, 98 patients diagnosed with ITP were evaluated at the Cleveland Clinic.[16] Of the 80 patients with available thyroid function tests, 16 (20%) had abnormal thyroid function. Six patients had clinically overt hyperthyroidism and 10 had hypothyroidism, of whom 7 had antibodies diagnostic of Hashimoto thyroiditis. Only 2 of the 16 (12.5%) patients had a simultaneous onset of thyroid disease and ITP. The median interval between the onset of the thyroid and hematological conditions was 84 months.[16]

In a study of 71 patients with ITP from the University of Southern California who were screened for thyroid disorders, 17 (23.9%) had a positive diagnosis.[37] Five patients (7%) had overt hyperthyroidism, 5 patients (7%) has subclinical hyperthyroidism. Four patients (5.6%) had overt hypothyroidism and 3 patients (17.6%) had subclinical hypothyroidism. Four patients were diagnosed with thyroid disorders before their ITP diagnosis, whereas 13 were diagnosed after the onset of ITP.[37] However, the diagnosis of subclinical thyroid disease in this patient cohort was enhanced by a routine screening protocol that included an assay for TSH.[37]

EFFECT OF TREATMENT OF THYROID DISEASE AND THE CLINICAL COURSE OF ITP

A review of the multiple case reports on the effect of thyroid disease and its treatment on the clinical course of ITP find no consistent effect on the disease. There are several reports of complete resolution of thrombocytopenia, even in highly refractory patients, following treatment of either hyper- or hypothyroidism. However, an equal number of reports find no improvement in thrombocytopenia after restitution of a euthyroid state.

Kohli and colleagues[17] described a woman with hypothyroidism due to Hashimoto thyroiditis, who presented with Guillain-Barré syndrome and ITP that was refractory to treatment with corticosteroids, intravenous immunoglobulin, and anti-RhD despite thyroid hormone treatment. The patient's platelet count stabilized only after a laparoscopic splenectomy.[17] This contrasts with the case report of a 52-year old-woman with chronic severe refractory thrombocytopenia whose platelet count remained less than 20×10^9/L over a period of 3 years despite treatment with corticosteroids, azathioprine, intravenous immunoglobulin, and splenectomy.[15] Only after the discovery of hypothyroidism and the successful correction of her hypothyroid state did she have a long-lasting and complete normalization of her platelet count.[15]

In contrast to the few reports regarding treatment of hypothyroidism in patients with ITP, a significant number of case reports and series suggest that untreated hyperthyroidism may be responsible for cases of ITP refractory to standard therapy. Herman and colleagues[14] reported a young woman with hyperthyroidism and ITP whose platelet count returned to normal after the successful treatment of hyperthyroidism. Their survey of the literature up until 1978 revealed 48 reports of hyperthyroidism and thrombocytopenia. The diseases coexisted in 37 patients and there was no apparent cause for thrombocytopenia in 28 patients. Eighteen of 22 patients adequately treated for hyperthyroidism had platelet counts return to normal. His group estimated that in 7% of patients with ITP, the platelet counts would respond to treatment of underlying thyrotoxicosis, and in many of these patients, the thrombocytopenia would be resistant to other forms of therapy.

Since 1978, another 16 patients have been reported in whom treatment of hyperthyroidism has either resulted in a complete hematologic remission of ITP or an improved response to standard ITP therapy.[2,20,22,23,26,31,36,38,39] This would contrast with only 5 reported patients in whom treatment of hyperthyroidism had no impact on the course of ITP.[19,20,22]

However, the largest published study evaluating the frequency of thyroid disease in patients with ITP suggests that there may have been a publication bias in previous reports on the effect of treatment of hyperthyroidism on the clinical course of ITP.[16] Sixteen patients with both diseases were identified, 6 with hyperthyroidism and 10 with hypothyroidism. The autoimmune nature of the thyroid disease was proven by antibody testing in 12 cases. Three patients, 1 with hyperthyroidism and 2 with hypothyroidism, had a transient increase in their platelet counts after therapy, which induced a euthyroid state. However, no durable remissions in thrombocytopenia were obtained by treatment of the thyroid disease.[16]

In a University of Southern California (USC) study of 71 patients with ITP, 17 were discovered to have clinically symptomatic (9 patients) or subclinical (8 patients) thyroid disease.[37] There was a trend for the patients with ITP and thyroid disease to have platelet counts less than 50, 000/mcL at the end of follow-up (4 of 17 [23.5%] versus 5 of 53 [9%], $P = .064$), despite receiving a similar numbers of individual therapies (2.82 vs 3.13). However, fewer patients with ITP and thyroid disease underwent splenectomy (3 of 17 vs 21 of 54, $P = .087$). Similar to the conclusions from the Cleveland Clinic Study,[16] the USC investigators concluded that although thyroid disorders are commonly observed in patients with ITP, they did not seem to significantly alter response to therapy or to the long-term outcome of the patients with regard to their thrombocytopenia.[37]

MECHANISMS CONNECTING THYROID DISEASE AND THROMBOCYTOPENIA
Decreased Platelet Survival/Accelerated Platelet Clearance

A mild thrombocytopenia ($>100 \times 10^9$/L,$<150 \times 10^9$/L) has been frequently observed in patients with Graves disease.[7] Panzer and colleagues[40] studied the platelet lifespan in patients with hyperthyroidism. For 15 patients with hyperthyroidism, the platelet count, mean platelet volume, and platelet kinetic studies of autologous 111-indium-labeled platelets and platelet-associated IgG and IgM were measured before and 3 weeks after the administration of antithyroid drugs when the patients were clinically euthyroid. Comparisons were made to 90 euthyroid controls. After 3 weeks of treatment, there was a statistically significant increase in the patients' platelet counts and decreases in the mean platelet volume, when compared with pretreatment values. All subjects had normal 111-indium platelet recovery. Platelet lifespan was significantly shorter in patients with hyperthyroidism compared with those of a control group,[40] even in patients with peripheral platelet counts in the normal range. There were no increases in platelet-associated immunoglobulins and the investigators concluded that the shortened platelet survival was metabolic in nature and not immunologically mediated.

The same investigators subsequently studied thrombopoietic activity in 15 patients with hyperthyroidism by determining the absolute and relative reticulated platelet counts.[41] In 10 patients with hyperthyroidism, there was an increase in the absolute reticulated platelet count when compared with normal subjects. In 14 patients, the reticulocyte percentage and absolute count decreased when the patients became euthyroid. These changes were statistically significant, but there was no statistical change in the total platelet count for the patients when compared with counts obtained before treatment of their hyperthyroidism. In patients with hyperthyroidism without ITP, the shortened platelet survival and increased platelet turnover seemed to be compensated for by an increase in thrombopoiesis.[41]

After noting an improvement in platelet counts with treatment, in approximately half the patients with Graves Disease, Kurata and coworkers[42] performed a series of animal experiments. Rats were injected with T3. The investigators found a treatment-associated decrease in the animals' platelet counts resulting from a shortened platelet survival. When platelets from the treated rats were transfused into untreated rats in the control group, platelet survival was normal. Platelets from untreated control rats transfused into the treated rats shortened platelet survival. There was a similar accelerated clearance of heat-damaged red blood cells in the T3-treated rats. The investigators hypothesized that thrombocytopenia in Graves disease may be the consequence of increased reticuloendothelial phagocytic activity.[42] If hyperthyroidism increases reticuloendothelial phagocytic activity by upregulation of Fc receptor expression or activity, it would, therefore, not be surprising that the concurrent presence of hyperthyroidism in patients with ITP could result in resistance to standard therapy.

Self-tolerance in Patients with ITP and Thyroid Disease

The increased prevalence of antiplatelet and antithyroid autoantibodies in patients with ITP and thyroid dysfunction compared with those with ITP alone seems to indicate a much more significant defect in immune regulation in these patients. Cordiano and colleagues[43] studied 3 groups for the presence and specificity of platelet and thyroid autoantibodies: 18 patients with autoimmune thyroid disease and ITP, 19 patients with autoimmune thyroid disease without thrombocytopenia, and 22 patients with ITP without findings of thyroid disease. Platelet-associated IgG or specific circulating platelet antibodies were detected in most patients with ITP, including patients with and without autoimmune thyroid disease (83% and 86%, respectively). In patients with autoimmune thyroid disease without thrombocytopenia, antiplatelet antibodies were detected in 2 of 19 patients (10%). There was no significant difference in the specificity of the antiplatelet autoantibodies detected in the patients with concurrent thyroid disease and ITP and the patients with ITP alone, with most antibodies directed against the common platelet glycoproteins Ib/IX or IIb/IIIa.[43] Thyroid autoantibodies were discovered in 89% of patients with ITP and autoimmune thyroid disease, in 95% of patients with autoimmune thyroid disease without thrombocytopenia, and only 18% of patients with primary ITP.[43] Other investigators have reported a somewhat higher incidence of antithyroid antibodies in patients with ITP without overt thyroid disease.[44] Altintas and colleagues[44] investigated the presence of antithyroglobulin and antimicrosomal antibodies in 74 patients with ITP without evident thyroid disease and in 162 control normal subjects. They found antithyroglobulin antibodies in 29 (39%) and antimicrosomal antibodies in 19 (26%), respectively in the patients with ITP. Antithyroglobulin antibodies were detected in 10% of control subjects. In addition, many of the same patients also had antigliadin and antiendomysium antibodies associated with celiac disease.[44] Neither of these studies offered information as to whether the presence of antithyroid antibodies was of clinical significance in the management of ITP.

In children, antithyroid antibodies have been reported, but at an apparent lower frequency than were discovered in patients with ITP.[45] Pratt and colleagues[45] evaluated 31 patients, 42% of whom had an acute course of ITP, 58% with a chronic course. Two children with acute ITP tested positive for antithyroid antibodies, as did 3 children with chronic ITP. None of these children had abnormal thyroid tests. In this small series, detection of antithyroid antibodies was not predictive of a chronic ITP; A larger study would be necessary to determine if the presence of antithyroid antibodies could be predictive of the development of chronic ITP in children.

Genetic Predisposition

A genetic predisposition to the coexistence of ITP and hyperthyroidism was suggested by a report on a family with 4 women who had ITP, of which 2 also had hyperthyroidism.[34] Evaluation of the patients' HLA phenotype disclosed antigens B8 and DR3.[34]

HLA B8 is the most frequently antigen reported in isolated ITP[46] and Graves disease.[35] However, no other systematic studies of HLA or other genetic analysis has been reported for patients with chronic ITP. In a case report of a black women diagnosed with Graves disease 20 years after having been diagnosed with ITP, HLA antigens A23, A28, and B17 were identified.[21] The time lapse between the diagnoses of the 2 disorders suggested a possible causal relationship between them or a possible racial difference in HLA relationships to the risk of developing both disorders. The importance of racial differences is supported by studies in which B8 antigens are more frequently identified in white patients with Graves disease as opposed to Bw35 antigens in Japanese patients.[35,47] Although recent HLA-typing studies have been less helpful in the genetic evaluation of ITP,[48] the evaluation of patients with both ITP and autoimmune thyroid disease could prove more productive.

SUMMARY

The American Society of Hematology Guidelines for ITP stated that the evaluation of thyroid function has "uncertain appropriateness" in adults with ITP. The only situation in which thyroid function evaluation is considered appropriate is before an elective splenectomy.[49] Later British guidelines on the investigation and management of ITP make no recommendation regarding screening for thyroid disease in patients with ITP.[50]

Several case reports and case series in the literature regarding an association between thyroid disease and ITP suggest that autoimmune thyroid disease is a frequent finding in patients with ITP. In view of the high incidence of antithyroid antibodies reported in several studies, screening patients for such antibodies would be appropriate. The detection of antithyroid antibodies should identify a patient population at greater risk of developing overt thyroid disease and, as such, these patients may be further screened with a TSH assay to detect subclinical thyroid disease.

The presence of thyroid disease appears not to have an impact on the overall management of patients with ITP. However, numerous case reports would suggest that patients with ITP and concurrent hyperthyroidism may be more refractory to standard ITP treatment, and control of the thyroid disease in these patients may improve ITP treatment outcome.

REFERENCES

1. Jackson AS. Acute hemorrhagic purpura associated with exophthalmic goiter. JAMA 1931;96:38–9.
2. Aggarwal A, Doolittle G. Autoimmune thrombocytopenic purpura associated with hyperthyroidism in a single individual. South Med J 1997;90:933–6.
3. Biro E, Szekanecz Z, Czirjak L, et al. Association of systemic and thyroid autoimmune diseases. Clin Rheumatol 2006;25:240–5.
4. Marder R, Mishail S, Adawi M, et al. Thyroid dysfunction in patients with systemic lupus erythematosus (SLE): relation to disease activity. Clin Rheumatol 2007;26: 1891–4.

5. Nakamura H, Usa T, Motomura M, et al. Prevalence of interrelated autoantibodies in thyroid diseases and autoimmune disorders. J Endocrinol Invest 2008;31: 861–5.
6. Cines DB, Bussel JB, Liebman HA, et al. The ITP syndrome: a diverse set of disorders with different immune mechanisms. Blood 2009;113:6511–21.
7. Brent GA. Graves' disease. N Engl J Med 2008;358:2594–605.
8. Dayan CM, Daniels GH. Chronic autoimmune thyroiditis. N Engl J Med 1996;335: 99–108.
9. Bartalena L, Tanada ML. Graves' ophthalmopathy. N Engl J Med 2009;360: 994–1001.
10. Helfand M, Redfern CC. Clinical guideline part 2 screening for thyroid disease: an update. Ann Intern Med 1998;129:144–58.
11. Rodeghiero F, Stasi R, Gernsheimer T, et al. Standardization of terminology, definitions, and outcome criteria in immune thrombocytopenic purpura of adults and children: report from an international working group. Blood 2009;113: 2386–93.
12. Segal BM, Weintraub MJ. Hashimoto's thyroiditis, myasthenia gravis, idiopathic thrombocytopenic purpura. Ann Intern Med 1976;85:761–3.
13. Crabtree GR, Lee JC, Corwell GG. Autoimmune thrombocytopenic purpura and Hashimoto's thyroiditis. Ann Intern Med 1975;83:371–2.
14. Herman J, Resnitzky P, Finch A. Association between thyrotoxicosis and thrombocytopenia. A case report and review of the literature. Isr J Med Sci 1978;14: 469–75.
15. Bowles KM, Turner GE, Wimperis JZ. Resolution of chronic severe refractory thrombocytopenia after treatment of hypothyroidism. J Clin Pathol 2004;57: 995–6.
16. Iochimescu AG, Makdissi A, Lichtin A, et al. Thyroid disease in patients with idiopathic thrombocytopenia: a cohort study. Thyroid 2007;17(11):1137–42.
17. Kohli R, Bleibel W, Bleibel H. Concurrent immune thrombocytopenic purpura and Guillain-Barre syndrome in a patient with Hashimoto's thyroiditis. Am J Hematol 2007;82:307–8.
18. Marshall JS, Weisberger AS, Levy RP, et al. Coexistent idiopathic thrombocytopenic purpura and hyperthyroidism. Ann Intern Med 1967;67:411–4.
19. Dunlap DB, McFarland KF, et al. Graves' disease and idiopathic thrombocytopenic purpura. Am J Med Sci 1974;268:107–11.
20. Adrouny A, Sandler RM, Carmel R. Variable presentation of thrombocytopenia in Graves' disease. Arch Intern Med 1982;142:1460–4.
21. Valenta L, Treadwell T, Berry R, et al. Idiopathic thrombocytopenic purpura and Graves disease. Am J Hematol 1982;12:69–72.
22. Jacobs P, Majoos F, Perrotta A. Hyperthyroidism and immune thrombocytopenia. Postgrad Med J 1984;60:657–61.
23. Hofbauer LC, Lorenz C, Spitzweg C, et al. Graves' disease associated with autoimmune thrombocytopenic purpura. Arch Intern Med 1997;12(157):1033–6.
24. Oren M, Cohen M. Immune thrombocytopenia, red cell aplasia, lupus, and hyperthyroidism. South Med J 1978;71:1577–8.
25. Kamei N, Yamane K, Yamashita Y, et al. Anti-Ku antibody-positive scleroderma-dermatomyositis overlap syndrome developing Graves' disease and immune thrombocytopenic purpura. Intern Med 2002;41:1199–203.
26. Azar M, Frates A, Rajput V. Idiopathic thrombocytopenic purpura (ITP) and hyperthyroidism: an unusual but critical association for clinicians. J Hosp Med 2008;3: 431–3.

27. Branehog I, Olsson KS, Weinfeld A, et al. Association of hyperthyroidism with idiopathic thrombocytopenic purpura and haemolytic anemia. Acta Med Scand 1979;205:125.
28. Lee FY, Ho CH, Chong LL. Hyperthyroidism and Evan's syndrome. A case report. J Formos Med Assoc 1985;84:256–60.
29. Ito M, Ninomiya N, Amino N, et al. [A case of Evans' syndrome combination of hyperthyroidism]. J Jpn Soc Intern Med 1985;74:1615 [in Japanese].
30. Lio S, Albin M, GirellinG, et al. Abnormal thyroid function test results in patients with Fisher-Evans syndrome. J Endocrinol Invest 1993;16:163–7.
31. Yashiro M, Nagoshi H, Kasuga Y, et al. Evans' syndrome associated with Graves' disease. Intern Med 1996;35:987–90.
32. Ikeda K, Maruyama Y, Yokoyama M, et al. Association of Graves' disease with Evans' syndrome in a patient with IgA nephropathy. Intern Med 2001;40:1004–10.
33. Lee AC, Li CH, Wong LM. Childhood thrombocytopenia associated with Graves' disease is distinct from idiopathic thrombocytopenic purpura. Pediatr Hematol Oncol 2003;20:39–42.
34. Bizzaro N. Familial association of autoimmune thrombocytopenia and hyperthyroidism. Am J Hematol 1992;39:294–8.
35. Grumet FC, Payne RD, Konishi J, et al. HL-A antigens as markers for disease susceptibility and autoimmunity in Graves' disease. J Clin Endocrinol Metab 1976;39:1115–9.
36. Sugimoto K, Sasaki M, Isobe Y, et al. Improvement of idiopathic thrombocytopenic purpura by antithyroid therapy. Eur J Haematol 2005;74:73–4.
37. Cheung EC, Naik R, Keng M, et al. Thyroid disorder-related immune thrombocytopenia: clinical and laboratory characteristics [abstract]. Blood 2008;112:4561.
38. Resnitzky P, Schonfeld S, et al. Effect of Graves' disease on idiopathic thrombocytopenic purpura. Arch Intern Med 1979;139:483–4.
39. Liechty RD. The thyrotoxicosis/thrombocytopenia connection. Surgery 1983;94: 966–8.
40. Panzer S, Haubenstock A, Minar E. Platelets in hyperthyroidism: studies on platelet counts, mean platelet volume, 111-indium-labeled platelet kinetics, and platelet-associated immunoglobulins G and M. J Clin Endocrinol Metab 1990; 70:491–6.
41. Stiegler G, Stohlawetz P, et al. Elevated numbers of reticulated platelets in hyperthyroidism: direct evidence for an increase of thrombopoiesis. Br J Haematol 1998;101:656–8.
42. Kurata Y, Nishioeda Y, Tsubakio T, et al. Thrombocytopenia in Graves' disease: effect of T3 on platelet kinetics. Acta Haematol 1980;63:185–90.
43. Cordiano I, Betterle C, Spadaccino CA, et al. Autoimmune thrombocytopenia (AITP) and thyroid autoimmune disease (TAD): overlapping syndromes? Clin Exp Immunol 1998;113:373–8.
44. Altintas A, Pasa S, Cil T, et al. Thyroid and celiac diseases autoantibodies in patients with adult chronic idiopathic thrombocytopenic purpura. Platelets 2008;19(4):252–7.
45. Pratt EL, Tarantino MD, Wagner D, et al. Prevalence of elevated anti-thyroid antibodies and antinuclear antibodies in children with immune thrombocytopenic purpura. Am J Hematol 2005;79:175–9.
46. Goebel KM, Hahn E, Havemann K. HLA matching in autoimmune thrombocytopenic purpura. Br J Haematol 1977;35:341–2.
47. Konishi J, Grumet FC, Payne RO, et al. HLA antigens in Japanese patients with Graves' disease and Hashimoto's disease. Diabete Metab 1976;2:163–4.

48. Gaiger A, Neumeister A, Heinz H, et al. HLA class I and II antigens in chronic idiopathic autoimmune thrombocytopenia. Ann Hematol 1994;68:299–302.

49. George JN, Woolf SH, Raskob GE, et al. Idiopathic thrombocytopenic purpura: a practice guideline developed by explicit methods for the American Society of Hematology. Blood 1996;88:3–40.

50. British Committee for Standards in Haematology, General Haematology Task Force. Guidelines for the investigation and management of idiopathic thrombocytopenic purpura in adults, children and in pregnancy. Br J Haematol 2003;120: 574–96.

Immune Thrombocytopenia in Lymphoproliferative Disorders

Carlo Visco, MD, Francesco Rodeghiero, MD*

KEYWORDS

- Immune thrombocytopenia • Chronic lymphocytic leukemia
- Hodgkin lymphoma • Non-Hodgkin lymphoma
- Lymphoproliferative disorders • ITP

Immune thrombocytopenia (ITP) includes different entities characterized by increased destruction or diminished production of platelets mediated by antibodies against platelet or megakaryocyte membrane antigens. According to the current nomenclature, ITP is defined as secondary (secondary ITP) when there is evidence of an underlying disease as opposed to primary (primary ITP) when no associated disorder can be demonstrated at the time of diagnosis.[1]

Lymphoproliferative disorders (LPDs) are recognized as a common cause of secondary ITP. Approximately 30% of secondary ITP cases are present on diagnosis of lymphoid tumors or develop during the course of the disease.[2,3] Among the different LPDs, ITP has the highest prevalence in chronic lymphocytic leukemia (CLL),[4] ranging between 2% and 5%.[5–8] It is far less frequent in non-Hodgkin lymphoma and Hodgkin lymphoma (HL), where its prevalence is invariably reported to be below 2%.[4,9–14]

Because of its rarity, the clinical behavior and response to treatment of secondary ITP in LPDs has been poorly investigated. A correlation between the survival of patients with LPDs and the occurrence of autoimmune phenomena directed against hematopoietic cells has been observed[4] but not confirmed.[12] Diagnosis of ITP associated with LPDs may be difficult at times, given that many confounding events are known to variably reduce the platelet count in addition to diffuse bone marrow infiltration by malignant lymphocytes. Moreover, reversible thrombocytopenia may be induced by the toxic effects of chemotherapy. The lack of sufficient sensitivity and specificity of platelet autoantibody tests (which parallel the direct Coomb test for

---

This work was supported in part by grants from the Associazione Vicentina per le Leucemie, i Linfomi e il Mieloma/Associazione Italiana Leucemie (Vicenza, Italy); Fondazione Progetto Ematologia (Vicenza, Italy); and Regione Veneto, Italy, through the Ricerca Sanitaria Finalizzata 2006 program.

Division of Hematology, Department of Cell Therapy and Hematology, San Bortolo Hospital, Via Rodolfi 37, Vicenza 36100, Italy
* Corresponding author.
E-mail address: rodeghiero@hemato.ven.it (F. Rodeghiero).

Hematol Oncol Clin N Am 23 (2009) 1261–1274
doi:10.1016/j.hoc.2009.08.006
0889-8588/09/$ – see front matter © 2009 Elsevier Inc. All rights reserved.

hemonc.theclinics.com

red blood cells in hemolytic anemias)[15,16] certainly hampers the interpretation of some acute thrombocytopenias. Reliable and standardized clinical criteria are needed to distinguish ITP from other immune and nonimmune causes of thrombocytopenia.

In contrast to primary ITP, patients with secondary ITP and LPDs are usually older and have lower initial platelet levels because of concomitant cytotoxic treatments. The specific therapy for ITP may negatively interfere with the chemotherapy program or aggravate the already present immunosuppression. A correct diagnosis and an adequate therapeutic approach may prevent life-threatening bleeding, avoid undue toxicity, and be life-saving.

The pathogenesis of secondary ITP is usually mediated by IgG autoantibodies that coat platelets, inducing their accelerated clearance by the spleen and the liver, or impair megakaryocyte platelet production, as in primary ITP. Although platelet-reactive antibodies may be responsible for platelet destruction in the course of LPDs, several other mechanisms have been described that may interfere with platelet production. Direct inhibition of megakaryocytopoiesis by cytotoxic T cells or by inhibitory cytokines and complement-mediated platelet destruction by IgM may explain the platelet decrease seen in different T- and B-cell neoplastic diseases. Dysregulation of the microenvironment induced by soluble factors secreted by malignant cells and the consequent T-cell dysfunction have been shown to be crucial for the emergence of autoreactive clones.[7,17] Furthermore, drugs commonly used in the treatment of LPDs (eg, fludarabine) have also been associated with an increased risk of developing ITP because of their different cytotoxic effects on T- and B-cell differentiation and survival.

ITP ASSOCIATED WITH CLL
Epidemiology and Diagnostic Criteria

Approximately one fourth of patients with CLL experience an autoimmune complication,[17] primarily autoimmune hemolytic anemia (AHA) or ITP. By pooling heterogeneous data from different series, it has been estimated that ITP complicates the course of CLL in about 2% of patients.[7,17] Recently, a higher prevalence of ITP (5%) was reported in a series of 1278 patients newly diagnosed with CLL consecutively referred to three major hematology institutions in Italy.[8] This estimate was based on standardized clinical criteria to exclude other causes of thrombocytopenia. Briefly, the diagnosis of ITP required all of the following criteria: rapid (<2 weeks) and severe fall (at least half of the initial level and below 100×10^9/L) of the platelet count; a normal or augmented number of megakaryocytes in the bone marrow; an absence of splenomegaly on physical examination; and no cytotoxic treatments in the last month. A lack of response to platelet transfusion (in patients without known refractoriness to platelet concentrates) or a rapid response (<1 week) to high-dose intravenous Ig (IVIg) were considered essential requirements for the diagnosis of ITP in patients with advanced Rai or Binet stage (3–4 or C) and extensive bone marrow involvement.

Biology

CLL is a mature B-cell neoplasm coexpressing the T-cell antigen CD5 and B-cell surface antigens CD19, CD20, and CD23. The biology of the disease is complex, and the cell from which CLL is derived has not been determined. The leukemia cells express immunoglobulins that may or may not have incurred somatic mutations in the immunoglobulin heavy chain variable region genes (IgVh), suggesting that CLL is more heterogeneous than previously suspected.[18]

CLL is typically characterized by profound immunosuppression, with T-cell function impairment and insufficient antibody production already manifest in the early phases of the disease. As a consequence, patients experience frequent infections, autoimmune cytopenias, and a relatively high rate of second tumors. T-cell functional defects may be caused by pathologic inhibitory cytokines (interleukin-10 and transforming growth factor-β) or by inappropriate interactions of normal T and B lymphocytes with CLL B cells. The altered function of the immune surveillance system and of regulatory T cells (T-reg) facilitates the emergence of B-cell clones producing autoantibodies. The inhibitory signals that the CLL B cells deliver to T-reg cells seem to prevent the elimination of nonneoplastic autoreactive T and B cells. Hence, the autoreactive antibodies are polyclonal and not secreted by the malignant clone.

Cytotoxic treatment may further complicate the homeostasis of the immune system. Fludarabine has been associated with the occurrence of ITP in the course of CLL and other chronic diseases, but cladribine and pentostatin have also been described to be associated with autoimmunity,[17,19] possibly caused by the profound T-cell suppression, toxic effects on T-reg cells, and altered CD4/CD8 ratio induced by these drugs. The same mechanism has been implicated in Campath-related ITP.[20]

IgVh DNA sequence analysis of CLL B cells has revealed a significantly higher risk for patients with unmutated cells to develop ITP.[21] Unlike their mutated counterparts, whose B-cell receptor is quiescent and unable to transmit external signals to the cell nucleus, unmutated CLL B cells usually remain responsive to external stimuli and are capable of binding multiple antigens, including autoantigens, which promote their survival and proliferation. Unmutated CLL B cells have an increased ability to phosphorylate p72 (Syk) and Zap-70 molecules in response to sIgM ligation by an antigen, providing evidence for an intact downstream signaling pathway of their B-cell receptor.[22] The more aggressive clinical behavior of unmutated CLL B cells might be related to frequent (auto) antigenic interactions with their B-cell receptor. The preferential occurrence of ITP and AHA and isolated positive direct antiglobulin tests in unmutated patients[23] suggests that unmutated cells also favor the emergence of autoimmune diseases.[24]

A bias toward the Vh1 gene family has recently been observed in patients with ITP and CLL (43%) compared with patients without ITP (21%; $P = .01$).[8] More interestingly, the Vh4 family, usually found in approximately 20% of CLL cases irrespective of mutational state,[25,26] was found in 22% of patients without ITP, as expected, but in only 4% of patients with ITP ($P = .02$).[21] The finding of a preferential Vh-gene distribution leads to the speculation of a possible antigen-driven process in ITP pathogenesis in these patients.

Clinical Impact

ITP seems to be equally distributed among the different CLL stages, with a median age of 68 years and a male predominance.[27] Unlike AHA, the occurrence of ITP seems not to be temporally related to tumor progression or recurrence, with most patients developing ITP after a median time of less than 2 years from diagnosis, whereas CLL is stable and patients have not initiated therapy.[5,8,11] Among patients with ITP associated with CLL, 8% have been reported to have experienced World Health Organization grade 4 bleeding episodes, and most of them died of this complication.[8] Bleeding complications, however, have not been systematically assessed thus far.

Both Rai and Binet staging classifications recognize a platelet count less than 100 × 10^9/L at CLL diagnosis as a very unfavorable prognostic factor, regardless of the etiology of the thrombocytopenia. Based on survival results from a few small series, the impact of ITP on overall CLL prognosis has been questioned,[6,28,29] supporting the idea that thrombocytopenia is an adverse prognostic marker only when reflecting extension of the disease.

In contrast, the occurrence of ITP itself was a strong negative prognostic factor for patients with CLL in a series of 1278 newly diagnosed patients with CLL. As shown in **Fig. 1**, patients with thrombocytopenia on CLL diagnosis did poorly regardless of the etiology of the low platelet count. Contrary to common belief, their prognosis was similar to patients with a low platelet count caused by tumor infiltration according to Rai and Binet classifications (**Fig. 2**). Multivariate analysis also indicated that the occurrence of ITP within 24 months of CLL diagnosis and its refractoriness to treatment had a further independent negative impact on overall survival.[8]

Treatment

Little is known about the treatment of ITP in the course of CLL. Some studies have reported that ITP of CLL can be successfully treated with steroids,[30] cyclosporin A,[31] or splenectomy,[28] with a variable duration of response. Furthermore, long-term responses have been described after treatment with cytotoxic agents[32,33] or anti-CD 20 monoclonal antibodies (rituximab).[34–36]

According to the authors' experience, when these patients are treated with conventional therapies used for primary ITP, a far less favorable response rate is observed.[8,37] In their patients a response to steroids occurred in 52% of patients, which is in the lower range of response rates to steroids reported for ITP (50%–75%). Furthermore, although approximately 80% of ITP patients usually respond to IVIg, only half of patients with ITP and CLL responded to IVIg alone. Splenectomy seemed effective, however, with 70% of patients experiencing a long-term response. A total of 14 (22%) patients were refractory to all administered treatments. This number is greater than what has been reported for adult ITP cohorts (9%).[38] Most patients require treatments directly targeted to the tumor.

Rituximab, which is known to be active in both CLL and ITP, needs to be further investigated in ITP associated with CLL, particularly in light of some promising preliminary results.[34,35] Rituximab therapy has also been reported to be effective in fludarabine-associated ITP, which is often refractory to conventional treatments and may be

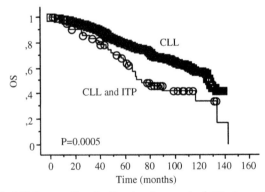

Fig. 1. Overall survival (OS) according to the development of ITP at any time. Survival curve of 64 patients with ITP and CLL compared with 1214 patients with CLL who did not develop ITP. (*From* Visco C, Ruggeri M, Evangelista ML, et al. Impact of immune thrombocytopenia on the clinical course of chronic lymphocytic leukemia. Blood 2008;111:1110–6; The American Society of Hematology; with permission.) Copyright © 2008 the American Society of Hematology.

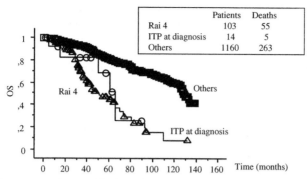

	Patients	Deaths
Rai 4	103	55
ITP at diagnosis	14	5
Others	1160	263

Fig. 2. Survival curves: patients with thrombocytopenia caused by tumor infiltration (*Rai* 4) or immune-mediated causes (*ITP*) at the time of CLL diagnosis are compared with other CLL patients (*Others*). Log-Rank test results were: P = .03 between Others and ITP, P = .47 between Rai 4 and ITP, and P<.0001 between Others and Rai 4. (*From* Visco C, Ruggeri M, Evangelista ML, et al. Impact of immune thrombocytopenia on the clinical course of chronic lymphocytic leukemia. Blood 2008;111:1110–6; The American Society of Hematology; with permission.) Copyright © 2008 the American Society of Hematology.

a life-threatening complication.[34,39] The most effective schedule is not clearly defined, and a lower dosage of 100 mg weekly for 4 weeks (compared with 375 mg/m^2 or higher), which has shown promising results in primary ITP,[40] deserves testing in patients with CLL and ITP. Rituximab may further deepen the immunosuppressed state, however, and favor potentially life-threatening infections.[41]

ITP ASSOCIATED WITH NON-HODGKIN'S LYMPHOMAS
Waldenström Macroglobulinemia

Some monoclonal proteins from patients with Waldenström macroglobulinemia (WM) possess antigen-binding activity for autologous or foreign antigens. Autoimmune phenomena, such as cold agglutinin hemolytic anemia, mixed cryoglobulinemia, and peripheral neuropathy, are well-recognized complications of WM. In a prospective cohort of patients with WM who were extensively investigated for the presence of autoimmune phenomena, about half of the serologic and clinical manifestations of autoimmunity were present at diagnosis, whereas others appeared during the course of the disease.[42] The prevalence of ITP in WM ranges between 3% and 9%,[42,43] and a platelet-associated monoclonal IgM has been shown to be related to the occurrence of ITP.[43–45] The size of the M-component was not correlated with ITP prevalence.[42]

Complement-mediated thrombocytopenia may appear in association with monoclonal IgM antiplatelet antibodies.[46] Together with antineoplastic drugs, plasmapheresis can be of value for temporarily treating selected patients with ITP and monoclonal gammopathy,[47] whereas splenectomy does not seem to be a good option.[46] Conventional treatments used for primary ITP do not seem to induce lasting remission of ITP secondary to WM.

Monoclonal Gammopathy of Undetermined Significance and Multiple Myeloma

Immune thrombocytopenia has only rarely been documented in patients with multiple myeloma.[48–50] A recent series reported a prevalence of 2.6% for secondary ITP in 228 patients with monoclonal gammopathy of undetermined significance. The monoclonal component was mostly of the IgG (71%) or IgM type (18%).[51] Patients with monoclonal gammopathy of undetermined significance–associated ITP were older than those with monoclonal gammopathy of undetermined significance without ITP, and no correlation was found between platelet response and variations in the M-component after B-cell clone directed therapies. Rituximab was tried in a single patient and was ineffective,[52] whereas others reported short-lived responses to IVIg or steroids.[49]

A shortened platelet half-life has been shown in patients with multiple myeloma,[53] although no correlation has been found between platelet survival and paraprotein concentration. An intravascular process of platelet activation and consumption has been postulated, either as a result of platelet defects related to the presence of the paraproteinemia or as a consequence of the high platelet autoantibody levels that increase the susceptibility of platelets to degradation. Elevated platelet-associated immunoglobulin has been reported in patients with myeloma and is believed to be secondary to nonspecific binding of serum IgG to platelets, usually not resulting in clinically significant thrombocytopenia.[54]

Marginal Zone Lymphoma

Secondary ITP has been reported quite frequently (in up to 5% of cases) in patients with marginal zone lymphoma (MZL) of the mucosa-associated lymphoid tissue or of the splenic type. A higher prevalence than other LPDs has also been reported for AHA and acquired coagulation disorders. These immune complications are typically found in patients without leukemic spread of the tumor or even preceding the diagnosis of lymphoma and seem to be associated with a higher risk of disease progression.[55–58] In most cases, the platelet count improved with antilymphoma therapy.[59,60] Refractoriness to steroids has frequently been reported.[57,58] Regression of ITP after mucosal resection of the lymphomatous lesion of the mucosa-associated lymphoid tissue type has been described.[61,62] The presence of monoclonal gammopathy of the IgM type, which is often encountered in this lymphoma subtype, might explain the more frequent finding of ITP in these patients.[63]

Other B-cell Lymphomas

Follicular lymphoma and diffuse large B-cell lymphoma, which represent the most frequent forms of non-Hodgkin lymphoma, have rarely been associated with secondary ITP.[4] Of note, an association with ITP has been occasionally described in aggressive lymphomas involving atypical extranodal organs (eg, kidney, heart, bladder, and mesentery).[64–66] Improvement of the platelet count was not always accomplished with chemotherapy. Most of the ITP cases occurring in patients with diffuse large B-cell lymphoma and follicular lymphoma have been described after patients received an autologous transplant. The prevalence of ITP in this setting seems to be lower than 2%.[67] Delayed immune reconstitution of T-regs and clonal expansion of CD8[+] T cells may contribute to the development of ITP in this setting, without an association with the underlying disease or the type of conditioning regimen.[68] Resolution of ITP is usually obtained by typical treatment, such as steroids or splenectomy, but ITP sometimes progressively resolves without specific treatment, possibly following immune reconstitution. Few cases have been reported of ITP associated with hairy cell leukemia,[69,70] sometimes triggered by treatment with purine analogs. The pathogenesis of thrombocytopenia in these patients is difficult to interpret because relevant splenomegaly is one of the presenting features. As already reported for other forms of low-grade lymphoma, refractoriness to steroids is frequent. In mantle cell lymphoma, the occurrence of ITP seems extremely rare.[9,71] Curiously, hairy cell leukemia and mantle cell lymphoma are the lymphoma subtypes most frequently associated with the occurrence of rituximab-related ITP, particularly when there is coexisting extensive bone marrow involvement or splenomegaly.[72–76]

The mechanisms responsible for this form of thrombocytopenia have not yet been defined. Opsonization of platelets by soluble CD20 and a cytokine release syndrome seem the most convincing pathogenic hypotheses, whereas autoimmunity can be ruled out by the timing of the phenomenon. The platelet decrease usually spontaneously recovers within a few days but may be accompanied by a significant hemorrhagic syndrome.[75,77]

T-cell LPDs

ITP is an extremely rare complication of peripheral T-cell lymphoma,[12] although some T-cell lymphoma subtypes have been frequently associated with autoimmune phenomena directed against hematopoietic cells. Both angioimmunoblastic T-cell lymphoma and hepatosplenic T-cell lymphoma may present with ITP, often associated with AHA,[78–82] and should be treated upfront with aggressive chemotherapy protocols because of their dismal prognosis. The underlying state of immunodeficiency that characterizes these aggressive diseases and predisposes these patients to severe infections may be relevant for the pathogenesis of autoimmune phenomena.

Autoimmune neutropenia and immune-mediated anemia are common findings in large granular T-lymphocyte leukemia (T-LGL), which is characterized by clonal expansion of mature $CD8^+$ T lymphocytes. Although severe thrombocytopenia has rarely been described in this condition,[83] mild thrombocytopenia is common.[84] Unlike other LPDs, the formation of autoantibodies is not implicated in peripheral platelet destruction in T-LGL because thrombocytopenia in these patients seems to derive from the suppression of megakaryopoiesis by LGL-mediated cytotoxicity. A defective Fas (CD95) apoptotic pathway has been related to the occurrence of autoimmunity in T-LGL, similar to what has been described for the autoimmune lymphoproliferative syndrome, an inherited disorder manifesting in childhood with autoimmune cytopenia, lymphadenopathy, and splenomegaly and characterized by the accumulation of double-negative ($CD3^+$, $CD4^-$, $CD8^-$) T cells. In both diseases leukemic lymphocytes constitutively express Fas and Fas-ligand but are resistant to Fas-induced apoptosis.[85] In addition, the accumulation of defective T cells interferes with immune tolerance. Treatment directed against the T-cell clone has been shown to resolve most immune complications. Methotrexate, cyclophosphamide, and cyclosporin A are the drugs most frequently adopted in this setting.[86]

ITP ASSOCIATED WITH HL

The prevalence of ITP in HL is around 0.5%. Nevertheless, many case reports have been described in the literature. In most cases, ITP occurred while lymphoma was in remission, after induction therapy had been completed, independent of the lymphoma activity.[11,13,87–91] The median time from the diagnosis of HL to the development of ITP is about 2 years,[13,87,88] although in rare instances ITP has been described at lymphoma presentation.[92–94] The response to specific conventional treatments for ITP is usually good, and the development of ITP does not seem to modify the prognosis of the underlying disease.[13,14,88] Although HL could be a predisposing condition, the characteristics, timing, and response to therapy of ITP associated with HL suggest that the underlying disease may have a minor influence on the development and course of the thrombocytopenia.

DISCUSSION

In the absence of an underlying disorder, most cases of acute-onset thrombocytopenia are grouped under the definition of primary ITP.[1] The wide variability in response to specific therapies and in the natural history of this disease suggests that primary ITP may not be a single entity and that certain cases may be triggered by underlying conditions that are not apparent, restricting the field of the pure idiopathic forms.[95] Among secondary forms, ITP associated with LPDs is of particular relevance for its clinical impact and less favorable response to conventional treatments.

The true prevalence of ITP in the course of LPDs is unknown because of the lack of standardized diagnostic criteria and the insufficient diagnostic power of platelet antibody testing. The increase in bone marrow megakaryocytes, rapidity of the platelet fall, and absence of a previous recent cytotoxic treatment remain the most reliable diagnostic criteria.[8,17] The recent demonstration of clonal $CD5^+/CD19^+$ B-cell populations in the bone marrow of 16% of patients with primary ITP by flow cytometry[96] is consistent with the hypothesis that some idiopathic cases might indeed be secondary to not yet clinically manifest LPDs. CLL is most frequently associated with ITP (2%–5% of cases). Unlike AHA, which has a very close relationship with CLL activity, ITP has a weak correlation with tumor activity.[5,8,11,27] Although some small series did not describe an adverse effect of ITP on the survival of patients with CLL,[6,28,29] a recent survey found ITP to be a strong adverse prognostic factor.[8] Patients with ITP at CLL diagnosis did poorly, and their prognosis was similar to patients with a low platelet count because of tumor infiltration (Rai 4, Binet C; see **Fig. 2**). The impaired survival of CLL patients with ITP might be caused by the strong association between ITP development and unmutated IgVh status (81% in the authors' series),[8] which is widely known to discriminate tumors with aggressive behavior. Furthermore, immunosuppressive treatments purposely administered to treat ITP may increase morbidity and mortality because of infection.[97]

The fact that ITP in the course of LPDs has different clinical characteristics and behavior than primary ITP is not surprising because it probably reflects the presence of different pathogenic mechanisms. Altered function of T-regs seems relevant in most of the cases of ITP arising in CLL, allowing the emergence of normal B-cell clones producing autoreactive antibodies against platelet antigens. Increasing evidence suggests that T-reg compartmentalization and trafficking may be modulated by chemokines and integrins secreted by the tumor.[98] In WM and at least some MZL, the tumor produces monoclonal IgM with antiplatelet activity, which induces complement-mediated platelet destruction, an exceptional occurrence in primary ITP. T-LGL instead represents a paradigm for T-cell–mediated direct toxicity to platelets and megakaryocytes in the bone marrow.

Conventional treatments for ITP, such as those based on steroids, IVIg, and in select cases splenectomy, should be attempted first to rapidly control the thrombocytopenia. To produce lasting results or in case of failure of conventional treatments, however, which occurs in around 50% of cases, treatment directed against the malignant clone may be ultimately required. **Table 1** summarizes the different therapeutic approaches and their correlation with the pathogenic background when ITP is associated with different LPDs.

Whatever the precise pathogenic mechanism causing ITP, whether mediated by autoreactive macroglobulins (WM, MZL) or by the cytotoxic effect of T cells (T-LGL) or when the malignant clone itself actively participates in the emergence of ITP (CLL), the most effective chemotherapy or immunotherapy against the tumor should be chosen. The second-generation thrombopoietin receptor agonists (romiplostim and eltrombopag) recently introduced for treatment of primary ITP, however, yield very good results in increasing platelet count in over 80% of patients, and despite failure of several previous treatments, including splenectomy, raise new hopes. Indeed, irrespective of the precise pathogenesis, autoimmune antibodies negatively interfering

Table 1
Biologic background, treatment options, and prognostic implications for ITP associated with LPDs

	Origin of Autoantibodies	Correlation to LPDs Presentation/ Activity/Tumor Burden	Effect of ITP Treatment	Effect of LPD Treatment	Prognostic Significance
CLL	Normal B cells	No	Weak	Good	Yes
WM/MGUS	Malignant B cells	No	No	Good/weak	Unknown
MZL	Both malignant and normal B cells	Not apparent	Weak	Good	Yes
T-LGL	Normal B cells	Yes	No	Good	Unknown
HL	Normal B cells	No	Good	Unknown	No
Other LPDs (DLBCL, FL, MCL, HCL)	Normal B cells	Yes	Unknown	Weak, may trigger ITP	Unknown

Abbreviations: CLL, chronic lymphocytic leukemia; DLBCL, diffuse large B-cell lymphoma; FL, follicular lymphoma; HCL, hairy cell leukemia; HL, Hodgkin lymphoma; LPD, lymphoproliferative disorder; MCL, mantle cell lymphoma; MGUS, monoclonal gammopathy of undetermined significance; MZL, marginal zone lymphoma; T-LGL, T-lymphocyte leukemia; WM, Waldenström macroglobulinemia.

with megakaryocyte platelet production are expected in most cases of ITP secondary to LPDs, not unlike what occurs in primary ITP. Ad hoc–designed prospective investigations are required to show the effectiveness of the agents for treatment of ITP associated with LPDs.

A more detailed understanding of the pathogenic mechanisms underlying the occurrence of ITP in different LPDs will drive targeted treatment decisions, avoiding unwarranted immunosuppression and bleeding complications.

REFERENCES

1. Rodeghiero F, Stasi R, Gernsheimer T, et al. Standardization of terminology, definitions and outcome criteria in immune thrombocytopenic purpura of adults and children: report from an international working group. Blood 2009;113(11): 2386–93.
2. Hegde UM, Zuiable A, Ball S, et al. The relative incidence of idiopathic and secondary autoimmune thrombocytopenia: a clinical and serological evaluation in 508 patients. Clin Lab Haematol 1985;7(1):7–16.
3. Liebman H. Other immune thrombocytopenias. Semin Hematol 2007;44(4 Suppl 5):S24–34.
4. Dührsen U, Augener W, Zwingers T, et al. Spectrum and frequency of autoimmune derangements in lymphoproliferative disorders: analysis of 637 cases and comparison with myeloproliferative diseases. Br J Haematol 1987;67(2): 235–9.
5. Hamblin TJ, Oscier DG, Young BJ. Autoimmunity in chronic lymphocytic leukaemia. J Clin Pathol 1986;39(7):713–6.

6. Kyasa MJ, Parrish RS, Schichman SA, et al. Autoimmune cytopenia does not predict poor prognosis in chronic lymphocytic leukemia/small lymphocytic lymphoma. Am J Hematol 2003;74(1):1–8.

7. Diehl LF, Ketchum LH. Autoimmune disease and chronic lymphocytic leukemia: autoimmune hemolytic anemia, pure red cell aplasia, and autoimmune thrombocytopenia. Semin Oncol 1998;25(1):80–97.

8. Visco C, Ruggeri M, Laura Evangelista M, et al. Impact of immune thrombocytopenia on the clinical course of chronic lymphocytic leukemia. Blood. 2008;111(3): 1110–6.

9. Hauswirth AW, Skrabs C, Schützinger C, et al. Autoimmune thrombocytopenia in non-Hodgkin's lymphomas. Haematologica 2008;93(3):447–50.

10. Váróczy L, Gergely L, Zeher M, et al. Malignant lymphoma-associated autoimmune diseases: a descriptive epidemiological study. Rheumatol Int 2002;22(6):233–7.

11. Jones SE. Autoimmune disorders and malignant lymphoma. Cancer 1973;31(5): 1092–8.

12. Grønbaek K, D'Amore F, Schmidt K. Autoimmune phenomena in non-Hodgkin's lymphoma. Leuk Lymphoma 1995;18(3–4):311–6.

13. Bradley SJ, Hudson GV, Linch DC. Idiopathic thrombocytopenic purpura in Hodgkin's disease: a report of eight cases. Clin Oncol (R Coll Radiol) 1993;5(6):355–7.

14. Xiros N, Binder T, Anger B, et al. Idiopathic thrombocytopenic purpura and autoimmune hemolytic anemia in Hodgkin's disease. Eur J Haematol 1988;40(5): 437–41.

15. Kelton JG, Murphy WG, Lucarelli A, et al. A prospective comparison of four techniques for measuring platelet-associated IgG. Br J Haematol 1989;71(1):97–105.

16. Warner MN, Moore JC, Warkentin TE, et al. A prospective study of protein-specific assays used to investigate idiopathic thrombocytopenic purpura. Br J Haematol 1999;104(3):442–7.

17. Hamblin TJ. Autoimmune complications of chronic lymphocytic leukemia. Semin Oncol 2006;33(2):230–9.

18. Hallek M, Cheson BD, Catovsky D, et al. Guidelines for the diagnosis and treatment of chronic lymphocytic leukemia: a report from the International Workshop on Chronic Lymphocytic Leukemia updating the National Cancer Institute-Working Group 1996 guidelines. Blood 2008;111(12):5446–56.

19. Leach M, Parsons RM, Reilly JT, et al. Autoimmune thrombocytopenia: a complication of fludarabine therapy in lymphoproliferative disorders. Clin Lab Haematol 2000;22(3):175–8.

20. Otton SH, Turner DL, Frewin R, et al. Autoimmune thrombocytopenia after treatment with Campath 1H in a patient with chronic lymphocytic leukaemia. Br J Haematol 1999;106(1):261–2.

21. Visco C, Giaretta I, Ruggeri M, et al. Un-mutated IgVH in chronic lymphocytic leukemia is associated with a higher risk of immune thrombocytopenia. Leukemia 2007;21(5):1092–3.

22. Mockridge CI, Potter KN, Wheatley I, et al. Reversible anergy of sIgM-mediated signaling in the two subsets of CLL defined by VH-gene mutational status. Blood 2007;109(10):4424–31.

23. Visco C, Giaretta I, Ruggeri M, et al. Rai and Binet classifications for chronic lymphocytic leukemia should recognize a role for immune thrombocytopenia, but not for autoimmune haemolytic anemia. Haematologica 2008;93(s1):36.

24. Hervé M, Xu K, Ng YS, et al. Unmutated and mutated chronic lymphocytic leukemias derive from self-reactive B cell precursors despite expressing different antibody reactivity. J Clin Invest 2005;115(6):1636–43.

25. Tobin G, Thunberg U, Karlsson K, et al. Subsets with restricted immunoglobulin gene rearrangement features indicate a role for antigen selection in the development of chronic lymphocytic leukemia. Blood 2004;104(9):2879–85.
26. Messmer BT, Albesiano E, Efremov DG, et al. Multiple distinct sets of stereotyped antigen receptors indicate a role for antigen in promoting chronic lymphocytic leukemia. J Exp Med 2004;200(4):519–25.
27. Barcellini W, Capalbo S, Agostinelli RM, et al. GIMEMA Chronic Lymphocytic Leukemia Group. Relationship between autoimmune phenomena and disease stage and therapy in B-cell chronic lymphocytic leukemia. Haematologica 2006;91(12):1689–92.
28. Rubinstein DB, Longo DL. Peripheral destruction of platelets in chronic lymphocytic leukemia: recognition, prognosis and therapeutic implications. Am J Med 1981; 71(4):729–732.
29. Kaden BR, Rosse WF, Hauch TW. Immune thrombocytopenia in lymphoproliferative diseases. Blood 1979;53(4):545–51.
30. Ebbe S, Wittels B, Dameshek W. Autoimmune thrombocytopenic purpura (ITP type) with chronic lymphocytic leukemia. Blood 1962;19:23–37.
31. Cortes J, O'Brien S, Loscertales J, et al. Cyclosporin A for the treatment of cytopenia associated with chronic lymphocytic leukemia. Cancer 2001;92(8):2016–22.
32. Carey RW, McGinnis A, Jacobson BM, et al. Idiopathic thrombocytopenic purpura complicating chronic lymphocytic leukemia. Arch Intern Med 1976; 136(1):62–6.
33. Aghai E, Quitt M, Lurie M, et al. Primary hepatic lymphoma presenting as symptomatic immune thrombocytopenic purpura. Cancer 1987;60(9):2308–11.
34. Hegde UP, Wilson WH, White T, et al. Rituximab treatment of refractory fludarabine-associated immune thrombocytopenia in chronic lymphocytic leukemia. Blood 2002;100(6):2260–2.
35. Zaja F, Vianelli N, Sperotto A, et al. Anti-CD20 therapy for chronic lymphocytic leukemia-associated autoimmune diseases. Leuk Lymphoma 2003;44(11): 1951–5.
36. Ammatuna E, Marino C, Mitra ME, et al. Successful treatment of steroid resistant autoimmune thrombocytopenia associated with chronic lymphocytic leukemia with alemtuzumab. Eur J Haematol 2004;73(3):225–6.
37. Cines DB, Blanchette VS. Immune thrombocytopenic purpura. N Engl J Med 2002;346(13):995–1008.
38. Portielje JE, Westendorp RG, Kluin-Nelemans HC, et al. Morbidity and mortality in adults with idiopathic thrombocytopenic purpura. Blood 2001;97(9):2549–54.
39. Fernandez MJ, Llopis I, Pastor E, et al. Immune thrombocytopenia induced by fludarabine successfully treated with rituximab. Haematologica 2003;88(2): ELT02.
40. Provan D, Butler T, Evangelista ML, et al. Activity and safety profile of low-dose rituximab for the treatment of autoimmune cytopenias in adults. Haematologica 2007;92(12):1695–8.
41. Carson KR, Evens AM, Richey EA, et al. Progressive multifocal leukoencephalopathy after rituximab therapy in HIV-negative patients: a report of 57 cases from the Research on Adverse Drug Events and Reports project. Blood 2009; 113(20):4834–40.
42. Jönsson V, Kierkegaard A, Salling S, et al. Autoimmunity in Waldenström's macroglobulinaemia. Leuk Lymphoma 1999;34(3–4):373–9.
43. Owen RG, Lubenko A, Savage J, et al. Autoimmune thrombocytopenia in Waldenström's macroglobulinemia. Am J Hematol 2001;66(2):116–9.

44. Stone MJ, Merlini G, Pascual V. Autoantibody activity in Waldenstrom's macroglobulinemia. Clin Lymphoma 2005;5(4):225–9.
45. Varticovski L, Pick AI, Schattner A, et al. Anti-platelet and anti-DNA IgM in Waldenström macroglobulinemia and ITP. Am J Hematol 1987;24(4):351–5.
46. Lehman HA, Lehman LO, Rustagi PK, et al. Complement-mediated autoimmune thrombocytopenia: monoclonal IgM antiplatelet antibody associated with lymphoreticular malignant disease. N Engl J Med 1987;316(4):194–8.
47. Patel TC, Moore SB, Pineda AA, et al. Role of plasmapheresis in thrombocytopenic purpura associated with Waldenström's macroglobulinemia. Mayo Clin Proc 1996;71(6):597–600.
48. Verdirame JD, Feagler JR, Commers JR. Multiple myeloma associated with immune thrombocytopenic purpura. Cancer 1985;56(5):1199–200.
49. Gupta V, Hegde UM, Parameswaran R, et al. Multiple myeloma and immune thrombocytopenia. Clin Lab Haematol 2000;22(4):239–42.
50. Falco P, Bertola A, Bringhen S, et al. Successful management of immune thrombocytopenic purpura with thalidomide in a patient with multiple myeloma. Hematol J 2004;5(5):456–7.
51. Rossi D, De Paoli L, Franceschetti S, et al. Prevalence and clinical characteristics of immune thrombocytopenic purpura in a cohort of monoclonal gammopathy of uncertain significance. Br J Haematol 2007;138(2):249–52.
52. Kuwana M, Iki S, Urabe A. The role of autoantibody-producing plasma cells in immune thrombocytopenic purpura refractory to rituximab. Am J Hematol 2007; 82(9):846–8.
53. Fritz E, Ludwig H, Scheithauer W, et al. Shortened platelet half-life in multiple myeloma. Blood 1986;68(2):514–20.
54. McGrath KM, Stuart JJ, Richards II F. Correlation between serum IgG, platelet membrane IgG, and platelet function in hypergammaglobulinaemic states. Br J Haematol 1979;42(4):585–91.
55. Thieblemont C, Felman P, Callet-Bauchu E, et al. Splenic marginal-zone lymphoma: a distinct clinical and pathological entity. Lancet Oncol 2003;4(2):95–103.
56. Magagnoli M, Balzarotti M, Castagna L, et al. Idiopathic thrombocytopenic purpura and splenic marginal-zone B-cell lymphoma: a casual correlation? Leuk Lymphoma 2003;44(9):1639–40.
57. Sakalli H, Akcali Z, Kayaselcuk F, et al. MALTOMA presenting with thrombocytopenia. Am J Clin Oncol 2005;28(3):321–2.
58. Bachmeyer C, Audouin J, Bouillot JL, et al. Immune thrombocytopenic purpura as the presenting feature of gastric MALT lymphoma. Am J Gastroenterol 2000; 95(6):1599–600.
59. Figueroa M, Gehlsen J, Hammond D, et al. Combination chemotherapy in refractory immune thrombocytopenic purpura. N Engl J Med 1993;328(17):1226–9.
60. Baudard M, Comte F, Conge AM, et al. Importance of [18F] fluorodeoxyglucose-positron emission tomography scanning for the monitoring of responses to immunotherapy in follicular lymphoma. Leuk Lymphoma 2007;48(2):381–8.
61. Kawashima T, Nishimura H, Akiyama H, et al. Primary pulmonary mucosa-associated lymphoid tissue lymphoma combined with idiopathic thrombocytopenic purpura and amyloidoma in the lung. J Nippon Med Sch 2005;72(6):370–4.
62. Noda M, Mori N, Nomura K, et al. Regression of idiopathic thrombocytopenic purpura after endoscopic mucosal resection of gastric mucosa associated lymphoid tissue lymphoma. Gut 2004;53(11):1698–700.
63. Murakami H, Irisawa H, Saitoh T, et al. Immunological abnormalities in splenic marginal zone cell lymphoma. Am J Hematol 1997;56(3):173–8.

64. Nakagawa H. A case of primary cardiac lymphoma complicated by idiopathic thrombocytopenic purpura. Nihon Kokyuki Gakkai Zasshi 2002;40(3):265–9 [in Japanese].

65. Tadokoro J, Gunji H, Handa T, et al. Primary renal non-Hodgkin's lymphoma presenting as immune thrombocytopenia. Rinsho Ketsueki 2001;42(1):41–6 [in Japanese].

66. Moriwaki Y, Naka M, Yamamoto T, et al. Malignant lymphoma in the mesentery with immune thrombocytopenia. Intern Med 1992;31(10):1185–9.

67. Hequet O, Salles G, Ketterer N, et al. Autoimmune thrombocytopenic purpura after autologous stem cell transplantation. Bone Marrow Transplant 2003;32(1):89–95.

68. Ashihara E, Shimazaki C, Hirata T, et al. Autoimmune thrombocytopenia following peripheral blood stem cell autografting. Bone Marrow Transplant 1993;12(3):297–9.

69. Hensel M, Ho AD. Successful treatment of a patient with hairy cell leukemia and pentostatin-induced autoimmune thrombocytopenia with rituximab. Am J Hematol 2003;73(1):37–40.

70. Virchis AE, Jan-Mohamed R, Kaczmarski KS, et al. Primary splenic hairy cell leukaemia variant presenting as immune thrombocytopenic purpura. Eur J Haematol 1998;61(4):288–91.

71. Kawachi Y, Ide M, Uchida T, et al. Idiopathic thrombocytopenic purpura associated with mantle cell lymphoma showing an increase in the platelet count receiving anti-CD20 antibody rituximab. Rinsho Ketsueki 2003;44(1):31–3 [in Japanese].

72. Otrock ZK, Mahfouz RA, Oghlakian GO, et al. Rituximab-induced acute thrombocytopenia: a report of two cases. Haematologica 2005;90(Suppl):ECR23.

73. Dhand S, Bahrain H. Rituximab-induced severe acute thrombocytopenia: a case report and review of literature. Cancer Invest 2008;26(9):913–5.

74. Ram R, Bonstein L, Gafter-Gvili A, et al. Rituximab-associated acute thrombocytopenia: an under-diagnosed phenomenon. Am J Hematol 2009;84(4):247–50.

75. Thachil J, Mukherje K, Woodcock B. Rituximab-induced haemorrhagic thrombocytopenia in a patient with hairy cell leukaemia. Br J Haematol 2006;135(2):273–4.

76. Shah C, Grethlein SJ. Case report of rituximab-induced thrombocytopenia. Am J Hematol 2004;75(4):263.

77. Rigamonti C, Volta C, Colombi S, et al. Severe thrombocytopenia and clinical bleeding associated with rituximab infusion in a lymphoma patient with massive splenomegaly without leukemic invasion. Leukemia 2001;15(1):186–7.

78. Motta G, Vianello F, Menin C, et al. Hepatosplenic gammadelta T-cell lymphoma presenting with immune-mediated thrombocytopenia and hemolytic anemia (Evans' syndrome). Am J Hematol 2002;69(4):272–6.

79. Yao M, Tien HF, Lin MT, et al. Clinical and hematological characteristics of hepatosplenic T gamma/delta lymphoma with isochromosome for long arm of chromosome 7. Leuk Lymphoma 1996;22(5–6):495–500.

80. Lin MT, Shen MC, Su IJ, et al. Peripheral T gamma/delta lymphoma presenting with idiopathic thrombocytopenic purpura-like picture. Br J Haematol 1991;78(2):280–2.

81. Suehiro S, Shiratsuchi M, Suehiro Y, et al. Angioimmunoblastic T cell lymphoma (AITL) with autoimmune thrombocytopenia. Rinsho Ketsueki 2002;43(9):841–5 [in Japanese].

82. Garderet L, Aoudjhane M, Bonte H, et al. Immune thrombocytopenic purpura: first symptom of gamma/delta T-cell lymphoma. Am J Med 2001;111(3):242–3.

83. Dhodapkar MV, Li CY, Lust JA, et al. Clinical spectrum of clonal proliferations of T-large granular lymphocytes: a T-cell clonopathy of undetermined significance? Blood 1994;84(5):1620–7.

84. Gentile TC, Wener MH, Starkebaum G, et al. Humoral immune abnormalities in T-cell large granular lymphocyte leukemia. Leuk Lymphoma 1996;23(3–4): 365–70.

85. Lamy T, Loughran TP Jr. Current concepts: large granular lymphocyte leukemia. Blood Rev 1999;13(4):230–40.

86. Rose MG, Berliner N. T-cell large granular lymphocyte leukemia and related disorders. Oncologist 2004;9(3):247–58.

87. Martinelli G, Zinzani PL, Magagnoli M, et al. Incidence and prognostic significance of idiopathic thrombocytopenic purpura in patients with Hodgkin's disease in complete hematological remission. Haematologica 1998;83(7):669–70.

88. Tahiliani RR, Banavali SD, Parikh PM, et al. Idiopathic thrombocytopaenic purpura in patients during remission of Hodgkin's disease. J Assoc Physicians India 1989;37(2):141–3.

89. Kedar A, Khan AB, Mattern JQ, et al. Autoimmune disorders complicating adolescent Hodgkin's disease. Cancer 1979;44(1):112–6.

90. Waddell CC, Cimo PL. Idiopathic thrombocytopenic purpura occurring in Hodgkin disease after splenectomy: report of two cases and review of the literature. Am J Hematol 1979;7(4):381–7.

91. Cohen JR. Idiopathic thrombocytopenic purpura in Hodgkin's disease: a rare occurrence of no prognostic significance. Cancer 1978;41(2):743–6.

92. Murphy WG, Allan NC, Perry DJ, et al. Hodgkin's disease presenting as idiopathic thrombocytopenic purpura. Postgrad Med J 1984;60(707):614–5.

93. Pedro-Botet J, Estruch R, Montserrat E, et al. Thrombocytopenic purpura as first manifestation of an inapparent Hodgkin's disease. Scand J Haematol 1986;36(4): 408–10.

94. Ertem M, Uysal Z, Yavuz G, et al. Immune thrombocytopenia and hemolytic anemia as a presenting manifestation of Hodgkin disease. Pediatr Hematol Oncol 2000;17(2):181–5.

95. Cines DB, Bussel JB, Liebman HA, et al. The ITP syndrome: pathogenic and clinical diversity. Blood 2009;113(26):6511–21.

96. Mittal S, Blaylock MG, Culligan DJ, et al. A high rate of CLL phenotype lymphocytes in autoimmune hemolytic anemia and immune thrombocytopenic purpura. Haematologica 2008;93(1):151–2.

97. Anaissie EJ, Kontoyiannis DP, O'Brien S, et al. Infections in patients with chronic lymphocytic leukemia treated with fludarabine. Ann Intern Med 1998;129(7): 559–66.

98. Wei S, Kryczek I, Zou W. Regulatory T-cell compartmentalization and trafficking. Blood 2006;108(2):426–31.

Infectious Causes of Chronic Immune Thrombocytopenia

Roberto Stasi, MD*, Fenella Willis, MD, Muriel S. Shannon, MD,
Edward C. Gordon-Smith, MD

KEYWORDS

- Immune thrombocytopenia • Infections • *H. pylori* • HCV
- HIV • Thrombopoietin

Primary immune thrombocytopenia (ITP), the most common cause of severe thrombocytopenia in otherwise healthy young adults, is a diagnosis of exclusion.[1–3] Thrombocytopenia may accompany or follow a variety of conditions from which ITP must be differentiated. Acute infections such as infectious mononucleosis, cytomegalovirus, rubella, mumps, and varicella may be associated with thrombocytopenia of varying severity that may be, at least in part, immune-mediated.[3] In children, symptoms of the primary viral disease are usually well established (1–4 weeks) before the onset of the thrombocytopenia, which is often abrupt and severe. The thrombocytopenia generally resolves spontaneously within 2 to 8 weeks, but in occasional individuals it may persist for months before remitting.[4] In adults, the most prevalent infections associated with thrombocytopenia are those from hepatitis C virus (HCV), human immunodeficiency virus (HIV), and *Helicobacter pylori*.[5] In typical cases the thrombocytopenia presents with an insidious onset, has no tendency to remit spontaneously (although its severity may parallel the stage of the infectious disease), and may closely mimic chronic ITP.[5]

The aim of this article is to provide an updated review of thrombocytopenia associated with chronic infections, focusing on the current understanding of the mechanisms leading to the thrombocytopenia and on the evolving therapeutic strategies.

HEPATITIS C VIRUS–ASSOCIATED THROMBOCYTOPENIA

HCV infection evolves toward a chronic state in approximately 85% of patients, as demonstrated by the persistence of HCV-RNA in serum.[6] However, severe and long-term complications of chronic HCV infection such as liver cirrhosis, end-stage liver disease, and hepatocellular carcinoma develop only in a proportion of infected

Department of Haematology, St George's Hospital, Blackshaw Road, London SW17 0QT, UK
* Corresponding author.
E-mail address: roberto.stasi@stgeorges.nhs.uk (R. Stasi).

Hematol Oncol Clin N Am 23 (2009) 1275–1297
doi:10.1016/j.hoc.2009.08.009
0889-8588/09/$ – see front matter © 2009 Elsevier Inc. All rights reserved.

hemonc.theclinics.com

patients, after a period that can exceed 10 to 20 years.[7] Chronic HCV infection has also been reported to be associated with the development of several extrahepatic alterations, including thrombocytopenia.[8] Thrombocytopenia may be present even in the absence of clinically evident liver disease or splenomegaly, and may be diagnosed as chronic idiopathic thrombocytopenic purpura.[9]

Epidemiology

HCV is now recognized as the most common viral infection causing chronic liver disease in humans worldwide.[10] Of these individuals, approximately 55% to 85% have chronic infection that might need curative treatment.[10] Thrombocytopenia either preexists and prevents the initiation of treatment with pegylated interferon (PEG-IFN) or develops as a consequence of PEG-IFN treatment, leading to dose modification in 19% of cases and discontinuation in 2% of cases.[11] In patients with cirrhosis, thrombocytopenia complicates antiviral treatment much more frequently than in patients with HCV infection without cirrhosis.[12]

Table 1 summarizes the results on the prevalence of HCV infection from several cross-sectional studies in adult ITP patients. The major series published to date evaluated 250 patients fulfilling the diagnostic criteria for ITP of the American Society of Hematology (ASH).[18] A positive serology was found in 76 (30%) of these patients. There were significant differences in demographic characteristics of HCV-positive patients when compared with HCV-negative ITP. HCV-positive patients were older (54.9 ± 8 years vs 40.3 ± 8 years, P<.001) and equally distributed between sexes in comparison with the female predominance in HCV-negative ITP. ITP was more frequent in Asian patients compared with the HCV-positive patients.

Whereas retrospective studies[19,20] suggest that the prevalence of ITP among HCV patients is greater than would be expected by chance, the prevalence of HCV-positive ITP patients in some cohorts may be indirectly related to the background prevalence of HCV infection reported in the general populations.[14,15,17,18] Chiao and colleagues[21] calculated the incidence rate of ITP among 120,691 HCV-infected and 454,905 matched HCV-uninfected United States veterans who received diagnoses during the period 1997 to 2004. Their results indicate that HCV infection is actually associated with an elevated risk of developing ITP (hazard ratio, 1.8; 95% confidence interval, 1.4–2.3) among both untreated and treated patients.

Table 1 Prevalence of HCV infection in adult ITP patients		
Study	**Total Number**	**Number Infected (%)**
Pawlotsly et al (1995)[13]	139[a]	14 (10)
Pivetti et al (1996)[14]	33	12 (36)
Garcia-Suarez et al (2000)[15]	51	13 (22)
Sakuraya et al (2002)[16]	79	11 (14)
Zhang et al (2003)[17]	247	33 (13)
Rajan et al (2005)[18]	250	76 (30)
Total	**799**	**159 (20)**

[a] Seven patients of this series had an associated autoimmune disorder. Study only included patients with platelet counts of less than 25 × 10^9/L.

Pathophysiology

A variety of pathogenic mechanisms are reported to be implicated in thrombocytopenia related to chronic HCV infection. These mechanisms include sequestration of platelets in the enlarged spleen secondary to portal hypertension (hypersplenism),[22] reduced hepatic production of the thrombopoietin,[23,24] bone marrow suppression by HCV[25] or interferon antiviral treatment,[26] and increased platelet destruction mediated by immune mechanisms involving antiplatelet autoantibodies and platelet-associated immune complexes.[27–30]

Although there is a higher prevalence of thrombocytopenia and antiplatelet antibodies in patients with liver disease caused by HCV than in patients with hepatitis B infection,[20] the pathogenic significance of antiplatelet antibodies is uncertain.[31] However, a recent study showed that HCV core envelope 1 can induce thrombocytopenia by molecular mimicry with an epitope on platelet surface integrin GPIIIa, GPIIIa49-66.[32]

Other studies have shown that HCV-RNA can be detected in washed platelets of infected individuals, particularly if thrombocytopenic.[28] Furthermore, there is a non-saturable binding of HCV to platelets.[27] High-affinity binding of HCV to platelet membrane with subsequent binding of anti-HCV antibody could theoretically lead to "innocent bystander" phagocytosis of platelets.[27] The improvement of thrombocytopenia after successful interferon therapy supports this kind of mechanism.

Clinical Manifestations

In one study from Japan[16] the platelet counts in HCV-positive patients were lower than in the HCV-negative patients (26 ± 9 vs $49 \pm 30 \times 10^9$/L, respectively; $P<.02$). In contrast, in an American series[18] fewer HCV-positive patients had severe thrombocytopenia, defined as platelet count 10×10^9/L or less (4% vs 46% for ITP, $P \leq .001$). However, 56 (74%) patients had a platelet count of 50×10^9/L or less. Symptoms and signs of thrombocytopenia were less frequent in HCV-positive ITP, but major bleeding was more frequent (25% vs 10%, $P = .0059$). Serum cryoglobulins and anticardiolipin antibodies were more frequent in HCV-positive ITP (90% and 62%, respectively), but rare in HCV-negative ITP (7% and 15%, $P \leq .001$ compared with HCV-positive ITP). In the French[13] and Chinese[17] studies the characteristics of ITP in HCV-positive patients did not differ from HCV-negative ones.

Treatment

Most case series of patients with HCV infection and chronic immune thrombocytopenia have reported a greater than 50% platelet response to steroids.[18,19,33,34] Response to splenectomy was not found to differ significantly between HCV-positive and HCV-negative patients in 2 studies describing patients with chronic ITP.[16,17]

Rajan and colleagues[18] noted that only a minority of HCV-positive patients received some form of treatment for thrombocytopenia (29 [38%] vs 158 [91%] for HCV-negative ITP). Of the 7 patients treated with prednisone (4 responded, 57%), 6 developed elevations of hepatic transaminases of greater than twice pretreatment levels while receiving prednisone. All 6 patients had a documented increase in HCV viral load. Two patients developed elevated serum bilirubin levels, with one patient developing overt jaundice. Treatment with either intravenous immunoglobulin (IVIG) or anti-RhD Ig proved effective in increasing platelet counts in both the HCV-seropositive and -seronegative patients. Of 5 HCV-positive patients treated with interferon-α (IFN-α), 4 responded with increased platelet counts. Responders to IFN-α could be distinguished from the nonresponder by a decrease in HCV quantitative RNA, hepatic transaminases, and cryoglobulins.[35] Considering the results of various studies,[15,25,35] approximately half of HCV-positive adult ITP patients treated with IFN-α responded with an increase in platelet count.

Research has focused on developing compounds specifically to stimulate thrombo-poietin (TPO) activity to prevent or treat thrombocytopenia in chronic liver diseases. Eltrombopag is a small-molecule nonpeptide oral platelet growth factor that acts as an agonist to the thrombopoietin receptor. A phase 2 multicenter, randomized trial of daily eltrombopag in patients with HCV-associated thrombocytopenia and compensated liver disease showed that after 4 weeks of therapy, platelet count increased to 100×10^9/L or more in 75%, 79%, and 95% of patients treated with 30 mg, 50 mg, and 75 mg eltrombopag, respectively, compared with no response in placebo patients (P<.001).[36] Significantly more patients in the eltrombopag treat-ment groups (36%, 53%, and 65% in the 30-mg, 50-mg, and 75-mg groups) completed 12 weeks of antiviral therapy compared with 6% of placebo patients, and 75% of these patients had platelet counts greater than baseline values at the end of the antiviral treatment phase. Because eltrombopag has shown remarkable activity in chronic ITP as well,[37] this agent seems to be an adequate candidate for the management of HCV-related chronic thrombocytopenia.

HUMAN IMMUNODEFICIENCY VIRUS–ASSOCIATED THROMBOCYTOPENIA

Thrombocytopenia was first linked to the acquired immune deficiency syndrome (AIDS) before the discovery of the HIV.[38–41] Isolated thrombocytopenia may actually be encountered as the initial presentation of HIV infection several years before the development of overt AIDS, and the early disease is clinically indistinguishable from classic ITP.[42]

Epidemiology

Before the use of highly active antiretroviral therapy (HAART), HIV-associated throm-bocytopenia (platelet count <150×10^9/L) was identified in approximately 5% to 30% of HIV-1 infected patients (**Table 2**).[50] Although patients may present with thrombocy-topenia at any time during the course of HIV infection, from asymptomatic infection to advanced AIDS, the incidence of thrombocytopenia seems to increase with progres-sive immunosuppression.[44,48] The finding of an increased incidence and severity of

Table 2 Incidence of thrombocytopenia in HIV infection		
Study	Total Number of HIV-Seropositive	Number of Thrombocytopenic (%)
Murphy et al (1987)[43]	105	11 (10.5%)
Kaslow et al (1987)[44]	1611	108 (6.7%)
Rossi et al (1990)[45]	657	72 (10.9%)
Peltier et al (1991)[46]	435	23 (5.5%)
Mientjes et al (1992)[47]	285	67 (23.5%)
Sloand et al (1992)[48]	1004	110 (11%)
Sullivan et al (1997)[49]	30214	2629 (8.7%)[a]
Total	**34311**	**3020 (8.8%)**

[a] Thrombocytopenia in this report was defined as platelets less than 50×10^9/L.

thrombocytopenia in HIV-infected injection drug users, when compared with HIV-infected homosexuals, has been reported by several investigators.[45–47,49,51,52] These differences may be explained, in part, by the finding of a higher incidence of coinfection with hepatitis C and underlying liver disease in HIV-infected intravenous drug users.[47,52–55] With widespread use of HAART in patients with early HIV infection, the more recent prevalence of thrombocytopenia in patients under active antiviral treatment is unknown. However, recent prospective data from the Women's Interagency HIV Study has documented a reduction in the incidence of anemia and neutropenia in HIV-infected women on HAART therapy.[56,57] Therefore, one could assume a similar improvement in the incidence of thrombocytopenia.

Pathophysiology

The thrombocytopenia associated with HIV infection recognizes several mechanisms, which can be present simultaneously. A study in 6 patients has shown that thrombocytopenia in HIV infection is caused by a combination of: (1) shortening of platelet life span by two-thirds and doubling of splenic platelet sequestration; and (2) ineffective platelet production despite a threefold TPO-driven expansion in marrow megakaryocyte mass.[58] The mechanism for the development of thrombocytopenia is dependent on the disease burden. HIV-associated thrombocytopenia of early HIV infection more often resembles classic ITP in which thrombocytopenia is mediated primarily by peripheral destruction, whereas patients with immunologic AIDS (CD4 lymphocytes <200/μL) have thrombocytopenia attributable predominantly to decreased platelet production and ineffective hematopoiesis.[59–61]

Accelerated platelet destruction is primarily related to immune complexes[62] and cross-reacting platelet antibodies.[63,64] Antibodies specific against an epitope of integrin subunit β3 (GPIIIa) on the surface of platelets, GPIIIa49-66, can be found in circulating immune complexes[65,66] and can cross-react with a peptide sharing a known epitope region with HIV-1 protein *nef*.[67] This antibody is unique in that it induces complement-independent platelet fragmentation in vitro by the generation of reactive oxygen species released through activation of 12-lipoxygenase and nicotinamide adenine dinucleotide phosphate–oxidase.[67–69] The talin head domain (talin-H), a cleavage product of talin that can be generated by platelet activation or HIV-1 protease, has also been identified as an immunodominant epitope of the antiplatelet antibody response in 3 patients with HIV-associated thrombocytopenia.[70] The role of antitalin antibodies in producing thrombocytopenia has not been investigated.

Ineffective platelet production has been linked to direct HIV cytopathic infection of the megakaryocyte.[71–76] Megakaryocytes express the CD4 receptor[75,77] and coreceptors[77] necessary for HIV infection. In vitro studies have demonstrated megakaryocyte internalization of HIV[72,73] and megakaryocytic expression of viral RNA.[78] Electron microscopy of megakaryocytes from HIV-infected individuals with thrombocytopenia clearly demonstrates ultrastructural abnormalities not encountered in noninfected patients; blebbing of the surface membrane and vacuolization of peripheral cytoplasm are the most common.[78] Other alterations in the bone marrow microenvironment may also contribute to poor platelet production.[79,80]

Secondary causes of thrombocytopenia during HIV infection are generally the result of underlying opportunistic infections, malignancy, medications, and comorbid conditions, resulting in hypersplenism (**Box 1**). Thrombotic thrombocytopenic purpura-hemolytic uremic syndrome (TTP-HUS) is a rare and potentially fatal cause of thrombocytopenia that must also be considered in the initial evaluation of HIV-infected patients with reduced platelet counts.

Box 1
Common causes of secondary thrombocytopenia in HIV-infected patients

Infections

    Bacterial

        Bacteremia/sepsis

        Bartonellosis

        Ehrlichiosis

    Parasitic

        Toxoplasma

        Babesia

        Leishmaniasis

    Mycobacterial

        Disseminated tuberculosis

        Disseminated *Mycobacterium avium* complex

    Viral

        Cytomegalovirus

        Epstein-Barr virus

        Rubella

    Fungal

        Histoplasmosis

        Coccidioidomycosis

        Other disseminated fungal infections

Malignancy

    Kaposi sarcoma

    Metastatic adenocarcinomas

    Non-Hodgkin lymphoma

    Chemotherapy-associated thrombocytopenia

    Hodgkin lymphoma

Medications

    Trimethoprim-sulfamethoxazole

    Ketoconazole

    Trimetrexate

    Ganciclovir

    Pyrimethamine

    Foscarnet

    Flucytosine

    Cidofovir

    Pentamidine

    Acyclovir

    Pyrazinamide

Interferon

Rifampin

Chemotherapeutic agents

Rifabutin

Valganciclovir

Secondary hypersplenism

Chronic viral hepatitis/cirrhosis

Other causes of hepatitis/cirrhosis

Thrombotic thrombocytopenic purpura

Disseminated intravascular coagulation

Clinical Manifestations

HIV-associated thrombocytopenia is rarely a serious clinical problem. In most cases, platelet counts remain greater than 50×10^9/L and the condition can be treated conservatively.[47–49] Bleeding is rare, unless the platelet count falls to less than 10×10^9/L. If this occurs, bleeding gums, extremity petechiae, and easy bruising are common presentations. However, menorrhagia in fertile women may sometimes be so massive as to require transfusion therapy. Only a few cases of fatal hemorrhage have been reported. Two studies reviewed hemorrhagic complications of HIV-infected hemophiliacs.[81,82] Finazzi and colleagues documented thrombocytopenia (platelets $<100 \times 10^9$/L) in 14 of 124 (11%) hemophiliacs, of which only one patient had a major hemorrhage.[82,83] In contrast, Ragni and colleagues[81] reported a platelet count of less than 100×10^9/L in 30 of 87 (36%) hemophiliacs, with 11 (13%) having a platelet count of less than 50×10^9/L. Nine of the 11 patients (82%) had major bleeding complications and 3 patients suffered fatal hemorrhages.[81]

Severe thrombocytopenia in patients with advanced HIV infection is frequently associated with additional cytopenias.[43–45] In a study of 52 HIV-infected injection drug users with thrombocytopenia, 4 patients (8%) with advanced HIV infection had a hypocellular bone marrow examination responsible for their pancytopenia.[60] HIV-infected injection drug users were also more likely to have antibodies to both hepatitis B and C, and have abnormal liver function studies.[47,51–55]

Treatment

Antiretroviral therapy is the first-line and most effective therapy for the thrombocytopenia associated with HIV infection. In fact, HIV-associated cytopenias have been shown to correlate with the degree of HIV viral replication as measured by plasma viral load,[84] and improve with effective antiretroviral therapies.[84–90] Zidovudine monotherapy was efficacious in increasing the platelet count in 60% to 70% of HIV thrombocytopenia patients when given in doses greater than 1 g/d.[85–87] Although other antiretroviral drugs as monotherapy have been shown to improve hematologic parameters in patients with advanced HIV infection,[91] their efficacy as monotherapy for the management of HIV thrombocytopenia has been less often demonstrated.[92] HAART likely is more effective than zidovudine monotherapy. One retrospective study compared patients with severe thrombocytopenia treated with zidovudine with those treated with HAART.[89] After 6 months, HAART therapy more frequently resulted in complete and sustained recovery of platelet counts. Responses were achieved even in those with zidovudine-resistant thrombocytopenia.

Responses to zidovudine and HAART may be more limited in HIV-infected injection drug users, possibly reflecting the impact of associated liver disease and HCV infection.[51,90,93] A prospective, placebo-controlled, double-blind, randomized trial of IFN-α enrolled 14 zidovudine refractory HIV-infected injection drug users.[93] Twelve patients had a statistically significant increase in their platelet counts by 4 weeks of therapy. Patients in this trial had elevated serum alanine aminotransferase, suggestive of underlying liver disease. Similar responses to IFN-α therapy alone have been reported in HIV-seronegative, HCV-infected patients,[15,18,35] suggesting a possible role of IFN-α in suppressing associated HCV infection in these HIV-infected patients. However, an open label trial of IFN-α in predominately homosexual men reported responses in 9 of 16 patients enrolled, with responses occurring as early as 2 weeks.[94] Such rapid responses preclude the possibility of improvement in the platelet counts due to suppression of concomitant HCV infection.

Because the beneficial effects of antiretroviral therapy may be seen after several weeks, during that time it may be necessary to support the platelet counts with other interventions. HIV-associated thrombocytopenia is generally responsive to the therapies used in classic ITP. Prednisone therapy can produce a major hematologic response in the platelet count (100×10^9/L) in over half the patients treated, although only a minority of patients will maintain platelet counts greater than 50×10^9/L after cessation of steroids.[41,95] There was no evidence of increased risk of infections or progressive immunosuppression with short-term prednisone treatment in these patients. IVIG and anti-RhD are equally effective in acutely increasing platelet counts in severely affected patients.[52,95,96] A cross-over study of comparing IVIG to anti-RhD in HIV-associated thrombocytopenia clearly demonstrated a longer duration of response to anti-RhD treatment.[95]

Splenectomy, which is safe and results in stable complete or partial remissions in 60% to 80% of patients,[38,39,41,52,60,61,95,97,98] should be reserved for patients with symptomatic thrombocytopenia after an adequate trial of antiretroviral therapy. A retrospective review of patients treated with splenic irradiation, as opposed to surgical splenectomy, failed to find evidence of efficacy for this procedure in the treatment of refractory HIV-associated thrombocytopenia.[99]

Thrombopoiesis stimulation was explored in a pilot clinical trial that administered recombinant human megakaryocyte growth and development factor (PEG-rHuMGDF) to 6 adult HIV-positive patients with thrombocytopenia.[100] All 6 responded; the elevated platelet counts were maintained through the 16 weeks of therapy and returned to pretreatment values 2 weeks after cessation of therapy. PEG-rHuMGDF and other first-generation thrombopoietic growth factors have not been developed further. The role of second-generation thrombopoietin receptor agonists, eltrombopag and romiplostim, has not yet been defined.

HELICOBACTER PYLORI–ASSOCIATED THROMBOCYTOPENIA

H. pylori, a Gram-negative bacterium, is recognized as the causative agent of active chronic gastritis and is the predominant cause of peptic ulceration (ie, gastric and duodenal ulcers).[101] *H. pylori* is also a cofactor in the development of both adenocarcinoma and mucosa-associated lymphoid tissue (MALT) lymphomas. Eradication of *H. pylori* infection can result in platelet responses in patients with chronic ITP, which has led to speculation on a causal role of the bacterium in the development of thrombocytopenia.

Epidemiology

H. pylori is estimated to infect the gastric mucosa of at least half of the world's population.[101] The prevalence of *H. pylori* infection in adult ITP patients does not seem different from that reported in the general healthy population matched for age and geographic area (**Table 3**). The detection method in these studies was predominantly the ^{13}C-urea breath test. Most studies were conducted in Japan, where the prevalence of the infection is greater than 70%,[127] or in Italy, where the *H. pylori* rate in the middle-aged adult general population is nearly 50%.[128]

Pathophysiology

Several hypotheses have been advanced. Molecular mimicry proposes that an *H. pylori* surface antigen evokes a host systemic immune response that produces antibodies cross-reactive with host platelets. The possible role of CagA-positive strains as a pathogenic candidate for ITP was recognized in 2 molecular studies.[109,129] In this

Table 3
Prevalence of *Helicobacter pylori* infection in adult ITP patients

Study	Total Number	Number Infected (%)
Gasbarrini et al (1998)[102]	18	11 (61)
Jarque et al (2001)[103]	56	40 (71)
Kohda et al (2002)[104]	40	25 (62)
Hino et al (2003)[105]	30	21 (70)
Hashino et al (2003)[106]	22	14 (64)
Ando et al (2003)[107]	61	50 (82)
Michel et al (2004)[108]	74	16 (22)
Takahashi et al (2004)[109]	20	15 (75)
Sato et al (2004)[110]	53	39 (74)
Ando et al (2004)[111]	20	17 (85)
Nomura et al (2004)[112]	42	28 (66)
Veneri et al (2005)[113]	52	34 (65)
Inaba et al (2005)[114]	35	25 (71)
Stasi et al (2005)[115]	137	64 (47)
Fujimura et al (2005)[116]	435	300 (69)
Suzuki et al (2005)[117]	36	25 (69)
Suvajdzic et al (2006)[118]	54	39 (72)
Sayan et al (2006)[119]	34	20 (59)
Asahi et al (2006)[120]	37	26 (70)
Kodama et al (2007)[121]	116	67 (58)
Campuzano-Maya (2007)[122]	32	29 (91)
Estrada-Gomez (2007)[123]	23	14 (61)
Satake (2007)[124]	38	12 (68)
Emilia et al (2007)[125]	75	38 (51)
Jackson et al (2008)[126]	22	4 (18)
Total	**1562**	**973 (62.3%)**

regard, it should be noted that most Japanese *H. pylori* strains are positive for CagA[83] and have the intact Cag pathogenicity island.[130] Further support to this hypothesis emerges from the results of an Italian study, showing that the prevalence of the *H. pylori* cagA gene was significantly higher in patients with ITP than in a control group.[125] A recent study suggests that *H. pylori* urease B can be involved in molecular mimicry, as antibodies against this bacterial enzyme could cross-react with human platelet GPIIIa and partly inhibit platelet aggregation.[131] Other putative targets of molecular mimicry are Lewis (Le) antigens, which are expressed by *H. pylori* in a strain-specific manner. Le antigens adsorb to platelets and might serve as targets for anti-Le antibodies in patients with an appropriate genetic background.[132]

A role for the lipopolysaccharide (LPS) of gram-negative bacteria has been suggested by recent laboratory experiments showing that in the presence of antiplatelet antibodies LPS can significantly enhance Fc-dependent platelet phagocytosis.[133] In addition, *H. pylori* eradication was associated with decreased phagocytic capacity and modulation of the inhibitory Fcγ receptor IIB (FcγRIIB) in peripheral blood monocytes.[134] These results may provide the explanation why thrombocytopenia worsens in some patients with ITP during infections and, alternatively, resolves in other patients with ITP who are treated with bacterial eradication therapy.

Other studies have shown that some strains of *H. pylori* bind von Willebrand factor (vWF) and induce glycoprotein Ib (GPIb)- and FcRIIa-dependent platelet aggregation in the presence of *H. pylori* antibodies.[135] Activation may promote platelet clearance and antigen presentation, which augments production of antibacterial antibodies. Somatic mutation may lead to the development of antibodies that either recognize bacterially derived factors that bind to platelets or cross-react with platelet antigens.[136]

Both *H. pylori* infection and ITP are associated with a polarized Th1-type phenotype.[137,138] It may accordingly be speculated that *H. pylori* infection creates an immunologic environment that facilitates the onset or persistence of ITP.[139]

The last 3 hypotheses are not mutually exclusive, and can account for the observation that clinical responses may occur as early as 1 week from initiation of eradication therapy, before antibody synthesis by plasma cells is affected.[120]

The importance of genetic factors emerged from the results of an Italian study, indicating that *H. pylori*–positive patients had a lower frequency of DRB1*03 and higher frequencies of DRB1*11, DRB1*14, and DQB1*03 relative to *H. pylori*–negative cases.[113]

Clinical Manifestations

H. pylori–infected ITP patients were found to be significantly older than *H. pylori*–uninfected patients.[5,140] This is not unexpected, as the prevalence of *H. pylori* infection in the general population increases with increasing with age.[101] In contrast, all prospective series failed to detect significant differences in other characteristics, such as sex and platelet count. A significant association between *H. pylori* infection and the presence of symptoms of dyspepsia has been reported by Michel and colleagues[108] but not by Stasi and colleagues.[115] A cross-sectional study by Fukui and colleagues[141] did not find any correlation between *H. pylori* infection and thrombocytopenia during pregnancy. In a retrospective Japanese study, the *H. pylori*–positive group was significantly older ($P<.005$) and had more cases of hyperplastic megakaryocytes in the bone marrow ($P = .01$) than patients without *H. pylori* infection.[116]

Treatment

In almost all studies eradication therapy consisted of the so-called triple therapy, a combination of amoxicillin, clarithromycin, and a proton pump inhibitor usually given for 1 or 2 weeks. Adverse events from eradication therapy have been described as mild, usually consisting of abdominal pain and diarrhea, and lead to discontinuation of treatment in less than 5% of cases.

An overall response rate (platelet count $\geq 30 \times 10^9$/L and at least a doubling of the basal count) of 52.7% in eradicated patients was noted using individual patient data from 25 series worlwide.[50] Responses were consistently high in Japan, of heterogeneous magnitude across European countries, and very low in the United States (**Table 4**). Further analysis shows that in almost every series in which there was a platelet response as a result of a successful eradication treatment, the *H. pylori* infection rate in patients with ITP was relatively higher than in those in which no association was found.[143] So in the United States, where the background prevalence of *H. pylori* is low, there are also low chances of obtaining a platelet response to eradication therapy; in Japan, where the prevalence of *H. pylori* in the general population is around 70%, eradication therapy produces platelet responses in a high proportion of cases. Of note, in most studies the mean platelet count was greater than 30×10^9/L, and relatively few patients with severe disease were investigated. The long-term results of *H. pylori* eradication have been reported recently by Italian[125] and Japanese[144] groups. In 29 of the 31 cases whose course could be followed up for 5 to 7 years, only 2 relapses occurred. The pretreatment factor that was more consistently associated with a platelet response to *H. pylori* eradication was a shorter ITP duration.[115,116] Patients with very low platelet counts ($<30 \times 10^9$/L) also seem to have fewer chances of response, although this issue has not been systematically addressed in most published reports.

In the only phase 3 trial, Suzuki and colleagues[117] evaluated the platelet count in a group of 25 *H. pylori*–positive chronic ITP patients who were randomized to receive treatment or no treatment for *H. pylori* infection. Response to the treatment was defined as complete (CR) if the platelet count was greater than 150×10^9/L, and partial (PR) if the platelet count increased by more than 50×10^9/L 6 months after the eradication therapy. The investigators found that the eradication of *H. pylori* infection in patients with ITP was associated with a platelet response: 46.2% in the eradication group (4 CR and 2 PR) and 0% in the noneradication group ($P<.01$). The platelet response was also significantly more common in patients with infection sustained by CagA-positive strains of *H. pylori* ($P = .04$). However, given the small number of patients recruited in the trial, these results should be interpreted with some caution.

The uncertainties regarding the actual role of standard eradication therapy warranted a prospective study in which 37 ITP patients were treated with triple therapy irrespective of the presence or absence of *H. pylori* infection.[120] With a therapeutic response defined as a platelet count greater than 100×10^9/L at 24 weeks, 16 of 26 *H. pylori*–positive patients (62%) were responders, whereas none of the *H. pylori*–negative patients was a responder. Besides, anti-GPIIb/IIIa antibody-producing B cells were significantly decreased at 12 and 24 weeks in *H. pylori*–positive responders ($P<.0001$) and, to a lesser extent, in nonresponders ($P = .02$), but not in *H. pylori*–negative patients. This study clearly supports the notion that platelet recovery after *H. pylori* eradication results from the disappearance of *H. pylori* itself, rather than from other *H. pylori*–independent mechanisms. It has been advanced that the increased platelet count in some patients who failed the *H. pylori* eradication or in those who received proton pump inhibitor monotherapy could have been mediated through a reduction in the quantity of *H. pylori* or a bacteriostatic effect of the regimen.[120]

MISCELLANEOUS INFECTIONS ASSOCIATED WITH THROMBOCYTOPENIA

A myriad of chronic infections can cause thrombocytopenia, but most of the time the associated clinical and laboratory features readily allow to discriminate them from ITP.

Table 4
Results of *H. pylori* eradication

Study	Bacterial Eradication (%)[a]	Platelet Response[a] (%)[b]	Follow-up Duration (months)[c]	No. of Relapsed Patients
Japan				
Kohda et al (2002)[104]	19/19 (100)	12 (63)	14.8 (9–39)	0
Hino et al (2003)[105]	18/21 (86)	8 (44)	37.8	NR
Hashino et al (2003)[106]	13/14 (93)	9 (69)	15	1
Ando et al (2003)[107]	27/29 (93)	16 (59)	11 (4–15)	1
Takahashi et al (2004)[109]	13/15 (87)	7 (54)	4	NR
Sato et al (2004)[110]	27/32 (84)	15 (56)	12	0
Ando et al (2004)[111]	15/17 (88)	10 (67)	24	0
Nomura et al (2004)[112]	12/28 (43)	12 (100)	NR	NR
Inaba et al (2005)[114]	25/25 (100)	11 (44)	NR	0
Fujimura et al (2005)[116]	161/207 (78)	88 (55)	12 (3–12)	NR
Suzuki et al (2005)[117]	22/25 (88)	6 (28)	6	NR
Asahi et al (2006)[120]	26/26 (100)	16 (61)	>12	0
Kodama et al (2007)[121]	44/52 (85)	27 (61)	NR	NR
Satake (2007)[124]	23/25 (92)	13 (57)	25.4* (6–48)	0
Subtotal	**445/535 (83.2)**	**250 (56.2)**		

Europe				
Gasbarrini et al (1998)[102]	8/11 (73)	NA	4	NR
Jarque et al (2001)[103]	23/32 (72)	3 (13)	21 (18–24)	2
Veneri et al (2005)[113]	32/34 (94)	18 (56)	24.2 (3–62)	1
Stasi et al (2005)[115]	52/52 (100)	16 (31)	25 (7–42)	6
Suvajdzic et al (2006)[118]	23/30 (77)	6 (26)	18 (14–32)	0
Emilia et al (2007)[125]	34/38 (89)	25 (74)	43.5 (18–90)	1
Subtotal	**172/197 (87.3)**	**68 (41.5)**		
North America				
Michel et al (2004)[108]	14/15 (93)	4 (29)	11.5 (3–18)	1
Ahn et al (2006)[142]	15/15 (100)	1 (7)	(6–24)	1
Jackson et al (2008)[126]	2/4 (50)	2 (100)	48.5	0
Subtotal	**31/34 (91)**	**7 (22.6)**		
Other countries				
Sayan et al (2006)[119]	18/20 (90)	11 (61)	11 (4–24)	0
Campuzano-Maya (2007)[122]	26/29 (90)	21 (81)	12.2	NR
Estrada-Gomez (2007)[123]	14/14 (100)	2 (14)	5 (2–7)	1
Subtotal	**58/63 (92.1)**	**34 (58.6)**		
Total	**706/829 (85.2)**	**369/698 (52.9)**		

Abbreviations: NR, not reported; NA, not assessable.
[a] Among patients who were successfully eradicated.
[b] Complete or partial response among patients with successful eradication.
[c] Median, with range in parantheses.
* Mean value.

Notable exceptions are cytomegalovirus (CMV) infection and malaria. The presence of CMV infection among asymptomatic or paucisymptomatic immunocompetent individuals with ITP is a rare finding[145] but is well described in the literature.[146] The mechanisms by which cytomegalovirus can cause thrombocytopenia include direct cytotoxicity, infection of the megakaryocytes, immune-mediated destruction, impairment of bone marrow stromal cells, and induction of specific or nonspecific autoantibodies resulting in antibody-mediated destruction of the platelets.[147,148] A review of 17 anecdotal cases suggests that the treatment schedule should include a short trial of corticosteroids as first-line therapy. Splenectomy should be avoided in those who fail to respond. Although observation is a reasonable option after failure of corticosteroids, intravenous immunoglobulin should be the treatment of choice in cases of severe bleeding, given its rapidity of action. As the overall outcome is favorable in CMV thrombocytopenia, usually within a few weeks, probably 1 or 2 infusions of intravenous immunoglobulin are sufficient.

Thrombocytopenia during plasmodium infection may appear even before fever, anemia, and splenomegaly become manifest.[149–151] The mechanism of thrombocytopenia in malaria is uncertain. Immune-mediated lysis, sequestration in the spleen, and a dyspoietic process in the marrow with diminished platelet production have all been postulated.[152] Platelet agglutination as a result of endothelial cell activation and release of activated vWF has also been suggested as a mechanism of thrombocytopenia during the early stages of infection.[153] Abnormalities in platelet structure and function have been described as a consequence of malaria, and in rare instances platelets can be invaded by malarial parasites themselves. Thrombocytopenia in malaria is rarely severe, and no particular precautions have to be observed. Treatment is focused on the eradication of the plasmodium.

SUMMARY

Chronic infections with HCV, HIV, and *H. pylori* may be associated with isolated thrombocytopenia and should be considered in the differential diagnosis of ITP. The thrombocytopenia in infection-associated ITP occurs via various potential mechanisms, including accelerated platelet clearance due to immune complex disease, cross-reactivity of antiplatelet glycoprotein antibodies and viral or bacterial antibodies, defective platelet production in HCV and HIV infections, and splenic sequestration of platelets secondary to portal hypertension and decreased production of thrombopoietin in HCV infection.

Serologic evaluation for HIV and HCV infection is indicated in patients with ITP because of the potentially adverse effect of prolonged corticosteroid usage on the underlying infection and the utility of antiviral therapy in treating both the underlying infection and the thrombocytopenia. *H. pylori* screening seems certainly worthwhile in Japan, a country with a high background prevalence of the infection, where significant response rates have been consistently reported. For countries such as the United States, in which both the prevalence of infection and the response rates to eradication therapy are low, testing for *H. pylori* infection remains controversial.

REFERENCES

1. George JN, Woolf SH, Raskob GE, et al. Idiopathic thrombocytopenic purpura: a practice guideline developed by explicit methods for the American Society of Hematology. Blood 1996;88(1):3–40.
2. British Committee for Standards in Haematology General Haematology Task Force. Guidelines for the investigation and management of idiopathic

thrombocytopenic purpura in adults, children and in pregnancy. Br J Haematol 2003;120(4):574–96.

3. Stasi R, Evangelista ML, Stipa E, et al. Idiopathic thrombocytopenic purpura: current concepts in pathophysiology and management. Thromb Haemost 2008;99(1):4–13.

4. Blanchette V, Bolton-Maggs P. Childhood immune thrombocytopenic purpura: diagnosis and management. Pediatr Clin North Am 2008;55(2):393–420, ix.

5. Liebman HA, Stasi R. Secondary immune thrombocytopenic purpura. Curr Opin Hematol 2007;14(5):557–73.

6. Nguyen TT, Sedghi-Vaziri A, Wilkes LB, et al. Fluctuations in viral load (HCV RNA) are relatively insignificant in untreated patients with chronic HCV infection. J Viral Hepat 1996;3(2):75–8.

7. Seeff LB. Natural history of chronic hepatitis C. Hepatology 2002;36(5 Suppl 1): S35–46.

8. Palekar NA, Harrison SA. Extrahepatic manifestations of hepatitis C. South Med J 2005;98(10):1019–23.

9. Pyrsopoulos NT, Reddy KR. Extrahepatic manifestations of chronic viral hepatitis. Curr Gastroenterol Rep 2001;3(1):71–8.

10. Armstrong GL, Wasley A, Simard EP, et al. The prevalence of hepatitis C virus infection in the United States, 1999 through 2002. Ann Intern Med 2006; 144(10):705–14.

11. Sulkowski MS. Management of the hematologic complications of hepatitis C therapy. Clin Liver Dis 2005;9(4):601–16, vi.

12. Bashour FN, Teran JC, Mullen KD. Prevalence of peripheral blood cytopenias (hypersplenism) in patients with nonalcoholic chronic liver disease. Am J Gastroenterol 2000;95(10):2936–9.

13. Pawlotsky JM, Bouvier M, Fromont P, et al. Hepatitis C virus infection and autoimmune thrombocytopenic purpura. J Hepatol 1995;23(6):635–9.

14. Pivetti S, Novarino A, Merico F, et al. High prevalence of autoimmune phenomena in hepatitis C virus antibody positive patients with lymphoproliferative and connective tissue disorders. Br J Haematol 1996;95(1):204–11.

15. Garcia-Suarez J, Burgaleta C, Hernanz N, et al. HCV-associated thrombocytopenia: clinical characteristics and platelet response after recombinant alpha2b-interferon therapy. Br J Haematol 2000;110(1):98–103.

16. Sakuraya M, Murakami H, Uchiumi H, et al. Steroid-refractory chronic idiopathic thrombocytopenic purpura associated with hepatitis C virus infection. Eur J Haematol 2002;68(1):49–53.

17. Zhang L, Li H, Zhao H, et al. Hepatitis C virus-related adult chronic idiopathic thrombocytopenic purpura: experience from a single Chinese center. Eur J Haematol 2003;70(3):196–7.

18. Rajan SK, Espina BM, Liebman HA. Hepatitis C virus-related thrombocytopenia: clinical and laboratory characteristics compared with chronic immune thrombocytopenic purpura. Br J Haematol 2005;129(6):818–24.

19. Pockros PJ, Duchini A, McMillan R, et al. Immune thrombocytopenic purpura in patients with chronic hepatitis C virus infection. Am J Gastroenterol 2002;97(8): 2040–5.

20. Nagamine T, Ohtuka T, Takehara K, et al. Thrombocytopenia associated with hepatitis C viral infection. J Hepatol 1996;24(2):135–40.

21. Chiao EY, Engels EA, Kramer JR, et al. Risk of immune thrombocytopenic purpura and autoimmune hemolytic anemia among 120 908 US veterans with hepatitis C virus infection. Arch Intern Med 2009;169(4):357–63.

22. Aster RH. Pooling of platelets in the spleen: role in the pathogenesis of "hypersplenic" thrombocytopenia. J Clin Invest 1966;45(5):645–57.
23. Peck-Radosavljevic M, Zacherl J, Meng YG, et al. Is inadequate thrombopoietin production a major cause of thrombocytopenia in cirrhosis of the liver? J Hepatol 1997;27(1):127–31.
24. Goulis J, Chau TN, Jordan S, et al. Thrombopoietin concentrations are low in patients with cirrhosis and thrombocytopenia and are restored after orthotopic liver transplantation. Gut 1999;44(5):754–8.
25. Iga D, Tomimatsu M, Endo H, et al. Improvement of thrombocytopenia with disappearance of HCV RNA in patients treated by interferon-alpha therapy: possible etiology of HCV-associated immune thrombocytopenia. Eur J Haematol 2005;75(5):417–23.
26. Peck-Radosavljevic M. Thrombocytopenia in liver disease. Can J Gastroenterol 2000;14(Suppl D):60D–6D.
27. Hamaia S, Li C, Allain JP. The dynamics of hepatitis C virus binding to platelets and 2 mononuclear cell lines. Blood 2001;98(8):2293–300.
28. de Almeida AJ, Campos-de-Magalhaes M, de Melo Marcal OP, et al. Hepatitis C virus-associated thrombocytopenia: a controlled prospective, virological study. Ann Hematol 2004;83(7):434–40.
29. Kajihara M, Kato S, Okazaki Y, et al. A role of autoantibody-mediated platelet destruction in thrombocytopenia in patients with cirrhosis. Hepatology 2003; 37(6):1267–76.
30. Doi T, Homma H, Mezawa S, et al. Mechanisms for increment of platelet associated IgG and platelet surface IgG and their implications in immune thrombocytopenia associated with chronic viral liver disease. Hepatol Res 2002;24(1):23.
31. Panzer S, Seel E, Brunner M, et al. Platelet autoantibodies are common in hepatitis C infection, irrespective of the presence of thrombocytopenia. Eur J Haematol 2006;77(6):513–7.
32. Zhang W, Nardi MA, Li Z, et al. Role of molecular mimicry of hepatitis C-virus (HCV) protein with platelet GPIIIa in hepatitis C-related immunologic thrombocytopenia. Blood 2009;113:4086–93.
33. Hernandez F, Blanquer A, Linares M, et al. Autoimmune thrombocytopenia associated with hepatitis C virus infection. Acta Haematol 1998;99(4):217–20.
34. Ramos-Casals M, Garcia-Carrasco M, Lopez-Medrano F, et al. Severe autoimmune cytopenias in treatment-naive hepatitis C virus infection: clinical description of 35 cases. Medicine (Baltimore) 2003;82(2):87–96.
35. Rajan S, Liebman HA. Treatment of hepatitis C related thrombocytopenia with interferon alpha. Am J Hematol 2001;68(3):202–9.
36. McHutchison JG, Dusheiko G, Shiffman ML, et al. Eltrombopag for thrombocytopenia in patients with cirrhosis associated with hepatitis C. N Engl J Med 2007;357(22):2227–36.
37. Bussel JB, Cheng G, Saleh MN, et al. Eltrombopag for the treatment of chronic idiopathic thrombocytopenic purpura. N Engl J Med 2007;357(22):2237–47.
38. Morris L, Distenfeld A, Amorosi E, et al. Autoimmune thrombocytopenic purpura in homosexual men. Ann Intern Med 1982;96(6 Pt 1):714–7.
39. Ratnoff OD, Menitove JE, Aster RH, et al. Coincident classic hemophilia and "idiopathic" thrombocytopenic purpura in patients under treatment with concentrates of antihemophilic factor (factor VIII). N Engl J Med 1983; 308(8):439–42.
40. Walsh CM, Nardi MA, Karpatkin S. On the mechanism of thrombocytopenic purpura in sexually active homosexual men. N Engl J Med 1984;311(10):635–9.

41. Walsh C, Krigel R, Lennette E, et al. Thrombocytopenia in homosexual patients. Prognosis, response to therapy, and prevalence of antibody to the retrovirus associated with the acquired immunodeficiency syndrome. Ann Intern Med 1985;103(4):542–5.
42. Karpatkin S. Autoimmune thrombocytopenias. Autoimmunity 2004;37(4):363–8.
43. Murphy MF, Metcalfe P, Waters AH, et al. Incidence and mechanism of neutropenia and thrombocytopenia in patients with human immunodeficiency virus infection. Br J Haematol 1987;66(3):337–40.
44. Kaslow RA, Phair JP, Friedman HB, et al. Infection with the human immunodeficiency virus: clinical manifestations and their relationship to immune deficiency. A report from the Multicenter AIDS Cohort Study. Ann Intern Med 1987;107(4):474–80.
45. Rossi G, Gorla R, Stellini R, et al. Prevalence, clinical, and laboratory features of thrombocytopenia among HIV-infected individuals. AIDS Res Hum Retroviruses 1990;6(2):261–9.
46. Peltier JY, Lambin P, Doinel C, et al. Frequency and prognostic importance of thrombocytopenia in symptom-free HIV-infected individuals: a 5-year prospective study. AIDS 1991;5(4):381–4.
47. Mientjes GH, van Ameijden EJ, Mulder JW, et al. Prevalence of thrombocytopenia in HIV-infected and non-HIV infected drug users and homosexual men. Br J Haematol 1992;82(3):615–9.
48. Sloand EM, Klein HG, Banks SM, et al. Epidemiology of thrombocytopenia in HIV infection. Eur J Haematol 1992;48(3):168–72.
49. Sullivan PS, Hanson DL, Chu SY, et al. Surveillance for thrombocytopenia in persons infected with HIV: results from the multistate Adult and Adolescent Spectrum of Disease Project. J Acquir Immune Defic Syndr Hum Retrovirol 1997;14(4):374–9.
50. Stasi R. Therapeutic strategies for hepatitis- and other infection-related immune thrombocytopenias. Semin Hematol 2009;46(1 Suppl 2):S15–25.
51. Burbano X, Miguez MJ, Lecusay R, et al. Thrombocytopenia in HIV-infected drug users in the HAART era. Platelets 2001;12(8):456–61.
52. Landonio G, Galli M, Nosari A, et al. HIV-related severe thrombocytopenia in intravenous drug users: prevalence, response to therapy in a medium-term follow-up, and pathogenetic evaluation. AIDS 1990;4(1):29–34.
53. Ciernik IF, Cone RW, Fehr J, et al. Impaired liver function and retroviral activity are risk factors contributing to HIV-associated thrombocytopenia. Swiss HIV Cohort Study. AIDS 1999;13(14):1913–20.
54. Quan CM, Krajden M, Grigoriew GA, et al. Hepatitis C virus infection in patients infected with the human immunodeficiency virus. Clin Infect Dis 1993;17(1):117–9.
55. Quaranta JF, Delaney SR, Alleman S, et al. Prevalence of antibody to hepatitis C virus (HCV) in HIV-1-infected patients (nice SEROCO cohort). J Med Virol 1994;42(1):29–32.
56. Berhane K, Karim R, Cohen MH, et al. Impact of highly active antiretroviral therapy on anemia and relationship between anemia and survival in a large cohort of HIV-infected women: Women's Interagency HIV Study. J Acquir Immune Defic Syndr 2004;37(2):1245–52.
57. Levine AM, Karim R, Mack W, et al. Neutropenia in human immunodeficiency virus infection: data from the women's interagency HIV study. Arch Intern Med 2006;166(4):405–10.
58. Cole JL, Marzec UM, Gunthel CJ, et al. Ineffective platelet production in thrombocytopenic human immunodeficiency virus-infected patients. Blood 1998;91(9):3239–46.

59. Ballem PJ, Belzberg A, Devine DV, et al. Kinetic studies of the mechanism of thrombocytopenia in patients with human immunodeficiency virus infection. N Engl J Med 1992;327(25):1779–84.

60. Landonio G, Nosari A, Spinelli F, et al. HIV-related thrombocytopenia: four different clinical subsets. Haematologica 1992;77(5):398–401.

61. Najean Y, Rain JD. The mechanism of thrombocytopenia in patients with HIV infection. J Lab Clin Med 1994;123(3):415–20.

62. Karpatkin S, Nardi M, Lennette ET, et al. Anti-human immunodeficiency virus type 1 antibody complexes on platelets of seropositive thrombocytopenic homosexuals and narcotic addicts. Proc Natl Acad Sci U S A 1988;85(24):9763–7.

63. Bettaieb A, Fromont P, Louache F, et al. Presence of cross-reactive antibody between human immunodeficiency virus (HIV) and platelet glycoproteins in HIV-related immune thrombocytopenic purpura. Blood 1992;80(1):162–9.

64. Hohmann AW, Booth K, Peters V, et al. Common epitope on HIV p24 and human platelets. Lancet 1993;342(8882):1274–5.

65. Nardi MA, Liu LX, Karpatkin S. GPIIIa-(49-66) is a major pathophysiologically relevant antigenic determinant for anti-platelet GPIIIa of HIV-1-related immunologic thrombocytopenia. Proc Natl Acad Sci U S A 1997;94(14):7589–94.

66. Karpatkin S, Nardi MA, Hymes KB. Sequestration of anti-platelet GPIIIa antibody in rheumatoid factor immune complexes of human immunodeficiency virus 1 thrombocytopenic patients. Proc Natl Acad Sci U S A 1995;92(6):2263–7.

67. Li Z, Nardi MA, Karpatkin S. Role of molecular mimicry to HIV-1 peptides in HIV-1-related immunologic thrombocytopenia. Blood 2005;106(2):572–6.

68. Nardi M, Tomlinson S, Greco MA, et al. Complement-independent, peroxide-induced antibody lysis of platelets in HIV-1-related immune thrombocytopenia. Cell 2001;106(5):551–61.

69. Li Z, Nardi MA, Wu J, et al. Platelet fragmentation requires a specific structural conformation of human monoclonal antibody against beta3 integrin. J Biol Chem 2008;283(6):3224–30.

70. Koefoed K, Ditzel HJ. Identification of talin head domain as an immunodominant epitope of the antiplatelet antibody response in patients with HIV-1-associated thrombocytopenia. Blood 2004;104(13):4054–62.

71. Zucker-Franklin D, Termin CS, Cooper MC. Structural changes in the megakaryocytes of patients infected with the human immune deficiency virus (HIV-1). Am J Pathol 1989;134(6):1295–303.

72. Zucker-Franklin D, Seremetis S, Zheng ZY. Internalization of human immunodeficiency virus type I and other retroviruses by megakaryocytes and platelets. Blood 1990;75(10):1920–3.

73. Sakaguchi M, Sato T, Groopman JE. Human immunodeficiency virus infection of megakaryocytic cells. Blood 1991;77(3):481–5.

74. Kunzi MS, Groopman JE. Identification of a novel human immunodeficiency virus strain cytopathic to megakaryocytic cells. Blood 1993;81(12):3336–42.

75. Sato T, Sekine H, Kakuda H, et al. HIV infection of megakaryocytic cell lines. Leuk Lymphoma 2000;36(3–4):397–404.

76. Sundell IB, Koka PS. Thrombocytopenia in HIV infection: impairment of platelet formation and loss correlates with increased c-Mpl and ligand thrombopoietin expression. Curr HIV Res 2006;4(1):107–16.

77. Kowalska MA, Ratajczak J, Hoxie J, et al. Megakaryocyte precursors, megakaryocytes and platelets express the HIV co-receptor CXCR4 on their surface: determination of response to stromal-derived factor-1 by megakaryocytes and platelets. Br J Haematol 1999;104(2):220–9.

78. Zucker-Franklin D, Cao YZ. Megakaryocytes of human immunodeficiency virus-infected individuals express viral RNA. Proc Natl Acad Sci U S A 1989;86(14): 5595–9.
79. Bahner I, Kearns K, Coutinho S, et al. Infection of human marrow stroma by human immunodeficiency virus-1 (HIV-1) is both required and sufficient for HIV-1-induced hematopoietic suppression in vitro: demonstration by gene modification of primary human stroma. Blood 1997;90(5):1787–98.
80. Moses A, Nelson J, Bagby GC Jr. The influence of human immunodeficiency virus-1 on hematopoiesis. Blood 1998;91(5):1479–95.
81. Ragni MV, Bontempo FA, Myers DJ, et al. Hemorrhagic sequelae of immune thrombocytopenic purpura in human immunodeficiency virus-infected hemophiliacs. Blood 1990;75(6):1267–72.
82. Finazzi G, Mannucci PM, Lazzarin A, et al. Low incidence of bleeding from HIV-related thrombocytopenia in drug addicts and hemophiliacs: implications for therapeutic strategies. Eur J Haematol 1990;45(2):82–5.
83. Maeda S, Ogura K, Yoshida H, et al. Major virulence factors, VacA and CagA, are commonly positive in *Helicobacter pylori* isolates in Japan. Gut 1998; 42(3):338–43.
84. Servais J, Nkoghe D, Schmit JC, et al. HIV-associated hematologic disorders are correlated with plasma viral load and improve under highly active antiretroviral therapy. J Acquir Immune Defic Syndr 2001;28(3):221–5.
85. Landonio G, Cinque P, Nosari A, et al. Comparison of two dose regimens of zidovudine in an open, randomized, multicentre study for severe HIV-related thrombocytopenia. AIDS 1993;7(2):209–12.
86. Oksenhendler E, Bierling P, Ferchal F, et al. Zidovudine for thrombocytopenic purpura related to human immunodeficiency virus (HIV) infection. Ann Intern Med 1989;110(5):365–8.
87. Cinque P, Landonio G, Lazzarin A, et al. Long-term treatment with zidovudine in patients with human immunodeficiency virus (HIV)-associated thrombocytopenia: modes of response and correlation with markers of HIV replication. Eur J Haematol 1993;50(1):17–21.
88. Aboulafia DM, Bundow D, Waide S, et al. Initial observations on the efficacy of highly active antiretroviral therapy in the treatment of HIV-associated autoimmune thrombocytopenia. Am J Med Sci 2000;320(2):117–23.
89. Carbonara S, Fiorentino G, Serio G, et al. Response of severe HIV-associated thrombocytopenia to highly active antiretroviral therapy including protease inhibitors. J Infect 2001;42(4):251–6.
90. Miguez MJ, Burbano X, Archer H, et al. Limited impact of highly active antiretroviral therapy in thrombocytopenia. J Acquir Immune Defic Syndr 2002;30(2):260–1.
91. Schacter LP, Rozencweig M, Beltangady M, et al. Effects of therapy with didanosine on hematologic parameters in patients with advanced human immunodeficiency virus disease. Blood 1992;80(12):2969–76.
92. Nasti G, Errante D, Tirelli U. Successful treatment of HIV-1-related, zidovudine resistant, thrombocytopenia with didanosine. Am J Hematol 1997;55(2):118–9.
93. Marroni M, Gresele P, Landonio G, et al. Interferon-alpha is effective in the treatment of HIV-1-related, severe, zidovudine-resistant thrombocytopenia. A prospective, placebo-controlled, double-blind trial. Ann Intern Med 1994; 121(6):423–9.
94. Northfelt DW, Charlebois ED, Mirda MI, et al. Continuous low-dose interferon-alpha therapy for HIV-related immune thrombocytopenic purpura. J Acquir Immune Defic Syndr Hum Retrovirol 1995;8(1):45–50.

95. Oksenhendler E, Bierling P, Farcet JP, et al. Response to therapy in 37 patients with HIV-related thrombocytopenic purpura. Br J Haematol 1987;66(4):491–5.

96. Scaradavou A, Woo B, Woloski BM, et al. Intravenous anti-D treatment of immune thrombocytopenic purpura: experience in 272 patients. Blood 1997; 89(8):2689–700.

97. Leissinger CA, Andes WA. Role of splenectomy in the management of hemophilic patients with human immunodeficiency virus-associated immunopathic thrombocytopenic purpura. Am J Hematol 1992;40(3):207–9.

98. Oksenhendler E, Bierling P, Chevret S, et al. Splenectomy is safe and effective in human immunodeficiency virus-related immune thrombocytopenia. Blood 1993; 82(1):29–32.

99. Marroni M, Sinnone MS, Landonio G, et al. Splenic irradiation versus splenectomy for severe, refractory HIV-related thrombocytopenia: effects on platelet counts and immunological status. AIDS 2000;14(11):1664–7.

100. Harker LA, Carter RA, Marzec UM, et al. Correction of thrombocytopenia and ineffective platelet production in patients infected with human immunodeficiency virus (HIV) by PEG-rHuMGDF therapy. Blood 1998;92(Suppl 1):707a.

101. Suerbaum S, Michetti P. *Helicobacter pylori* infection. N Engl J Med 2002; 347(15):1175–86.

102. Gasbarrini A, Franceschi F, Tartaglione R, et al. Regression of autoimmune thrombocytopenia after eradication of *Helicobacter pylori*. Lancet 1998; 352(9131):878.

103. Jarque I, Andreu R, Llopis I, et al. Absence of platelet response after eradication of *Helicobacter pylori* infection in patients with chronic idiopathic thrombocytopenic purpura. Br J Haematol 2001;115(4):1002–3.

104. Kohda K, Kuga T, Kogawa K, et al. Effect of *Helicobacter pylori* eradication on platelet recovery in Japanese patients with chronic idiopathic thrombocytopenic purpura and secondary autoimmune thrombocytopenic purpura. Br J Haematol 2002;118(2):584–8.

105. Hino M, Yamane T, Park K, et al. Platelet recovery after eradication of *Helicobacter pylori* in patients with idiopathic thrombocytopenic purpura. Ann Hematol 2003;82(1):30–2.

106. Hashino S, Mori A, Suzuki S, et al. Platelet recovery in patients with idiopathic thrombocytopenic purpura after eradication of *Helicobacter pylori*. Int J Hematol 2003;77(2):188–91.

107. Ando K, Shimamoto T, Tauchi T, et al. Can eradication therapy for *Helicobacter pylori* really improve the thrombocytopenia in idiopathic thrombocytopenic purpura? Our experience and a literature review. Int J Hematol 2003;77(3): 239–44.

108. Michel M, Cooper N, Jean C, et al. Does *Helicobater pylori* initiate or perpetuate immune thrombocytopenic purpura? Blood 2004;103(3):890–6.

109. Takahashi T, Yujiri T, Shinohara K, et al. Molecular mimicry by *Helicobacter pylori* CagA protein may be involved in the pathogenesis of *H. pylori*-associated chronic idiopathic thrombocytopenic purpura. Br J Haematol 2004; 124(1):91–6.

110. Sato R, Murakami K, Watanabe K, et al. Effect of *Helicobacter pylori* eradication on platelet recovery in patients with chronic idiopathic thrombocytopenic purpura. Arch Intern Med 2004;164(17):1904–7.

111. Ando T, Tsuzuki T, Mizuno T, et al. Characteristics of *Helicobacter pylori*-induced gastritis and the effect of *H. pylori* eradication in patients with chronic idiopathic thrombocytopenic purpura. Helicobacter 2004;9(5):443–52.

112. Nomura S, Inami N, Kanazawa S. The effects of *Helicobacter pylori* eradication on chemokine production in patients with immune thrombocytopenic purpura. Eur J Haematol 2004;72(4):304–5.

113. Veneri D, De Matteis G, Solero P, et al. Analysis of B- and T-cell clonality and HLA class II alleles in patients with idiopathic thrombocytopenic purpura: correlation with *Helicobacter pylori* infection and response to eradication treatment. Platelets 2005;16(5):307–11.

114. Inaba T, Mizuno M, Take S, et al. Eradication of *Helicobacter pylori* increases platelet count in patients with idiopathic thrombocytopenic purpura in Japan. Eur J Clin Invest 2005;35(3):214–9.

115. Stasi R, Rossi Z, Stipa E, et al. *Helicobacter pylori* eradication in the management of patients with idiopathic thrombocytopenic purpura. Am J Med 2005; 118(4):414–9.

116. Fujimura K, Kuwana M, Kurata Y, et al. Is eradication therapy useful as the first line of treatment in *Helicobacter pylori*-positive idiopathic thrombocytopenic purpura? Analysis of 207 eradicated chronic ITP cases in Japan. Int J Hematol 2005;81(2):162–8.

117. Suzuki T, Matsushima M, Masui A, et al. Effect of *Helicobacter pylori* eradication in patients with chronic idiopathic thrombocytopenic purpura-a randomized controlled trial. Am J Gastroenterol 2005;100(6):1265–70.

118. Suvajdzic N, Stankovic B, Artiko V, et al. *Helicobacter pylori* eradication can induce platelet recovery in chronic idiopathic thrombocytopenic purpura. Platelets 2006;17(4):227–30.

119. Sayan O, Akyol Erikci A, Ozturk A. The efficacy of *Helicobacter pylori* eradication in the treatment of idiopathic thrombocytopenic purpura—the first study in Turkey. Acta Haematol 2006;116(2):146–9.

120. Asahi A, Kuwana M, Suzuki H, et al. Effects of a *Helicobacter pylori* eradication regimen on antiplatelet autoantibody response in infected and uninfected patients with idiopathic thrombocytopenic purpura. Haematologica 2006; 91(10):1436–7.

121. Kodama M, Kitadai Y, Ito M, et al. Immune response to CagA protein is associated with improved platelet count after *Helicobacter pylori* eradication in patients with idiopathic thrombocytopenic purpura. Helicobacter 2007;12(1):36–42.

122. Campuzano-Maya G. Proof of an association between *Helicobacter pylori* and idiopathic thrombocytopenic purpura in Latin America. Helicobacter 2007; 12(3):265–73.

123. Estrada-Gomez RA, Parra-Ortega I, Martinez-Barreda C, et al. *Helicobacter pylori* infection and thrombocytopenia: a single-institution experience in Mexico. Rev Invest Clin 2007;59(2):112–5.

124. Satake M, Nishikawa J, Fukagawa Y, et al. The long-term efficacy of *Helicobacter pylori* eradication therapy in patients with idiopathic thrombocytopenic purpura. J Gastroenterol Hepatol 2007;22(12):2233–7.

125. Emilia G, Luppi M, Zucchini P, et al. *Helicobacter pylori* infection and chronic immune thrombocytopenic purpura: long-term results of bacterium eradication and association with bacterium virulence profiles. Blood 2007;110(12):3833–41.

126. Jackson SC, Beck P, Buret AG, et al. Long term platelet responses to *Helicobacter pylori* eradication in Canadian patients with immune thrombocytopenic purpura. Int J Hematol 2008;88(2):212–8.

127. Graham DY, Kimura K, Shimoyama T, et al. *Helicobacter pylori* infection in Japan: current status and future options. Eur J Gastroenterol Hepatol 1994; 6(Suppl 1):S1–4.

128. Russo A, Eboli M, Pizzetti P, et al. Determinants of *Helicobacter pylori* seroprevalence among Italian blood donors. Eur J Gastroenterol Hepatol 1999;11(8): 867–73.

129. Franceschi F, Christodoulides N, Kroll MH, et al. *Helicobacter pylori* and idiopathic thrombocytopenic purpura. Ann Intern Med 2004;140(9):766–7.

130. Maeda S, Yoshida H, Ikenoue T, et al. Structure of cag pathogenicity island in Japanese *Helicobacter pylori* isolates. Gut 1999;44(3):336–41.

131. Bai Y, Wang Z, Bai X, et al. Cross-reaction of antibody against *Helicobacter pylori* urease B with platelet glycoprotein IIIa and its significance in the pathogenesis of immune thrombocytopenic purpura. Int J Hematol 2009;89(2):142–9.

132. Gerhard M, Rad R, Prinz C, et al. Pathogenesis of *Helicobacter pylori* infection. Helicobacter 2002;7(Suppl 1):17–23.

133. Semple JW, Aslam R, Kim M, et al. Platelet-bound lipopolysaccharide enhances Fc receptor-mediated phagocytosis of IgG-opsonized platelets. Blood 2007; 109(11):4803–5.

134. Asahi A, Nishimoto T, Okazaki Y, et al. *Helicobacter pylori* eradication shifts monocyte Fcgamma receptor balance toward inhibitory FcgammaRIIB in immune thrombocytopenic purpura patients. J Clin Invest 2008;118(8):2939–49.

135. Byrne MF, Kerrigan SW, Corcoran PA, et al. *Helicobacter pylori* binds von Willebrand factor and interacts with GPIb to induce platelet aggregation. Gastroenterology 2003;124(7):1846–54.

136. Cines DB. ITP: time to "bug off"? Blood 2007;110(12):3818–9.

137. Stasi R, Del Poeta G, Stipa E, et al. Response to B-cell depleting therapy with rituximab reverts the abnormalities of T-cell subsets in patients with idiopathic thrombocytopenic purpura. Blood 2007;110(8):2924–30.

138. Guo C, Chu X, Shi Y, et al. Correction of Th1-dominant cytokine profiles by high-dose dexamethasone in patients with chronic idiopathic thrombocytopenic purpura. J Clin Immunol 2007;27(6):557–62.

139. McCrae KA. *Helicobacter pylori* and ITP: many questions, few answers. Blood 2004;103(3):751–2.

140. Franchini M, Cruciani M, Mengoli C, et al. Effect of *Helicobacter pylori* eradication on platelet count in idiopathic thrombocytopenic purpura: a systematic review and meta-analysis. J Antimicrob Chemother 2007;60(2):237–46.

141. Fukui O, Shimoya K, Shimizu T, et al. *Helicobacter pylori* infection and platelet counts during pregnancy. Int J Gynaecol Obstet 2005;89(1):26–30.

142. Ahn ER, Tiede MP, Jy W, et al. Platelet activation in *Helicobacter pylori*-associated idiopathic thrombocytopenic purpura: eradication reduces platelet activation but seldom improves platelet counts. Acta Haematol 2006;116(1):19–24.

143. Stasi R, Sarpatwari A, Segal JB, et al. Effects of eradication of *Helicobacter pylori* infection in patients with immune thrombocytopenic purpura: a systematic review. Blood 2009;113(6):1231–40.

144. Tsumoto C, Tominaga K, Okazaki H, et al. Long-term efficacy of *Helicobacter pylori* eradication in patients with idiopathic thrombocytopenic purpura: 7-year follow-up prospective study. Ann Hematol 2009;88:789–93.

145. Levy AS, Bussel J. Immune thrombocytopenic purpura: investigation of the role of cytomegalovirus infection. Br J Haematol 2004;126(4):622–3.

146. Alliot C, Barrios M. Cytomegalovirus-induced thrombocytopenia in an immunocompetent adult effectively treated with intravenous immunoglobulin: a case report and review. Hematology 2005;10(4):277–9.

147. Crapnell K, Zanjani ED, Chaudhuri A, et al. In vitro infection of megakaryocytes and their precursors by human cytomegalovirus. Blood 2000;95(2):487–93.

148. Toyoda M, Petrosian A, Jordan SC. Immunological characterization of anti-endo-thelial cell antibodies induced by cytomegalovirus infection. Transplantation 1999;68(9):1311–8.
149. Ladhani S, Khatri P, El-Bashir H, et al. Imported malaria is a major cause of thrombocytopenia in children presenting to the emergency department in east London. Br J Haematol 2005;129(5):707–9.
150. Kumar A, Shashirekha. Thrombocytopenia—an indicator of acute vivax malaria. Indian J Pathol Microbiol 2006;49(4):505–8.
151. Jeremiah ZA, Uko EK. Depression of platelet counts in apparently healthy children with asymptomatic malaria infection in a Nigerian metropolitan city. Platelets 2007;18(6):469–71.
152. Jadhav UM, Patkar VS, Kadam NN. Thrombocytopenia in malaria–correlation with type and severity of malaria. J Assoc Physicians India 2004;52:615–8.
153. de Mast Q, Groot E, Lenting PJ, et al. Thrombocytopenia and release of activated von Willebrand factor during early *Plasmodium falciparum* malaria. J Infect Dis 2007;196(4):622–8.

Immune Thrombocytopenia in Pregnancy

Evi Stavrou, MD[a], Keith R. McCrae, MD[a,b],*

KEYWORDS

- Thrombocytopenia • Pregnancy
- Thrombotic thrombocytopenic purpura • Preeclampsia
- Immune thrombocytopenia • Microangiopathic

Thrombocytopenia complicates up to 10% of all pregnancies, and may result from a number of causes (**Table 1**). Some of these are unique to pregnancy, whereas others may occur with increased frequency during gestation,[1–7] and still others bear no relationship to pregnancy per se. Although some thrombocytopenic disorders are not associated with adverse pregnancy outcomes, others are associated with significant maternal or neonatal morbidity and mortality. The time of onset of these disorders during pregnancy and their clinical manifestations often overlap, making the diagnosis challenging.

Immune thrombocytopenia (ITP) is one of the thrombocytopenic disorders that may complicate pregnancy and its management. This article focuses on the clinical characteristics and management of ITP in pregnancy, and also includes brief discussions on additional thrombocytopenic disorders that may occur in pregnancy and potentially be confused with ITP.

ITP IN PREGNANCY
Clinical Features

ITP[8] occurs in 1 or 2 of every 1000 pregnancies,[9] and accounts for 5% of cases of pregnancy-associated thrombocytopenia. Despite its rarity compared with gestational thrombocytopenia, ITP is the most common cause of isolated thrombocytopenia in the first and early second trimesters.[3,6,9–11] The pathophysiology of ITP has been classically believed to reflect the accelerated clearance of platelets coated by IgG antiplatelet autoantibodies. These antibodies recognize specific epitopes

[a] Division of Hematology-Oncology, Case Western Reserve University School of Medicine, 10900 Euclid Avenue, Cleveland, OH 44106, USA
[b] Case Western Reserve University School of Medicine, 2103 Cornell Road, WRB 2-132, Cleveland, OH 44106, USA
* Corresponding author. Case Western Reserve University School of Medicine, 2103 Cornell Road, WRB 2-132, Cleveland, OH 44106.
E-mail address: keith.mccrae@case.edu (K.R. McCrae).

Hematol Oncol Clin N Am 23 (2009) 1299–1316
doi:10.1016/j.hoc.2009.08.005
0889-8588/09/$ – see front matter © 2009 Elsevier Inc. All rights reserved.

hemonc.theclinics.com

Table 1
Causes of pregnancy-associated thrombocytopenia

Isolated Thrombocytopenia	Thrombocytopenia Associated with Systemic Disorders
Gestational (incidental)	Microangiopathic
Immune (ITP)	Preeclampsia
Drug induced	HELLP syndrome
HIT (with or without thrombosis)	HUS
Inherited	TTP
Type IIb von Willebrand disease	Disseminated intravascular coagulation
	Acute fatty liver of pregnancy
	Collagen vascular diseases
	Systemic lupus erythematosus
	Antiphospholipid syndrome
	Others
	Viral infections
	HBV
	EBV
	CMV
	Nutritional deficiencies
	Hypersplenism
	Bone marrow dysfunction

Abbreviations: CMV, cytomegalovirus; EBV, Epstein-Barr virus; HBV, hepatitis B virus; HIT, heparin-induced thrombocytopenia; HUS, hemolytic uremic syndrome; ITP, immune thrombocytopenia; TTP, thrombotic thrombocytopenic purpura.

expressed on platelet glycoproteins, such as glycoprotein IIb/IIIa, or less commonly glycoproteins Ib/IX or Ia/IIa.[12] These antibody-coated platelets are then removed following binding to macrophage Fcγ receptors, primarily in the spleen.[9,13–16] Some antiplatelet antibodies may also directly activate complement.[17] Recent studies indicate, however, that several other mechanisms also contribute to the pathogenesis of ITP, including diminished platelet production,[18,19] caused at least in part by antibodies that cross react with megakaryocytes,[19] and alterations in T-cell subsets, in particular loss of regulatory T cells.[20] Whether the role of any of these mechanisms is of particular importance in the setting of pregnancy has not been determined.

The presentation of ITP in pregnancy is much like that in the nonpregnant individual. Patients may be diagnosed following the detection of asymptomatic thrombocytopenia on routine testing, or less commonly with more severe thrombocytopenia accompanied by bruising, bleeding, and petechiae. ITP that predates pregnancy may either worsen or remain quiescent during gestation.[21,22] One study that reviewed the experience of 92 women with ITP during 119 pregnancies over an 11-year period found that women with previously diagnosed ITP were less likely to require therapy for ITP than those with newly diagnosed ITP.[23]

Diagnosis

As in the nonpregnant state, the diagnosis of ITP is a clinical diagnosis of exclusion. The likelihood that a patient suffers from ITP rather than incidental thrombocytopenia of pregnancy increases as the platelet count decreases; however, no specific platelet count below which incidental thrombocytopenia may be excluded has been defined. Furthermore, because many patients with apparent incidental thrombocytopenia have elevated levels of platelet-associated IgG, platelet antibody tests do not differentiate these syndromes.[24] In a large study using the monoclonal antibody-specific immobilization of platelet-antigens assay (MAIPA), less than 7% of thrombocytopenic pregnant women were found to have autoantibodies, and there was no significant difference in the prevalence of autoantibodies between thrombocytopenic and non-thrombocytopenic pregnant women.[24-27] The most useful means of differentiating these syndromes is, by definition, the antenatal history.[28,29] A history of prior thrombocytopenia, underlying autoimmune disease, or severe thrombocytopenia (<50,000/μL) makes the diagnosis of ITP more likely. In the absence of a platelet count before pregnancy, significant thrombocytopenia in the first trimester, with a declining platelet count as gestation progresses, is most consistent with ITP. In contrast, mild thrombocytopenia developing in the second or third trimester and not associated with hypertension or proteinuria most likely represents incidental thrombocytopenia.[11]

Other relevant questions that should be assessed when evaluating a pregnant patient with thrombocytopenia include whether prior deliveries were complicated by excessive bleeding, and whether the infant had thrombocytopenia or bleeding complications. The physical examination should focus on excluding secondary causes of thrombocytopenia. For example, elevated blood pressure or the onset of peripheral edema or weight gain may suggest thrombocytopenia complicating a pregnancy-associated hypertensive disorder.[30] In addition, symptoms potentially consistent with the early development of the HELLP syndrome, such as vague right upper quadrant pain, increasing malaise, or unrelenting cephalgia, should be specifically sought.[31,32] Finally, all thrombocytopenic pregnant patients should be carefully evaluated for the presence of risk factors for HIV and hepatitis C virus (HCV) infection.[33]

Laboratory investigation of the pregnant patient with suspected ITP should include a complete blood count and platelet count. Examination of the peripheral blood film is essential to exclude not only pseudothrombocytopenia, but other thrombocytopenic disorders, such as thrombotic thrombocytopenic purpura (TTP) or preeclampsia, in which the peripheral blood film may reveal increased numbers of fragmented red cells.[30] Other studies that should be considered include liver enzyme tests, urinalysis, and HIV and HCV testing. Bone marrow examination is not recommended unless other hematologic abnormalities (other than mild pregnancy-associated anemia) or unusual findings on physical examination are identified. As in nonpregnant individuals, a lack of response to standard ITP therapy in a pregnant patient with thrombocytopenia should prompt consideration of a bone marrow examination.

Maternal Management During Gestation

The clinical management of pregnancy-associated ITP is a complex task, requiring close collaboration between the obstetrician and hematologist. Pregnant women with ITP require careful monitoring, and should be seen monthly in the first and second trimester, every 2 weeks after 28 weeks, and weekly after 36 weeks. Visits should involve routine obstetric care with emphasis on blood pressure, weight, urine dipstick analysis for protein, and serial platelet counts. Decisions concerning the need for therapy are determined primarily by the patient's symptoms, particularly whether active bleeding is present, although the absolute platelet count should be considered as term approaches due to the potential need for epidural anesthesia. The American Society of Hematology (ASH) and British Committee for Standards in Hematology General Hematology Task Force (BCSH) guidelines consider treatment to be appropriate for severe thrombocytopenia or thrombocytopenia associated with bleeding. There is no evidence, however, to support the opinion that platelet counts should be kept higher in the asymptomatic pregnant woman than in other thrombocytopenic patients.[34] More aggressive treatment is recommended later in pregnancy to prepare the patient for labor and delivery, which often is accompanied by the use of epidural anesthesia.

Treatment has been recommended for women with a platelet count below 10,000/μL at any time during pregnancy, or below 30,000/μL in the second or third trimester or when associated with bleeding.[16,35–37] There is lack of consensus in regard to treatment of patients with a platelet count of less than 30,000/μL but no bleeding in the first trimester, reflecting the desire to avoid exposure of such patients to corticosteroids during pregnancy.[16,37,38] Although treatment of the pregnant woman with ITP generally does not differ significantly from that of nonpregnant individuals, there are some unique considerations.[39–42] Because of their efficacy and low cost, many consider corticosteroids to be first-line treatment for ITP in pregnancy.[10,14,36] The mechanisms of action of corticosteroids are caused, at least in part, by the inhibition of phagocytosis of opsonized platelets and impairment of autoantibody production.[11,43] The typical therapeutic dose of prednisone is 1 mg/kg/d (based on the prepregnancy weight), which after achieving a response is gradually titrated to the lowest effective dose. The many adverse effects of corticosteroids are amplified during pregnancy, however, and pregnancy-specific toxicities, such as gestational diabetes, weight gain, acceleration of bone loss, hypertension, and possibly placental abruption and premature labor, must be recognized.[7,38] Furthermore, some studies have associated the use of corticosteroids in the first trimester with congenital anomalies, such as orofacial clefts.[44,45] Appreciation of such toxicities might suggest that in the patient in whom therapy is indicated but not urgent, initiation of corticosteroid therapy at a low dose (perhaps 20–30 mg/d of prednisone) should be considered. Alternatively, others have suggested that intravenous immunoglobulin (IVIg) should be the first-line therapy for pregnancy-associated ITP, especially when a long duration of therapy may not be required.[11]

Treatment with high-dose (ie, 2 g/kg over 2–5 days) IVIg is an effective means of raising the platelet count rapidly. Although the therapeutic effects of IVIg likely reflect a number of mechanisms, a critical requirement for FcRγ IIb, an inhibitory FcRγ receptor, has been defined in animal models.[46] Compared with corticosteroids, IVIg is less likely to induce toxicities, such as hypertension.[23,34] ASH guidelines consider IVIg to be an appropriate first-line agent for severe thrombocytopenia, or thrombocytopenic bleeding in the third trimester.[47] Responses to IVIg tend to be transient, however, and multiple courses of therapy may be required at significant cost and patient inconvenience. A subset of patients who fail to respond satisfactorily to corticosteroids or IVIg alone may respond to high doses of these agents when administered in combination (methylprednisolone, 1g, IVIg, 1–2 g/kg).[2,10]

Splenectomy may be considered as another option for patients who fail to adequately respond to corticosteroids or IVIg. Remission of ITP is initially achieved in approximately 75% of pregnant women who undergo splenectomy.[48] If required, splenectomy should be performed in the second trimester, because surgery earlier in pregnancy may induce premature labor, and later in pregnancy splenectomy may be technically difficult because of obstruction of the surgical field by the gravid uterus.[2,4] Laparoscopic splenectomy can be safely performed in pregnant women.[49] **Table 2** summarizes the antepartum management of pregnant women with ITP.

In patients who develop severe ITP refractory to steroids and IVIg, and who are beyond the optimal second trimester window for splenectomy, intravenous anti-D has been used successfully. In one report, six of eight women who received anti-D in their second and third trimester had partial responses, with no major maternal or fetal complications, and no evidence of hydrops.[47] Experience with this agent in pregnancy is limited, however, and its safety in this setting has not been clearly established.

Other agents used to treat ITP in the nonpregnant population, namely cytotoxic and immunosuppressive agents, are potential teratogens.[50–52] For this reason, danazol,

Table 2
Medical management of ITP in pregnancy: ASH and BCSH guidelines

	ASH	BCSH
Treatment indications	Platelets <10,000/μL Platelets 10,000–30,000/μL in 2nd or 3rd trimester Bleeding	Platelets <20,000/μL, unless deliver imminent
IVIg	Initial treatment: 3rd trimester and platelets <10,000/μL Initial treatment: platelets 10,000–30,000/μL and bleeding After steroid failure: platelets <10,000/μL After steroid failure: platelets 10,000–30,000/μL and bleeding After steroid failure: 3rd trimester, platelets 10,000–30,000/μL, asymptomatic	Oral corticosteroids and IVIg have similar responses as in nonpregnant state
Splenectomy	2nd trimester, platelets <10,000/μL, bleeding	If essential, in the second trimester Laparoscopic approach advantageous
Safe platelet count for delivery	50,000/μL	Vaginal delivery: 50,000/μL Cesarean section: 80,000/μL Epidural anesthesia: 80,000/μL

Abbreviations: ASH, American Society of Hematology; BSCH, British Committee for Standards in Haematology; ITP, immune thrombocytopenia; IVIg, intravenous immune-globulin.

cyclophosphamide, and vinca alkaloids should be avoided in pregnancy. Azathioprine is a possible exception that has been used safely in pregnant patients with renal transplants.[53–55] Neonatal hematologic and immune impairment have been reported in some exposed infants, however, and azathioprine remains a category D agent. Rituximab has been used in several pregnant patients with lymphoma. No major fetal malformations have been associated with its use,[56] although infants born to mothers treated with this agent may experience abnormal B-lymphocyte development in their first year of life. In a few case reports, immunologic recovery was observed at 6 months of life with no infection-related complications.[57] Because of the lack of sufficient evidence of safety, most recommend that rituximab be avoided in the treatment of pregnancy-associated ITP.[58] In general, the use of cytotoxic and immunosuppressive agents should be limited to severe cases refractory to other treatments. These agents should be used in the second and third trimesters only and each case should be considered individually.

There is very little experience with either of the thrombopoietic agents in pregnancy, and both are considered category C for this indication. A pregnancy registry has been developed for patients who become pregnant while taking either Eltrombopag or Romiplostim. Likewise, it is not known whether either of these agents is excreted in human milk, and their safety in nursing mothers has not been established.

Management of Parturition: Fetal and Maternal Considerations

In managing delivery of the pregnant patient with ITP, some unique issues must be considered. In terms of maternal management, the primary consideration is achieving a platelet count sufficient to minimize maternal hemorrhage not only during vaginal delivery, but in case of cesarean section. Epidural anesthesia is also commonly used during parturition, and adequate hemostasis is required to minimize the risk of any resulting neurologic complications that might arise. The ASH guidelines (**Table 3**) suggest that a maternal platelet count of 50,000/μL is sufficient for vaginal delivery and cesarean section. The BCSH guidelines recommend that a platelet count of 80,000/μL be attained for cesarean delivery and for epidural anesthesia, based on a retrospective review in which epidural anesthesia was successfully delivered with no neurologic complications in 30 thrombocytopenic women with platelet counts between 69,000 and 98,000/μL.[59] Although no prospective, randomized data are available to address this issue definitively, most experts consider a platelet count in the range of 80,000/μL adequate for epidural anesthesia and either vaginal delivery or cesarean section in the parturient. Because this may be significantly higher than the therapeutic platelet count range targeted earlier in pregnancy, additional therapy may be required in some pregnant patients as term approaches.

Unique considerations also exist with respect to the fetal platelet count and the risk of intracranial hemorrhage during delivery. Maternal IgG is actively transported to the fetal circulation subsequent to its binding to Fcγ receptors on the syncytiotrophoblast cells of the placenta.[60–62] These maternal platelet-reactive antibodies may cross react with antigens on fetal platelets, leading to the development of fetal thrombocytopenia, which is associated with an increased risk for hemorrhage during delivery. In a large meta-analysis that reviewed series containing 10 or more patients in whom fetal platelet counts were determined, 288 live-born infants were identified. Platelet counts below 50,000/μL were observed in 10.1% of these infants, whereas platelet counts below 20,000/μL occurred in 4.2%.[63]

The most feared consequence of fetal thrombocytopenia is the risk of intracranial hemorrhage, which in theory has been expected to be increased by head trauma occurring during passage of the fetus through the birth canal during vaginal delivery. Despite this concern, the risk of fetal intracranial hemorrhage in the offspring of patients with ITP is very low. In the meta-analysis noted in the preceding paragraph, no cases of fetal

Table 3
Management of delivery in patients with pregnancy-associated ITP: ASH and BCSH guidelines

	ASH	BCSH
Cordocentesis or fetal scalp sampling	Not necessarily required Unnecessary in women without known ITP	Not recommended
Cesarean section	In selected circumstances Appropriate if fetal platelet count is <20,000/μL Not indicated if fetal platelet count unknown Not indicated if maternal platelet count >50,000/μL	Obstetric indications only
Safe platelet count for delivery	Vaginal delivery: 50,000/μL Cesarean section: 50,000/μL	Vaginal delivery: 50,000/μL Cesarean section: 80,000/μL Epidural anesthesia: 80,000/μL

Abbreviations: ASH, American Society of Hematology; BSCH, British Committee for Standards in Haematology; ITP, immune thrombocytopenia; IVIg, intravenous immune-globulin.

intracranial hemorrhage were observed.[63] In another large observational study, the incidence of intracranial hemorrhage was below 1%.[38] In this report, the course of 284 mothers with ITP and their 286 newborn infants was described.[38] Neonatal thrombocytopenia (platelet count <100,000/μL) was diagnosed in 22.6% of the offspring, although only 6.3% experienced bleeding events, and there were no episodes of intracranial hemorrhage. There was no correlation between platelet counts or the ITP status of the mothers and the development of neonatal thrombocytopenia, an observation that has been reported in almost all studies that have examined this issue. Indeed, there is no consistent or reproducible correlation between the fetal platelet count at delivery and a number of maternal characteristics including the severity of maternal thrombocytopenia,[10,11] or the level of circulating maternal antiplatelet IgG.[29] Evidence suggests that, of all parameters studied, the most reliable predictor of neonatal thrombocytopenia is a history of thrombocytopenia at delivery in a prior sibling.[64]

Because of the inability to predict neonatal thrombocytopenia based on maternal clinical characteristics, invasive procedures, such as fetal scalp sampling during labor or percutaneous umbilical blood sampling, have been developed. Fetal scalp vein sampling is technically difficult; platelet counts obtained through this procedure have not been shown to correlate with the platelet count at delivery[65] and may falsely predict thrombocytopenia, possibly caused by clotting of blood during sampling. In contrast, percutaneous umbilical blood sampling is often able to yield accurate platelet counts, but is associated with complication rates of up to 2%, approximately half of which may necessitate emergent delivery and ultimately result in pregnancy loss.[65–67] The risks of fetal platelet count determination are at the least equal to and likely exceed that of fetal intracranial hemorrhage, negating its clinical use.[34,47,66,68]

Although it was previously believed that cesarean section reduced the risk of fetal intracranial hemorrhage during delivery of offspring of patients with ITP, studies over the last two decades have demonstrated that this does not seem to be the case.[11,47] In one study, 31 pregnancies in 25 women with ITP over a 10-year period were reviewed.[69] Fourteen infants were born vaginally, and 18 by cesarean, with no complications in any, despite platelet counts below 100,000/μL in five infants, and below 50,000/μL in two.[69] These authors also reviewed literature reports of 474 infants born to mothers with ITP, finding that platelet counts below 50,000/μL occurred in 15%, and intracranial hemorrhage in 3%. No association of intracranial hemorrhage with the mode of delivery was observed.[69] In another retrospective review of 601 infants of mothers with ITP, severe neonatal thrombocytopenia was reported in 72 (12%), with relatively equal numbers of these babies being delivered by vaginal delivery (N = 307) or cesarean section (N = 247). Six infants developed intracranial hemorrhage, two of which were delivered by cesarean section. Four of these six infants had severe neonatal thrombocytopenia.[29,65,66,69–80] Given the fact that neonatal intracranial hemorrhage is an extremely rare complication of maternal ITP,[65] and that cesarean deliveries may be associated with significant maternal morbidity, it is generally recommended that cesarean section be performed solely for maternal indications.

Following delivery, serial platelet counts should be obtained in all newborns at birth and during the first week postpartum, because the onset of thrombocytopenia caused by maternal antiplatelet IgG may be delayed. In a study of 61 infants born to ITP mothers, 66% of neonates experienced a further fall in their platelet counts after birth, with 54% reaching their nadir by day 2. The platelet count stabilized or began to rise by day 7 in all infants.[75] ASH guidelines suggest that infants with a platelet count below 20,000/μL, or those with hemorrhage, receive treatment. IVIg at a dose of 1 g/kg is effective in inducing a prompt rise in the platelet count; the concurrent use of corticosteroids is controversial because of a possible predisposition to neonatal sepsis. Imaging of the brain with ultrasonography, CT, or MRI should be performed in all newborns with platelet counts of less than 50,000/μL to exclude the possibility of occult intracranial hemorrhage that may require prompt intervention. Finally, women with ITP should not be discouraged from breast-feeding, because there has been no firm association established between breast-feeding and neonatal thrombocytopenia.[43]

OTHER CAUSES OF THROMBOCYTOPENIA IN PREGNANCY

The differential diagnosis of ITP in a pregnant patient is wide, certainly much larger than in the nonpregnant setting. Determining the appropriate diagnosis with the greatest degree of certainty is essential to initiating appropriate therapy. An understanding of other causes of thrombocytopenia in pregnancy is useful in differentiating these from ITP, and is discussed briefly next.

Gestational Incidental Thrombocytopenia

Population-based studies demonstrate that a physiologic decline in the platelet count of approximately 10% occurs during uncomplicated pregnancy, with the decline being greatest in the third trimester.[81] Despite this decrease, however, the platelet count usually remains in the normal range throughout gestation.[3,10] Gestational or "incidental" thrombocytopenia of pregnancy may represent a more severe variant of this physiologic thrombocytopenia, although its pathogenesis is not well defined.

Gestational thrombocytopenia is the most common cause of thrombocytopenia in pregnancy, affecting 5% of all pregnancies and accounting for more than 75% of cases of pregnancy-associated thrombocytopenia.[4,6,10,25,82–84] This disorder usually develops in the late second or third trimester and generally affects women with no prior history of ITP or autoimmune disease. It is characterized by mild thrombocytopenia not accompanied by abnormal physical findings, such as hypertension, that would implicate other causes of thrombocytopenia. Although no absolute value of the platelet count below which gestational thrombocytopenia can be excluded has been defined, the ASH and the BCSH suggest that at platelet counts below 70,000/μL or 80,000/μL, respectively, gestational thrombocytopenia becomes increasingly less likely and other causes of thrombocytopenia should be more strongly considered.[36,37]

Gestational thrombocytopenia is not associated with an increased incidence of pregnancy-related complications or the delivery of thrombocytopenic offspring.[2,4,6,25,82,83] Evaluation of healthy pregnant women with no history of prior thrombocytopenia and a platelet count greater than 70,000/μL may be limited to a physical examination and a thorough inspection of the peripheral blood film.[35] Confirmation of a normal platelet count before pregnancy may also be very useful in diagnosing this disorder.[37] Some of the more severe cases of gestational thrombocytopenia cannot be reliably distinguished from mild cases of ITP,[1,23] because platelet counts in these two disorders overlap and patients with either disorder may be otherwise asymptomatic.

Preeclampsia and the HELLP Syndrome

Preeclampsia affects 3% to 14% of pregnancies and is the most common medical disorder of pregnancy.[85] In contrast to ITP, preeclampsia usually occurs in the third trimester[85,86] affecting women less than 20 or greater than 30 years of age.[87,88] The criteria for preeclampsia include hypertension (systolic blood pressure ≥140 mm

Hg, diastolic blood pressure $\geq$ 90 mm Hg) and proteinuria (>300 mg protein/24 hours) developing after 20 weeks of gestation.[88] A genetic role in the development of preeclampsia is likely, but remains incompletely defined[89]; some studies demonstrate paternal and maternal genetic influences.[89]

Thrombocytopenia develops in approximately 50% of patients with preeclampsia, and may precede other manifestations.[10] Despite this complex constellation of symptoms, thrombocytopenia may occasionally be the presenting manifestation of preeclampsia, and preeclampsia should be considered in patients presenting with isolated thrombocytopenia, particularly during the later stages of pregnancy. The mechanisms of thrombocytopenia in patients with preeclampsia and thrombocytopenia are uncertain, but the presence of normal to increased numbers of megakaryocytes in these patients suggests that this results from a compensated thrombocytolytic state.[90]

The pathogenesis of preeclampsia is poorly understood, but several studies have demonstrated that it is initiated and mediated by factors within the placenta.[91–93] Placentation, the process by which fetal trophoblasts invade the endometrium and remodel the uterine vasculature, seems to be disordered.[94–96] Abnormalities in the expression of cell adhesion molecules,[97] vascular endothelial growth factor, and vascular endothelial growth factor receptors by trophoblasts have been described.[10] The net result of such a process is the development of fetoplacental ischemia,[92] which leads to impaired release and metabolism of prostaglandins.[4] The diminished production of prostacyclin (PGI_2), PGE_2, and the augmented production of thromboxane and prostaglandin $F_2\alpha$ has been reported to contribute to the development of hypertension, reduced placental flow, and platelet activation.[91,98]

The HELLP syndrome is often considered to be a variant of preeclampsia. It occurs in about 0.5% to 0.9% of all pregnancies and in 10% to 20% of cases with severe preeclampsia.[99,100] Like preeclampsia, most cases occur in the third trimester with about 10% occurring before week 27, and 20% beyond gestational week 37.[101] This disorder occurs primarily in white, multiparous women above the age of 25 years who present with nausea, malaise, and right upper quadrant pain or epigastric pain.[32,102,103] The triad of microangiopathic hemolytic anemia (MAHA), abnormal liver function (AST $\geq$70 U/L), and thrombocytopenia with a platelet count less than 100,000/μL constitutes the diagnostic criteria of HELLP.[104] Other signs suggestive of hemolysis include an elevated lactate dehydrogenase ($\geq$600 IU/L) and increased bilirubin levels ($\geq$1.2 mg/dL). Unlike preeclampsia, proteinuria is generally minimal or absent.[105] Despite their similarities, HELLP is associated with significantly greater maternal and fetal morbidity and mortality than preeclampsia.[106] This symptom profile should generally allow one to distinguish HELLP from ITP with relative certainty, although as with preeclampsia, thrombocytopenia may be an early presenting feature of HELLP.

The overall approach to management of either of these syndromes involves medical stabilization of the patient, followed by delivery of the fetus.[105–107] Because most cases of preeclampsia and HELLP develop after 34 weeks of gestation, by which time the fetal lung has adequately matured,[79] immediate delivery is considered to be the definite treatment. Therapy in the setting of severe thrombocytopenia and bleeding may require platelet transfusion; however, because the mechanism of thrombocytopenia in these cases is accelerated platelet destruction, survival of transfused platelets is short.[106]

Thrombotic Thrombocytopenic Purpura and the Hemolytic Uremic Syndrome

TTP and hemolytic uremic syndrome (HUS) are characterized by MAHA and thrombocytopenia. Although neither disease is unique to pregnancy, the incidence of these disorders is clearly increased in pregnant women.

TTP is characterized by a pentad of findings that include MAHA; thrombocytopenia; neurologic abnormalities (including confusion, headache, weakness, and in some cases seizures); fever; and renal dysfunction.[4,10] This complete set of symptoms occurs in only 40% of patients, and more than 70% have only the triad of MAHA, thrombocytopenia, and neurologic changes at the time of diagnosis.[4,108] The clinical manifestations of HUS are similar, although often predominated by renal abnormalities as opposed to neurologic abnormalities in patients with TTP.[109] In a patient exhibiting the full spectrum of abnormalities associated with TTP or HUS, distinction from ITP should be straightforward, although as with preeclampsia and HELLP, thrombocytopenia may be a predominant early finding that should lead the clinician to look for accompanying manifestations, such as MAHA, renal dysfunction, and subtle neurologic abnormalities. Discriminating features between these disorders are listed in **Table 4**.

The pathogenesis of TTP involves the congenital or acquired deficiency of the von Willebrand factor–cleaving protease[109–113] ADAMTS13. Levels of ADAMTS13 are markedly decreased in patients with TTP, usually secondary to antibodies against the protease,[112,114] or more rarely, a congenital deficiency caused by mutation of the ADAMTS13 gene.[110] HUS may present with a variety of manifestations, with one variant occurring after *Escherichia coli* O157:H7 gastroenteritis, primarily in children.[115] In adults, however, HUS occurs most commonly in association with pregnancy, with more than 90% of cases developing in the postpartum period.[116]

Miscellaneous Causes of Thrombocytopenia in Pregnancy

In addition to the disorders described previously, other obstetric entities, such as amniotic fluid embolism,[117] placental abruption,[118] uterine rupture,[119] and retention of a dead fetus,[120] may be associated with disseminated intravascular coagulation, which can induce a consumptive thrombocytopenia.

Acute fatty liver of pregnancy typically presents in primiparas between gestational weeks 30 and 38,[121] with a 1- to 2-week history of malaise, anorexia, nausea, vomiting, epigastric or right upper quadrant pain, mental status changes, and cholestatic liver abnormalities. Laboratory examination reveals hemoconcentration, metabolic acidosis, mild thrombocytopenia, and low-grade disseminated intravascular coagulation with low serum fibrinogen, low antithrombin, and prolonged prothrombin time.[109,121]

Although not unique to pregnancy, drug-induced thrombocytopenia should always be considered when evaluating a pregnant patient with low platelet counts. Of note, acute cocaine ingestion has been associated with a syndrome resembling HELLP, and may be accompanied by the transient development of profound thrombocytopenia.[122]

Pseudothrombocytopenia, an in vitro artifact attributable to platelet clumping caused by EDTA-dependent antiplatelet antibodies, may be transferred from the mother to fetus because of transplacental passage of the antibodies.

Systemic lupus erythematosus is the collagen-vascular disorder most commonly compromising pregnancy.[123] Thrombocytopenia occurs in approximately 15% to 26% of patients with systemic lupus erythematosus, and results from increased peripheral platelet destruction induced by antiplatelet antibodies or circulating immune complexes (secondary ITP).[124] In addition, approximately 25% of patients with systemic lupus erythematosus have antiphospholipid antibodies, which have been associated with both thrombocytopenia[125] and preeclampsia.[126]

HIV or hepatitis C–associated thrombocytopenia should be considered in any pregnant woman and may be initially diagnosed during pregnancy. Finally, type IIb von

Table 4
Differential diagnosis of pregnancy-associated thrombocytopenia

	MAHA	Thrombocytopenia	Coagulopathy	Hypertension	Renal Disease	CNS Disease	Peak Time of Onset
ITP	—	+/+++	—	—	—	—	1st–2nd trimester
Gestational "incidental"	—	+	—	—	—	—	2nd–3rd trimester
Preeclampsia	+	+	±	+++	+	+	3rd trimester
HELLP	++	+++	+	±	+	±	3rd trimester
HUS	++	++	±	±	+++	±	Postpartum
TTP	+++	+++	±	±	+/±	+++	2 trimester, term
SLE	+	+	±	±	+/++	+	Anytime
AFLP	+	+/±	+++	±	±	+	3rd trimester

Abbreviations: AFLP, acute fatty liver of pregnancy; CNS, central nervous system; HUS, hemolytic uremic syndrome; MAHA, microangiopathic hemolytic anemia; SLE, systemic lupus erythematosus; TTP, thrombotic thrombocytopenic purpura; ±, variably present; +, mild; ++, moderate; +++, severe.

Data from McCrae, KR. Thrombocytopenia in pregnancy: differential diagnosis, pathogenesis and management. Blood Rev 2003;17:10.

Willebrand disease is an unusual cause of thrombocytopenia in pregnancy, in which the estrogen-rich environment induces an increased production of von Willebrand factor, which in the case of the type IIb von Willebrand disease variant may further accelerate platelet clearance.[127,128]

SUMMARY

ITP is an uncommon, but important cause of thrombocytopenia in pregnancy. Although most commonly presenting in the first trimester, ITP may present at any point during gestation. Although ITP is associated with a significant incidence of neonatal thrombocytopenia, it is generally not associated with major morbidity if properly managed. IVIg and low-dose corticosteroids comprise the mainstays of treatment in ITP, but high doses of corticosteroids or prolonged corticosteroid therapy are associated with significant toxicity in the pregnant patient and should be avoided. Despite the development of severe thrombocytopenia in approximately 5% to 10% of the offspring of patients with ITP, the incidence of neonatal intracranial hemorrhage in these individuals is extremely low. Invasive procedures for establishing the fetal platelet count are associated with a degree of risk that likely exceeds that of fetal intracranial hemorrhage, and are not indicated in most cases. Moreover, delivery by cesarean section has not been shown to decrease the risk of neonatal intracranial hemorrhage compared with vaginal delivery, and the mode of delivery in pregnant patients with ITP should be solely dictated by maternal factors.

The diagnosis of ITP in pregnancy is complicated by a wide differential diagnosis that includes several other disorders that can cause thrombocytopenia in this setting. Gestational or incidental thrombocytopenia remains the most common cause of thrombocytopenia in pregnancy, accounting for approximately 75% of cases, and may be impossible to distinguish from mild ITP. Gestational thrombocytopenia is not associated, however, with adverse maternal or fetal outcomes. Preeclampsia, the HELLP syndrome, and TTP-HUS are other disorders that may cause thrombocytopenia in pregnancy. These disorders are generally not difficult to distinguish from ITP, but in some individuals the presenting feature may be thrombocytopenia, and these disorders should be considered in any pregnant patient with a low platelet count. Meticulous attention to accurate diagnosis of these disorders generally allows them to be separated from ITP, and is critical for their successful management.

REFERENCES

1. McCrae K. Thrombocytopenia in pregnancy. In: Michelson A, editor. Platelets. New York: Elsevier; 2006.
2. McCrae KR. Thrombocytopenia in pregnancy: differential diagnosis, pathogenesis, and management. Blood Rev 2003;17(1):7–14.
3. McCrae KR, Bussel JB, Mannucci PM, et al. Platelets: an update on diagnosis and management of thrombocytopenic disorders. Hematology Am Soc Hematol Educ Program 2001;100:282–305.
4. McCrae KR, Cines DB. Thrombotic microangiopathy during pregnancy. Semin Hematol 1997;34(2):148–58.
5. McMinn JR, George JN. Evaluation of women with clinically suspected thrombotic thrombocytopenic purpura-hemolytic uremic syndrome during pregnancy. J Clin Apher 2001;16(4):202–9.
6. Crowther MA, Burrows RF, Ginsberg J, et al. Thrombocytopenia in pregnancy: diagnosis, pathogenesis and management. Blood Rev 1996;10(1):8–16.

7. Kelton JG. Idiopathic thrombocytopenic purpura complicating pregnancy. Blood Rev 2002;16(1):43–6.
8. Cines DB, Bussel JB, Liebman HA, et al. The ITP syndrome: pathogenic and clinical diversity. Blood 2009;113(26):6511–21.
9. Provan D, Newland A. Idiopathic thrombocytopenic purpura in adults. J Pediatr Hematol Oncol 2003;25(Suppl 1):S34–8.
10. McCrae KR, Samuels P, Schreiber AD. Pregnancy-associated thrombocytopenia: pathogenesis and management. Blood 1992;80(11):2697–714.
11. Gill KK, Kelton JG. Management of idiopathic thrombocytopenic purpura in pregnancy. Semin Hematol 2000;37(3):275–89.
12. McMillan R. Immune-mediated thrombocytopenias: focus on chronic immune thrombocytopenic purpura. Semin Hematol 2007;44(4 Suppl 5):S1–2.
13. Baldini M. Idiopathic thrombocytopenic purpura. N Engl J Med 1966;274(24): 1360–7.
14. Cines DB, Blanchette VS. Immune thrombocytopenic purpura. N Engl J Med 2002;346(13):995–1008.
15. Harrington WJ, Minnich V, Hollingsworth JW, et al. Demonstration of a thrombocytopenic factor in the blood of patients with thrombocytopenic purpura. J Lab Clin Med 1951;38(1):1–10.
16. Cines DB, McMillan R. Management of adult idiopathic thrombocytopenic purpura. Annu Rev Med 2005;56:425–42.
17. Cines DB, Schreiber AD. Immune thrombocytopenia: use of a Coombs antiglobulin test to detect IgG and C3 on platelets. N Engl J Med 1979;300(3): 106–11.
18. Chang M, Nakagawa PA, Williams SA, et al. Immune thrombocytopenic purpura (ITP) plasma and purified ITP monoclonal autoantibodies inhibit megakaryocytopoiesis in vitro. Blood 2003;102(3):887–95.
19. McMillan R, Wang L, Tomer A, et al. Suppression of in vitro megakaryocyte production by antiplatelet autoantibodies from adult patients with chronic ITP. Blood 2004;103(4):1364–9.
20. McMillan R. The pathogenesis of chronic immune thrombocytopenic purpura. Semin Hematol 2007;44(4 Suppl 5):S3–11.
21. Devendra K, Koh LP. Pregnancy in women with idiopathic thrombocytopaenic purpura. Ann Acad Med Singapore 2002;31(3):276–80.
22. Won YW, Moon W, Yun YS, et al. Clinical aspects of pregnancy and delivery in patients with chronic idiopathic thrombocytopenic purpura (ITP). Korean J Intern Med 2005;20(2):129–34.
23. Webert KE, Mittal R, Sigouin C, et al. A retrospective 11-year analysis of obstetric patients with idiopathic thrombocytopenic purpura. Blood 2003; 102(13):4306–11.
24. Boehlen F, Hohlfeld P, Extermann P, et al. Maternal antiplatelet antibodies in predicting risk of neonatal thrombocytopenia. Obstet Gynecol 1999;93(2):169–73.
25. Shehata N, Burrows R, Kelton JG. Gestational thrombocytopenia. Clin Obstet Gynecol 1999;42(2):327–34.
26. Sainio S, Kekomaki R, Riikonen S, et al. Maternal thrombocytopenia at term: a population-based study. Acta Obstet Gynecol Scand 2000;79(9):744–9.
27. Samuels P, Main EK, Tomaski A, et al. Abnormalities in platelet antiglobulin tests in preeclamptic mothers and their neonates. Am J Obstet Gynecol 1987;157(1):109–13.
28. Burrows RF, Kelton JG. Incidentally detected thrombocytopenia in healthy mothers and their infants. N Engl J Med 1988;319(3):142–5.

29. Samuels P, Bussel JB, Braitman LE, et al. Estimation of the risk of thrombocytopenia in the offspring of pregnant women with presumed immune thrombocytopenic purpura. N Engl J Med 1990;323(4):229–35.

30. Pridjian G, Puschett JB. Preeclampsia. Part 1: clinical and pathophysiologic considerations. Obstet Gynecol Surv 2002;57(9):598–618.

31. O'Brien JM, Barton JR. Controversies with the diagnosis and management of HELLP syndrome. Clin Obstet Gynecol 2005;48(2):460–77.

32. Barton JR, Sibai BM. Diagnosis and management of hemolysis, elevated liver enzymes, and low platelets syndrome. Clin Perinatol 2004;31(4):807–33, vii.

33. Nardi M, Karpatkin S. Antiidiotype antibody against platelet anti-GPIIIa contributes to the regulation of thrombocytopenia in HIV-1-ITP patients. J Exp Med 2000;191(12):2093–100.

34. Ajzenberg N, Dreyfus M, Kaplan C, et al. Pregnancy-associated thrombocytopenia revisited: assessment and follow-up of 50 cases. Blood 1998;92(12):4573–80.

35. Letsky EA, Greaves M. Guidelines on the investigation and management of thrombocytopenia in pregnancy and neonatal alloimmune thrombocytopenia. Maternal and Neonatal Haemostasis Working Party of the Haemostasis and Thrombosis Task Force of the British Society for Haematology. Br J Haematol 1996;95(1):21–6.

36. George JN, Woolf SH, Raskob GE, et al. Idiopathic thrombocytopenic purpura: a practice guideline developed by explicit methods for the American Society of Hematology. Blood 1996;88(1):3–40.

37. British Committee for Standards in Haematology General Haematology Task Force. Guidelines for the investigation and management of idiopathic thrombocytopenic purpura in adults, children and in pregnancy. Br J Haematol 2003;120(4):574–96.

38. Fujimura K, Harada Y, Fujimoto T, et al. Nationwide study of idiopathic thrombocytopenic purpura in pregnant women and the clinical influence on neonates. Int J Hematol 2002;75(4):426–33.

39. Kelton JG. Management of the pregnant patient with idiopathic thrombocytopenic purpura. Ann Intern Med 1983;99(6):796–800.

40. Carloss HW, McMillan R, Crosby WH. Management of pregnancy in women with immune thrombocytopenic purpura. JAMA 1980;244(24):2756–8.

41. Moise KJ Jr. Autoimmune thrombocytopenic purpura in pregnancy. Clin Obstet Gynecol 1991;34(1):51–63.

42. Kessler I, Lancet M, Borenstein R, et al. The obstetrical management of patients with immunologic thrombocytopenic purpura. Int J Gynaecol Obstet 1982;20(1):23–8.

43. Christiaens GC, Nieuwenhuis HK, von dem Borne AE, et al. Idiopathic thrombocytopenic purpura in pregnancy: a randomized trial on the effect of antenatal low dose corticosteroids on neonatal platelet count. Br J Obstet Gynaecol 1990;97(10):893–8.

44. Kallen B. Maternal drug use and infant cleft lip/palate with special reference to corticoids. Cleft Palate Craniofac J 2003;40(6):624–8.

45. Pradat P, Robert-Gnansia E, Di Tanna GL, et al. First trimester exposure to corticosteroids and oral clefts. Birth Defects Res A Clin Mol Teratol 2003;67(12):968–70.

46. Teeling JL, Jansen-Hendriks T, Kuijpers TW, et al. Therapeutic efficacy of intravenous immunoglobulin preparations depends on the immunoglobulin G dimers: studies in experimental immune thrombocytopenia. Blood 2001;98(4):1095–9.

47. Cines DB, Bussel JB. How I treat idiopathic thrombocytopenic purpura (ITP). Blood 2005;106(7):2244–51.

48. Bussel JB. Splenectomy-sparing strategies for the treatment and long-term maintenance of chronic idiopathic (immune) thrombocytopenic purpura. Semin Hematol 2000;37(1 Suppl 1):1–4.

49. Griffiths J, Sia W, Shapiro AM, et al. Laparoscopic splenectomy for the treatment of refractory immune thrombocytopenia in pregnancy. J Obstet Gynaecol Can 2005;27(8):771–4.

50. Bar Oz B, Hackman R, Einarson T, et al. Pregnancy outcome after cyclosporine therapy during pregnancy: a meta-analysis. Transplantation 2001;71(8):1051–5.

51. Cote CJ, Meuwissen HJ, Pickering RJ. Effects on the neonate of prednisone and azathioprine administered to the mother during pregnancy. J Pediatr 1974;85(3): 324–8.

52. Herold M, Schnohr S, Bittrich H. Efficacy and safety of a combined rituximab chemotherapy during pregnancy. J Clin Oncol 2001;19(14):3439.

53. Marushak A, Weber T, Bock J, et al. Pregnancy following kidney transplantation. Acta Obstet Gynecol Scand 1986;65(6):557–9.

54. Brown JH, Maxwell AP, McGeown MG. Outcome of pregnancy following renal transplantation. Ir J Med Sci 1991;160(8):255–6.

55. Bar J, Stahl B, Hod M, et al. Is immunosuppression therapy in renal allograft recipients teratogenic? A single-center experience. Am J Med Genet A 2003; 116A(1):31–6.

56. Ojeda-Uribe M, Gilliot C, Jung G, et al. Administration of rituximab during the first trimester of pregnancy without consequences for the newborn. J Perinatol 2006;26(4):252–5.

57. Klink DT, van Elburg RM, Schreurs MW, et al. Rituximab administration in third trimester of pregnancy suppresses neonatal B-cell development. Clin Dev Immunol 2008;2008:271363.

58. Kimby E, Sverrisdottir A, Elinder G. Safety of rituximab therapy during the first trimester of pregnancy: a case history. Eur J Haematol 2004;72(4):292–5.

59. Beilin Y, Zahn J, Comerford M. Safe epidural analgesia in thirty parturients with platelet counts between 69,000 and 98,000 mm(-3). Anesth Analg 1997;85(2): 385–8.

60. Schlamowitz M. Membrane receptors in the specific transfer of immunoglobulins from mother to young. Immunol Commun 1976;5(6):481–500.

61. Leach L, Eaton BM, Firth JA, et al. Immunogold localisation of endogenous immunoglobulin-G in ultrathin frozen sections of the human placenta. Cell Tissue Res 1989;257(3):603–7.

62. Stuart SG, Simister NE, Clarkson SB, et al. Human IgG Fc receptor (hFcRII; CD32) exists as multiple isoforms in macrophages, lymphocytes and IgG-transporting placental epithelium. EMBO J 1989;8(12):3657–66.

63. Burrows RF, Kelton JG. Pregnancy in patients with idiopathic thrombocytopenic purpura: assessing the risks for the infant at delivery. Obstet Gynecol Surv 1993; 48(12):781–8.

64. Christiaens GC, Nieuwenhuis HK, Bussel JB. Comparison of platelet counts in first and second newborns of mothers with immune thrombocytopenic purpura. Obstet Gynecol 1997;90(4 Part 1):546–52.

65. Payne SD, Resnik R, Moore TR, et al. Maternal characteristics and risk of severe neonatal thrombocytopenia and intracranial hemorrhage in pregnancies complicated by autoimmune thrombocytopenia. Am J Obstet Gynecol 1997;177(1): 149–55.

66. Garmel SH, Craigo SD, Morin LM, et al. The role of percutaneous umbilical blood sampling in the management of immune thrombocytopenic purpura. Prenat Diagn 1995;15(5):439–45.

67. Christiaens GC. Immune thrombocytopenic purpura in pregnancy. Baillieres Clin Haematol 1998;11(2):373–80.

68. Song TB, Lee JY, Kim YH, et al. Low neonatal risk of thrombocytopenia in pregnancy associated with immune thrombocytopenic purpura. Fetal Diagn Ther 1999;14(4):216–9.

69. Cook RL, Miller RC, Katz VL, et al. Immune thrombocytopenic purpura in pregnancy: a reappraisal of management. Obstet Gynecol 1991;78(4):578–83.

70. Territo M, Finklestein J, Oh W, et al. Management of autoimmune thrombocytopenia in pregnancy and in the neonate. Obstet Gynecol 1973;41(4):579–84.

71. Jones RW, Asher MI, Rutherford CJ, et al. Autoimmune (idiopathic) thrombocytopenic purpura in pregnancy and the newborn. Br J Obstet Gynaecol 1977; 84(9):679–83.

72. Scott JR, Cruikshank DP, Kochenour NK, et al. Fetal platelet counts in the obstetric management of immunologic thrombocytopenic purpura. Am J Obstet Gynecol 1980;136(4):495–9.

73. Moise KJ Jr, Carpenter RJ Jr, Cotton DB, et al. Percutaneous umbilical cord blood sampling in the evaluation of fetal platelet counts in pregnant patients with autoimmune thrombocytopenia purpura. Obstet Gynecol 1988;72(3 Pt 1): 346–50.

74. Scioscia AL, Grannum PA, Copel JA, et al. The use of percutaneous umbilical blood sampling in immune thrombocytopenic purpura. Am J Obstet Gynecol 1988;159(5):1066–8.

75. Burrows RF, Kelton JG. Low fetal risks in pregnancies associated with idiopathic thrombocytopenic purpura. Am J Obstet Gynecol 1990;163(4 Pt 1):1147–50.

76. Kelton JG, Inwood MJ, Barr RM, et al. The prenatal prediction of thrombocytopenia in infants of mothers with clinically diagnosed immune thrombocytopenia. Am J Obstet Gynecol 1982;144(4):449–54.

77. Moutet A, Fromont P, Farcet JP, et al. Pregnancy in women with immune thrombocytopenic purpura. Arch Intern Med 1990;150(10):2141–5.

78. Karpatkin M, Porges RF, Karpatkin S. Platelet counts in infants of women with autoimmune thrombocytopenia: effects of steroid administration to the mother. N Engl J Med 1981;305(16):936–9.

79. Laros RK, Sweet RL. Management of idiopathic thrombocytopenic purpura during pregnancy. Am J Obstet Gynecol 1975;122(2):182–91.

80. Wahbeh CJ, Eden RD, Killam AP, et al. Pregnancy and immune thrombocytopenic purpura. Am J Obstet Gynecol 1984;149(2):238–40.

81. Verdy E, Bessous V, Dreyfus M, et al. Longitudinal analysis of platelet count and volume in normal pregnancy. Thromb Haemost 1997;77(4):806–7.

82. Burrows RF, Kelton JG. Fetal thrombocytopenia and its relation to maternal thrombocytopenia. N Engl J Med 1993;329(20):1463–6.

83. Burrows RF, Kelton JG. Thrombocytopenia at delivery: a prospective survey of 6715 deliveries. Am J Obstet Gynecol 1990;162(3):731–4.

84. Matthews JH, Benjamin S, Gill DS, et al. Pregnancy-associated thrombocytopenia: definition, incidence and natural history. Acta Haematol 1990;84(1):24–9.

85. Cunningham FG, Lindheimer MD. Hypertension in pregnancy. N Engl J Med 1992;326(14):927–32.

86. Lindheimer MD, Katz AI. Hypertension in pregnancy. N Engl J Med 1985; 313(11):675–80.

87. Rauramo L. The incidence of eclampsia in Finland, 1927–1958. Pathol Microbiol 1961;24:435–43.
88. Sibai BM. Diagnosis and management of gestational hypertension and preeclampsia. Obstet Gynecol 2003;102(1):181–92.
89. Esplin MS, Fausett MB, Fraser A, et al. Paternal and maternal components of the predisposition to preeclampsia. N Engl J Med 2001;344(12):867–72.
90. Romero R, Duffy TP. Platelet disorders in pregnancy. Clin Perinatol 1980;7(2): 327–48.
91. Romero R, Lockwood C, Oyarzun E, et al. Toxemia: new concepts in an old disease. Semin Perinatol 1988;12(4):302–23.
92. Redman CW. Current topic: pre-eclampsia and the placenta. Placenta 1991; 12(4):301–8.
93. Lindheimer MD, Katz AI. Preeclampsia: pathophysiology, diagnosis, and management. Annu Rev Med 1989;40:233–50.
94. Brosens I, Dixon HG, Robertson WB. Fetal growth retardation and the arteries of the placental bed. Br J Obstet Gynaecol 1977;84(9):656–63.
95. De Wolf F, Brosens I, Renaer M. Fetal growth retardation and the maternal arterial supply of the human placenta in the absence of sustained hypertension. Br J Obstet Gynaecol 1980;87(8):678–85.
96. Meekins JW, Pijnenborg R, Hanssens M, et al. A study of placental bed spiral arteries and trophoblast invasion in normal and severe pre-eclamptic pregnancies. Br J Obstet Gynaecol 1994;101(8):669–74.
97. Zhou Y, Damsky CH, Chiu K, et al. Preeclampsia is associated with abnormal expression of adhesion molecules by invasive cytotrophoblasts. J Clin Invest 1993;91(3):950–60.
98. Bussolino F, Benedetto C, Massobrio M, et al. Maternal vascular prostacyclin activity in pre-eclampsia. Lancet 1980;2(8196):702.
99. Geary M. The HELLP syndrome. Br J Obstet Gynaecol 1997;104(8):887–91.
100. Karumanchi SA, Maynard SE, Stillman IE, et al. Preeclampsia: a renal perspective. Kidney Int 2005;67(6):2101–13.
101. Magann EF, Martin JN Jr. Twelve steps to optimal management of HELLP syndrome. Clin Obstet Gynecol 1999;42(3):532–50.
102. Audibert F, Friedman SA, Frangieh AY, et al. Clinical utility of strict diagnostic criteria for the HELLP (hemolysis, elevated liver enzymes, and low platelets) syndrome. Am J Obstet Gynecol 1996;175(2):460–4.
103. Padden MO. HELLP syndrome: recognition and perinatal management. Am Fam Physician 1999;60(3):829–36, 839.
104. Stone JH. HELLP syndrome: hemolysis, elevated liver enzymes, and low platelets. JAMA 1998;280(6):559–62.
105. Weinstein L. Syndrome of hemolysis, elevated liver enzymes, and low platelet count: a severe consequence of hypertension in pregnancy. Am J Obstet Gynecol 1982;142(2):159–67.
106. Sibai BM. The HELLP syndrome (hemolysis, elevated liver enzymes, and low platelets): much ado about nothing? Am J Obstet Gynecol 1990;162(2):311–6.
107. Thiagarajah S, Bourgeois FJ, Harbert GM Jr, et al. Thrombocytopenia in preeclampsia: associated abnormalities and management principles. Am J Obstet Gynecol 1984;150(1):1–7.
108. Ridolfi RL, Bell WR. Thrombotic thrombocytopenic purpura: report of 25 cases and review of the literature. Medicine (Baltimore) 1981;60(6):413–28.
109. Sibai BM. Imitators of severe pre-eclampsia/eclampsia. Clin Perinatol 2004; 31(4):835–52, vii–viii.

110. Levy GG, Nichols WC, Lian EC, et al. Mutations in a member of the ADAMTS gene family cause thrombotic thrombocytopenic purpura. Nature 2001; 413(6855):488–94.

111. Mayer SA, Aledort LM. Thrombotic microangiopathy: differential diagnosis, pathophysiology and therapeutic strategies. Mt Sinai J Med 2005;72(3):166–75.

112. Furlan M, Robles R, Galbusera M, et al. von Willebrand factor-cleaving protease in thrombotic thrombocytopenic purpura and the hemolytic-uremic syndrome. N Engl J Med 1998;339(22):1578–84.

113. Sanchez-Luceros A, Farias CE, Amaral MM, et al. von Willebrand factor-cleaving protease (ADAMTS13) activity in normal non-pregnant women, pregnant and post-delivery women. Thromb Haemost 2004;92(6):1320–6.

114. Tsai HM, Lian EC. Antibodies to von Willebrand factor-cleaving protease in acute thrombotic thrombocytopenic purpura. N Engl J Med 1998;339(22): 1585–94.

115. Karmali MA, Petric M, Lim C, et al. The association between idiopathic hemolytic uremic syndrome and infection by verotoxin-producing Escherichia coli. J Infect Dis 1985;151(5):775–82.

116. McCrae KR, Sadler JE, Cines DB. Thrombotic thrombocytopenic purpura and the hemolytic uremic syndrome. In: Hoffman R, Benz EJJ, Shattil SJ, editors. Hematology: basic principles and practice. Philadelphia: Elsevier, Churchill, Livingstone; 2005. p. 2287.

117. Bick RL. Disseminated intravascular coagulation and related syndromes: a clinical review. Semin Thromb Hemost 1988;14(4):299–338.

118. Ratnoff OD, Pritchard JA, Colopy JE. Hemorrhagic states during pregnancy. N Engl J Med 1955;253(3):97–102.

119. Purdie FR, Nieto JM, Summerson DJ, et al. Rupture of the uterus with DIC. Ann Emerg Med 1983;12(3):174–6.

120. Bick RL. Syndromes of disseminated intravascular coagulation in obstetrics, pregnancy, and gynecology: objective criteria for diagnosis and management. Hematol Oncol Clin North Am 2000;14(5):999–1044.

121. Knox TA, Olans LB. Liver disease in pregnancy. N Engl J Med 1996;335(8): 569–76.

122. Abramowicz JS, Sherer DM, Woods JR Jr. Acute transient thrombocytopenia associated with cocaine abuse in pregnancy. Obstet Gynecol 1991;78(3 Pt 2): 499–501.

123. Gimovsky ML, Montoro M. Systemic lupus erythematosus and other connective tissue diseases in pregnancy. Clin Obstet Gynecol 1991;34(1):35–50.

124. Budman DR, Steinberg AD. Hematologic aspects of systemic lupus erythematosus: current concepts. Ann Intern Med 1977;86(2):220–9.

125. Weiner CP. The mechanism of reduced antithrombin III activity in women with preeclampsia. Obstet Gynecol 1988;72(6):847–9.

126. Schiff E, Peleg E, Goldenberg M, et al. The use of aspirin to prevent pregnancy-induced hypertension and lower the ratio of thromboxane A2 to prostacyclin in relatively high risk pregnancies. N Engl J Med 1989;321(6):351–6.

127. Cunningham FG, Gant NF. Prevention of preeclampsia–a reality? N Engl J Med 1989;321(9):606–7.

128. Lockwood CJ, Peters JH. Increased plasma levels of ED1+ cellular fibronectin precede the clinical signs of preeclampsia. Am J Obstet Gynecol 1990;162(2): 358–62.

Intravenous Immunoglobulin and Anti-RhD Therapy in the Management of Immune Thrombocytopenia

Nichola Cooper, MA, MD, MRCP, MRCPath

KEYWORDS

- IVIG • IV anti-D • ITP • Thrombocytopenia • FcRIIb
- Immunemodulation

Intravenous immunoglobulin (IVIG) and intravenous (IV) anti-D are frequently used in the treatment of immune thrombocytopenia (ITP). Because of their speed of action, they can be used instead of or in conjunction with steroids as first-line therapy. Alternatively, they can be used as second-line therapy in those who do not go into an immediate remission. Responses are rapid but limited and further treatment is usually required. Although some patients go into remission after many months of treatment, it is not thought that either product induces a cure but instead allows patients the time to restore tolerance and establish a normal platelet count. Both are steroid-sparing agents that are reasonably well tolerated and useful in the period of persistent ITP when patients may still go into remission. Because of their speed of activity and predictability of responses, they are also useful before planned procedures, such as surgery. Side effects are different for the two products, and adverse events, although rare, can be significant in their nature. Experimental data from human and murine studies suggest that despite their similarities, the mechanisms of action of IVIG and anti-D are likely different.

This article explores the activity of IVIG and IV anti-D in patients with ITP and discusses the use of each product in different circumstances, the proposed mechanisms of actions, and the side effects and toxicity profile for each agent.

INTRAVENOUS IMMUNOGLOBULIN
Activity

IVIG was first used for the management of patients with inherited hypogammaglobulinemia in the 1950s. It is prepared from large pools of plasma, typically from more than

Department of Haematology, Hammersmith Hospital, Imperial Health Care NHS Trust, Du Cane Road, London W12 OHS, UK
E-mail address: n.cooper@imperial.ac.uk

Hematol Oncol Clin N Am 23 (2009) 1317–1327
doi:10.1016/j.hoc.2009.09.002
0889-8588/09/$ – see front matter © 2009 Elsevier Inc. All rights reserved.

hemonc.theclinics.com

10,000 healthy blood donors. After observing the resolution of ITP in two children treated routinely with IVIG for agammaglobulinemia, Imbach and colleagues[1] first used IVIG in children with ITP in the early 1980s.[2] The majority of the children responded to this initial dose—0.4 g/kg daily for 5 days—and further studies examined its use in children and adults. These studies confirmed between 65% and 80% platelet responses in adults with ITP.[3,4] Later studies showed more rapid responses after the same dose given over 2 days rather than 5[5] and subsequently Godeau and colleagues[6] found that 1 g/kg on 1 day was just as effective as 2 g/kg over 2 days. Two of 6 patients in this study who did not respond to a single dose of 1 g/kg responded to a 2-g/kg regime, allowing Godeau and colleagues[6] to propose that individuals should be treated with a single dose of 1 g/kg, which can be repeated on day 3 if no response is seen.

Despite good immediate responses, however, the duration of response remains limited. Repeated doses are often required and, if used in this manner, may allow patients to avoid splenectomy[7,8]; hence, they are useful in the period of ITP described as persistent ITP. Because of its quick and predictable mode of action, IVIG is also useful before surgical procedures. IVIG is costly, however, and it is a blood product; thus, it has theoretic risks of blood-transmitted infections and is reasonably resource intensive, requiring day-care attendance. Therefore, in patients requiring continued use, alternative potentially curative agents may be more appropriate.

Intravenous Immunoglobulin in Secondary Immune Thrombocytopenia

IVIG may be particularly useful in patients with common variable immunodeficiency (CVID) and associated autoimmunity. In approximately 20% of patients with CVID, autoimmunity in the form of ITP or autoimmune hemolytic anemia is the presenting feature.[9] In some patients, regular prophylaxis of IVIG at standard dose may prevent further autoimmune relapses.[10] IVIG is also useful in patients with lupus-related ITP and in patients with HIV-related ITP. Treatment of the underlying disorder, however, is usually required to maintain responses.

Intravenous Immunoglobulin in Pregnancy

IVIG is useful in ITP during pregnancy. It is well tolerated with no adverse events to neonates. It does not necessarily affect fetal and neonatal platelet counts, however.

Intravenous Immunoglobulin in Pediatrics

IVIG has established efficacy children with ITP. Early studies showed that intermittent use can allow children to avoid splenectomy.[11] After a randomized controlled study of different doses of IVIG, anti-D, and prednisone, Blanchette and colleagues describe that a single dose of 0.8 g/kg is considered sufficient for management of thrombocytopenia in children. In this same study, platelet increment was significantly faster after the 0.8-g/kg IVIG group than after steroids ($P<.05$).[12] In a later study, children treated with corticosteroids were 26% less likely to have a platelet increment at 48 hours than those treated with IVIG.[13] The use of IVIG early on in the management of ITP in childhood may also influence the progression of the disease. Using data from registry I of the Intercontinental Cooperative ITP Study Group, including a total of 1984 children with ITP, a matched-pairs analysis comparing children with thrombocytopenia 6 months after diagnosis with children whose platelet count was greater than 150×10^9/L, children initially treated with IVIG were more likely to have a normal platelet count at 6 months than children not receiving IVIG. When a lower platelet count was chosen ($<50 \times 10^9$/L at 6 months), a similar finding showed those with counts less than 50×10^9/L at 6 months were more likely to have been treated with steroids than with IVIG ($P = .02$).[14]

Toxicity and Side Effects of Intravenous Immunoglobulin

IVIG is generally well tolerated. Adverse effects occur in approximately 5% of patients, including headaches, chills, myalgia, fatigue, arthralgia, and back pain. Headaches may be severe and rarely may cause acute septic meningitis within 72 hours of the administration of IVIG. Symptoms usually resolve spontaneously and may be prevented by use of nonsteroidal anti-inflammatory drugs. More serious adverse events, such as intravascular hemolysis, renal failure, strokes, and myocardial infarctions, have been reported. These are rare, however, and usually occur in patients with pre-existing risks factors, such as in elderly patients and patients with diabetes or impaired renal function. In these patients, administration over a longer period of time (3–5 days) may be advisable. Transmission of viruses remains a theoretic risk with the use of blood products. Despite transmission of hepatitis C associated with the use of IVIG in the 1990s,[15,16] no transmissions of hepatitis, HIV, or Creutzfeldt-Jakob disease have been reported since.

INTRAVENOUS ANTI-D
Activity

IV anti-D is a pooled IgG product taken from the plasma of RhD− donors who have been immunized to the D antigen. In the 1980s, Salama and colleagues hypothesized that low levels of anti–red blood cell (RBC) antibodies contained in the IVIG preparations might cause substitution of antibody-coated RBCs for the antibody-coated platelets and result in FcR blockade, resulting in the increase in platelet counts seen after IVIG. To prove this hypothesis, they injected Rh+ ITP patients with anti-D. In the majority of patients, the platelet count increased.[17] This prompted several studies designed to assess the efficacy and safety of anti-D in adults and children with ITP.[18,19] The largest of these studies was reported by Scaradavou and colleagues in 1997: 261 patients (124 children and 137 adults) were treated with anti-D between 1987 and 1994 with ITP (n = 156) or HIV-related thrombocytopenia (n = 105) and included patients with acute (n = 75) or chronic ITP (n = 186). The study showed anti-D to be safe, with response rates of 70%. Responses were greater in children and in HIV+ patients and the platelet effects lasted more than 21 days in 50% of responders.[20] In a small number of patients, these early studies showed minimal or no responses in patients who had undergone splenectomy or in patients who are Rh−. Later studies showed that higher doses of anti-D, such as 75 µg/kg, results in a greater median day 1 and day 7 platelet count compared with 50 µg/kg,[21] with no corresponding increase in the fall in hemoglobin. The duration of effect of anti-D is also greater after the higher dose (median 46 days after 75 µg/kg compared with median 21 days after 50 µg/kg) and results in effects equivalent to IVIG. Tarantino and colleagues[22] described similar findings in children (described later) with similar time to response on the higher dose of anti-D (75 µg/kg) compared with IVIG, with increased (but tolerable) infusion reactions at the higher dose. Infusion reactions can be ameliorated with the use of steroids (usually 50 mg prednisolone), antihistamine, and paracetemol premedication.[21,23] This may in part be related to increased interleukin (IL)-10 levels on patients treated with prednisolone.[23]

Similarly to IVIG, anti-D can be used as first-line therapy or as a maintenance regime whenever the platelet count falls to below a specified level. Using this approach, many patients can avoid splenectomy and may even go into a long-term remission (**Fig. 1**).[24]

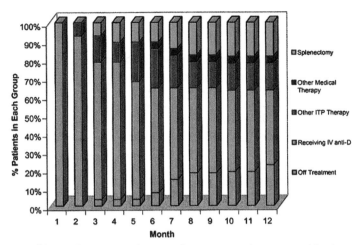

Fig. 1. The use of intermittent IV anti-D can allow some patients to avoid splenectomy and some patients to improve their counts enough to stop treatment. Twenty-eight RhD+ patients with ITP—duration 1 to 12 months—were treated with IV anti-D whenever their platelets fell to less than 30×10^9/L. Each bar chart represents 1 month on study. Over time, several patients came off treatment altogether (*pink*); some patients underwent splenectomy (*orange*); some required other therapy, such as prednisone, danazol, or IVIG (*intermediate blue*); one patient received chemotherapy for breast cancer (*dark blue*); and the remaining patients continued on intermittent anti-D (*light blue*). (*From* Cooper N, Woloski BM, Fodero EM, et al. Does treatment with intermittent infusions of intravenous anti-D allow a proportion of adults with recently diagnosed immune thrombocytopenic purpura to avoid splenectomy? Blood 2002;99:1922–7; with permission.) Copyright © 2002 the American Society of Hematology.

Although there is no direct evidence of induction of a cure, immune modulation is known to occur after IVIG and IV anti-D.

Anti-D in Secondary Immune Thrombocytopenia

Several studies have shown greater efficacy of IV anti-D in individuals with HIV-related thrombocytopenia. Scaradavou reported nine Rh+ nonsplenectomized HIV-positive patients with thrombocytopenia treated sequentially in random order with IVIG and IV anti-D, receiving each treatment for 3 months. IV anti-D resulted in a mean peak platelet count of 77×10^9/L compared with a mean peak to 29×10^6/L after IVIG ($P = .07$). The mean duration of response was also longer, with a mean duration of response of 41 days after anti-D compared with mean 19 days response after IVIG. No changes in CD4 counts or viral loads were reported.[25] Although there was a small number of patients in this study, this confirms previous results.[20,26]

Anti-D in Pregnancy

As with IVIG, anti-D is useful in ITP during pregnancy, although published series remain limited. Michel and colleagues reported eight Rh+ pregnant women treated with anti-D during second and third trimesters of pregnancy. The response rate was 75%, it was well tolerated, and a hemoglobin fall of greater than 2 g/dL occurred only once. Fetal hydrops did not occur in any individual and although the direct antiglobulin test was positive in three of seven newborns, none was anemic or jaundiced.[27] A second report in 2009 describes 10 patients treated with anti-D during pregnancy. No disseminated intravascular coagulation (DIC), no renal failure, and no neonatal hemolysis was reported, and only one child had jaundice, which resolved with phototherapy.[28]

Anti-D in Pediatrics

Anti-D is well established in pediatric ITP. Scaradavou and colleagues[20] described better responses in children than in adults and Tarantino and colleagues[22] described single-dose anti-D (75 μg/kg) as effective as IVIG in newly diagnosed ITP in children. Responses occurred in 50%, 72%, and 77% of patients treated with anti-D50, anti-D75, and IVIG, respectively **(Fig. 2)** Headaches and chills were less frequent in patients receiving 50 μg/kg IV anti-D.

Toxicity and Side Effects of Anti-D

Large cohort studies suggest anti-D is reasonably safe and well tolerated. In 2000, however, Gaines[29] reported 15 patients with acute hemoglobinemia or hemaglobinuria after IV anti-D reported to the Food and Drug Administration (FDA). Eleven of these 15 patients experienced additional complications: seven had clinically compromising anemia (six required transfusion with packed RBCs), and eight had onset or exacerbation of renal insufficiency, with two undergoing dialysis. Two patients died from pulmonary edema and respiratory distress. Postmarketing surveillance led to six further patients reported to the FDA as having DIC after anti-D; one child recovered without complications whereas five adults died (FDA surveillance from October 1999 to November 2004). The five deaths occurred up to 10 days from infusion of IV anti-D, four associated with renal failure with two on dialysis. There was a median fall in the hemoglobin of 7.2 g/dL (range 3.0 to 10 g/dL).[30] These five deaths and the previously described morbidity are thought to have occurred on an approximate denominator of 121,389 patients treated with anti-D. These events are, therefore, rare, although unpredictable and devastating in their severity. The use of prednisolone increases IL-10 production in patients treated with IV anti-D and is associated with a lower incidence of infusion reactions.[23] Although not formally assessed, avoiding anti-D in patients with renal impairment; in those with other causes of a cytokine storm, such as sepsis; and in those with evidence of pre-existing hemolysis and the prophylactic use of steroid-containing premedication may allow safer use of this therapy.

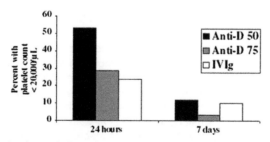

Fig. 2. Use of IV anti-D (75 μg/kg) works as quickly as IVIG (0.8 g/dL) in children with ITP. One hundred four children were treated with IV anti-D at two doses (50 μg/kg or 75 μg/kg) or IVIG (0.8 g/kg). At 24 hours, 50%, 72%, and 77% of patients in the anti-D50, anti-D75, and IVIG groups, respectively, had achieved a platelet count greater than 20×10^9/L (P = .03). By day 7, responses in the three groups were equal. (*From* Tarantino MD, Young G, Bertolone SJ, et al. Acute ITP Study Group. Single-dose of anti-D immune globulin at 75 microg/kg is as effective as intravenous immune globulin at rapidly raising the platelet count in newly diagnosed immune thrombocytopenic purpura in children. J Pediatr 2006;148(4):489–94; with permission.)

HOW DO INTRAVENOUS IMMUNOGLOBULIN AND INTRAVENOUS ANTI-D WORK?
Intravenous Immunoglobulin

FcγR blockade

Prolonged in vivo clearance of radiolabeled, antibody-sensitized, RBCs in nonsplenectomized patients treated with IVIG was first described in 1982.[31] This was confirmed in other human[11,32] and animal models[33] and led to an assumption that IVIG blocks the monocyte/macrophage-mediated destruction of antibody-coated platelets.

Subsequent human and animal studies suggested that blockade of the activating receptors FcγII/III may be critical to responses. Treatment of patients with ITP with an antibody specific for FcγRII/III resulted in a transient platelet increment,[34] and in a mouse model, antibodies that block FcγRII/III ameliorates murine ITP.[35] This same anti-FcγRII/III antibody in mice prevents the clearance of IgG-sensitized RBCs.[36] Further evidence of a role for the FcγRII/IIIa receptor was demonstrated when dimers of IVIG (which have stronger efficacy to FcγRII/III) were shown more effective than monomers in treating ITP in mice.[37] In humans, a monoclonal antibody to FcγRIII successfully treated thrombocytopenia in patients with HIV-related ITP,[38,39] and a humanized anti-FcγRIII antibody (GMA161) can transiently increase the platelet count in patients who failed IVIG therapy.

Involvement of inhibitory receptors

There is mounting evidence against the FcγR-activating receptor blockade hypothesis, however. In 1984, platelet responses were described to the F(ab')$_2$ fragments of IVIG, which have little FcγR-binding activity.[40,41] Subsequently, seminal work by Samuelsson and colleagues showed that IVIG is not effective at treating thrombocytopenia in mice deficient in the inhibitory low-affinity IgG receptor, FcγRIIb.[42] Crow and colleagues,[43,44] in addition to confirming the requirement for the FcγRIIb receptor in the responses to IVIG, show that mononuclear phagocyte system (MPS) blockade continues to occur in mice deficient in FcγRIIb, even when thrombocytopenia is not corrected, suggesting that IVIG does not function via MPS blockade or that RBC clearance may occur by different mechanisms than platelet clearance in murine ITP.

Upregulation of FcγRIIb: macrophages or dendritic cells?

How the FcγRIIb receptor is involved in the platelet responses to IVIG is not clear but up-regulation of FcγRIIb by receptor activation or other intermediary effects appears crucial.

Work from Ravetch's group showed dependence of colony-stimulating factor 1 and suggested a two-step model where colony-stimulating factor 1–dependent macrophages interact with IVIG and lead to the induction of FcγRIIb expression on effector macrophages.[45] Further work from the same group shows that glycosylation of IVIG is crucial for anti-inflammatory activity and suggests that the reason such high doses of IVIG are required lies in the small percentage (1%–2%) of IgGs with fully processed glycan.[46] In some manner, splenic marginal zone macrophages that express dendritic cell (DC)-SIGN, which specifically interacts with sialylated Fc's mediate this effect, although the specific steps remain unclear. The end result is up-regulation of the inhibitory FcγRIIb on macrophages.[47]

In a different model Siragam and colleagues propose that IVIG works via activation of DCs. In a mouse model, they demonstrate that priming of CD11c$^+$ DCs with IVIG is required to abrogate thrombocytopenia in ITP.[48] In this model, they show that FcγRIIb does not need to be expressed by the primed DCs but does need to be expressed in the recipient mouse (ie, primed DCs from FcγRIIb−/− mice still ameliorated ITP whereas primed wild-type DCs did not ameliorate ITP in FcγRIIb−/− mice). This group speculates that IVIG primes the DCs via activation of FcγRs—through an unknown signal—causing interaction with phagocytic macrophages, resulting in an anti-inflammatory effect involving up-regulation of FcγRIIb on macrophages and inhibition of platelet clearance.[49] Further work from the same group suggests this mechanism is only beneficial in autoimmune states with low levels of immune complexes, where DCs are not continually stimulated.

Other mechanisms

Several studies have described changes in cytokine levels after IVIG, including IL-6, IL-8, tumor necrosis factor (TNF)-α, IL-1 receptor antagonist (IL-1RA), and IL-10. Although considered initially to contribute to the immunomodulatory effect, this may be a bystander effect from the effect on the DC. The effect of IVIG on T cells is being explored. Even early studies showed cellular changes, including changes in the ratio of activating and suppressive T cells.[50]

Anti-D

FcR blockade

Salamas' original theory was that antibody-coated red cells would competitively compete with antibody-coated platelets and result in MPS blockade. These experiments were successful and the hypothesis of FcR blockade is supported by the fact that anti-D is not effective in RhD− individuals[26,51] or in most patients in whom the spleen has been removed,[19] although this is not conclusive with some activity in individuals post splenectomy.[52] Fewer data are available to explore the mechanism of effect of anti-D compared with that of IVIG.

Cytokine modulation

Several studies have described cytokine changes after IV anti-D, including increases in IL-6, TNF-α, MCP-1, IL-10, and transforming growth factor-beta.[23,53,54] Cytokine levels were significantly higher after anti-D than after IVIG in one study, suggesting a different mechanism of effect. In this same study, changes in cytokines were influenced by the FcγRIIa genotype, with higher levels of IL-6, MCP-1, and TNF-α in the high-affinity receptor, HH,[23] suggesting that anti-D exerts its effect via the activating Fcγ receptors. In addition to increases in the cytokines (discussed previously), Coopamah and colleagues[55] also describe increases in IL-1RA after anti-D and describe induction of monocyte and granulocyte production of IL-1RA in vitro with a subsequent inhibition of phagocytosis, suggesting that the downstream effects of anti-D are to inhibit phagocytosis of the antibody-coated platelet. Crow and colleagues,[56] however, showed that although a monoclonal antibody also induced IL-1RA increases in mice, this antibody also increased the platelet count in mice without the receptor for IL-1RA, suggesting that at least some of the cytokine production after anti-D may be a bystander effect rather than a cause of the platelet increase.

Activating receptors

In a murine model of ITP, RBC-specific antibodies ameliorated the thrombocytopenia in wild-type and in Fcγllb−/− mice, suggesting a different mechanism of action to IVIG. This study also describes down-regulation of activating FcγRIIIa on splenic macrophages[57] in association with an increase in the platelet count. Much lower doses of anti-D are required to treat ITP in humans, and a similar finding is found in mice, with anti-RBC doses 1000× less than the doses of IVIG required for a similar effect.

Further work is required to understand the activity of anti-D in ITP, which has a different activity from that of IVIG.

SUMMARY

IVIG and IV anti-D are useful treatments for the management of ITP. Although steroids remain the standard of care in newly diagnosed patients, IVIG and IV anti-D can be used when steroids are contradicted. In children, where there is a suggestion that acute use of IVIG may result in longer-term results and where anti-D is well tolerated, either therapy may be more appropriately used. In patients who do not go in to an immediate remission and where it is anticipated that remission may still occur and steroid-sparing agents are required, both IVIG and IV anti-D may be used as maintenance treatment to keep platelet counts at a "safe" level. Side effects to both treatments remain tolerable and despite reports of severe hemolysis and five deaths from hemolysis or renal failure after anti-D, these reports remain rare, and, although vigilance to effects is required, it is likely that long-term adverse events are less significant than with long-term steroids. In addition, in certain diseases, such as HIV, anti-D may be more efficacious and in CVID, IVIG is likely to be more useful.

Finally, the mechanism of action of both of these therapies sheds light on the activity of activating and inhibitory receptors in the pathology of ITP. With better understanding of the roles of these receptors in disease, more specific targets can be used in the management of ITP. So far, attempts in this direction, with antibodies to FcγRIII showing some efficacy and a syc kinase inhibitor that targets signaling pathways downstream of FcγRIIa and FcγRIIb showing some efficacy in mice and humans,[58] have been of moderate success.

REFERENCES

1. Imbach P, Barandun S, Baumgartner C, et al. High-dose intravenous gammaglobulin therapy of refractory, in particular idiopathic thrombocytopenia in childhood. Helv Paediatr Acta 1981;36:81–6.
2. Wagner HP, Barandun S, Hirt A, et al. High-dose immunoglobulin infusions in idiopathic thrombopenic purpura. Presse Med 1983;12:2612–4 [in French].
3. Bussel JB, Hilgartner MW. The use and mechanism of action of intravenous immunoglobulin in the treatment of immune haematologic disease. Br J Haematol 1984; 56:1–7.
4. Bussel JB, Szatrowski TP. Uses of intravenous gammaglobulin in immune hematologic disease. Immunol Invest 1995;24:451–6.
5. Kurlander R, Coleman RE, Moore J, et al. Comparison of the efficacy of a two-day and a five-day schedule for infusing intravenous gamma globulin in the treatment of immune thrombocytopenic purpura in adults. Am J Med 1987;83:17–24.
6. Godeau B, Lesage S, Divine M, et al. Treatment of adult chronic autoimmune thrombocytopenic purpura with repeated high-dose intravenous immunoglobulin. Blood 1993;82:1415–21.
7. Bussel JB. Splenectomy-sparing strategies for the treatment and long-term maintenance of chronic idiopathic (immune) thrombocytopenic purpura. Semin Hematol 2000;37:1–4.
8. Bussel JB, Pham LC, Aledort L, et al. Maintenance treatment of adults with chronic refractory immune thrombocytopenic purpura using repeated intravenous infusions of gammaglobulin. Blood 1988;72:121–7.
9. Cunningham-Rundles C. Autoimmune manifestations in common variable immunodeficiency. J Clin Immunol 2008;28(Suppl 1):S42–5.

10. Michel M, Chanet V, Galicier L, et al. Autoimmune thrombocytopenic purpura and common variable immunodeficiency: analysis of 21 cases and review of the literature. Medicine (Baltimore) 2004;83:254–63.

11. Bussel JB, Schulman I, Hilgartner MW, et al. Intravenous use of gammaglobulin in the treatment of chronic immune thrombocytopenic purpura as a means to defer splenectomy. J Pediatr 1983;103:651–4.

12. Blanchette V, Imbach P, Andrew M, et al. Randomised trial of intravenous immunoglobulin G, intravenous anti-D, and oral prednisone in childhood acute immune thrombocytopenic purpura. Lancet 1994;344:703–7.

13. Beck CE, Nathan PC, Parkin PC, et al. Corticosteroids versus intravenous immune globulin for the treatment of acute immune thrombocytopenic purpura in children: a systematic review and meta-analysis of randomized controlled trials. J Pediatr 2005;147:521–7.

14. Tamminga R, Berchtold W, Bruin M, et al. Possible lower rate of chronic ITP after IVIG for acute childhood ITP an analysis from registry I of the Intercontinental Cooperative ITP Study Group (ICIS). Br J Haematol 2009;146:180–4.

15. Lefrere JJ, Loiseau P, Martinot-Peignoux M, et al. Infection by hepatitis C virus through contaminated intravenous immune globulin: results of a prospective national inquiry in France. Transfusion 1996;36:394–7.

16. Pawlotsky JM, Bouvier M, Deforges L, et al. Chronic hepatitis C after high-dose intravenous immunoglobulin. Transfusion 1994;34:86–7.

17. Salama A, Kiefel V, Amberg R, et al. Treatment of autoimmune thrombocytopenic purpura with rhesus antibodies (anti-Rh0(D)). Blut 1984;49:29–35.

18. Becker T, Kuenzlen E, Salama A, et al. Treatment of childhood idiopathic thrombocytopenic purpura with Rhesus antibodies (anti-D). Eur J Pediatr 1986;145:166–9.

19. Salama A, Kiefel V, Mueller-Eckhardt C. Effect of IgG anti-Rho(D) in adult patients with chronic autoimmune thrombocytopenia. Am J Hematol 1986;22:241–50.

20. Scaradavou A, Woo B, Woloski BM, et al. Intravenous anti-D treatment of immune thrombocytopenic purpura: experience in 272 patients. Blood 1997;89:2689–700.

21. Newman GC, Novoa MV, Fodero EM, et al. A dose of 75 microg/kg/d of i.v. anti-D increases the platelet count more rapidly and for a longer period of time than 50 microg/kg/d in adults with immune thrombocytopenic purpura. Br J Haematol 2001;112:1076–8.

22. Tarantino MD, Young G, Bertolone SJ, et al. Single dose of anti-D immune globulin at 75 microg/kg is as effective as intravenous immune globulin at rapidly raising the platelet count in newly diagnosed immune thrombocytopenic purpura in children. J Pediatr 2006;148:489–94.

23. Cooper N, Heddle NM, Haas M, et al. Intravenous (IV) anti-D and IV immunoglobulin achieve acute platelet increases by different mechanisms: modulation of cytokine and platelet responses to IV anti-D by FcgammaRIIa and FcgammaRIIIa polymorphisms. Br J Haematol 2004;124:511–8.

24. Cooper N, Woloski BM, Fodero EM, et al. Does treatment with intermittent infusions of intravenous anti-D allow a proportion of adults with recently diagnosed immune thrombocytopenic purpura to avoid splenectomy? Blood 2002;99:1922–7.

25. Scaradavou A, Cunningham-Rundles S, Ho JL, et al. Superior effect of intravenous anti-D compared with IV gammaglobulin in the treatment of HIV-thrombocytopenia: results of a small, randomized prospective comparison. Am J Hematol 2007;82:335–41.

26. Bussel JB, Graziano JN, Kimberly RP, et al. Intravenous anti-D treatment of immune thrombocytopenic purpura: analysis of efficacy, toxicity, and mechanism of effect. Blood 1991;77:1884–93.

27. Michel M, Novoa MV, Bussel JB. Intravenous anti-D as a treatment for immune thrombocytopenic purpura (ITP) during pregnancy. Br J Haematol 2003;123: 142–6.

28. Cromwell C, Tarantino M, Aledort LM. Safety of anti-D during pregnancy. Am J Hematol 2009;84:261–2.

29. Gaines AR. Acute onset hemoglobinemia and/or hemoglobinuria and sequelae following Rh(o)(D) immune globulin intravenous administration in immune thrombocytopenic purpura patients. Blood 2000;95:2523–9.

30. Gaines AR. Disseminated intravascular coagulation associated with acute hemoglobinemia or hemoglobinuria following Rh(0)(D) immune globulin intravenous administration for immune thrombocytopenic purpura. Blood 2005;106: 1532–7.

31. Fehr J, Hofmann V, Kappeler U. Transient reversal of thrombocytopenia in idiopathic thrombocytopenic purpura by high-dose intravenous gamma globulin. N Engl J Med 1982;306:1254–8.

32. Newland AC, Macey MG. Immune thrombocytopenia and Fc receptor-mediated phagocyte function. Ann Hematol 1994;69:61–7.

33. Siragam V, Brinc D, Crow AR, et al. Can antibodies with specificity for soluble antigens mimic the therapeutic effects of intravenous IgG in the treatment of autoimmune disease? J Clin Invest 2005;115:155–60.

34. Clarkson SB, Bussel JB, Kimberly RP, et al. Treatment of refractory immune thrombocytopenic purpura with an anti-Fc gamma-receptor antibody. N Engl J Med 1986;314:1236–9.

35. Song S, Crow AR, Freedman J, et al. Monoclonal IgG can ameliorate immune thrombocytopenia in a murine model of ITP: an alternative to IVIG. Blood 2003; 101:3708–13.

36. Kurlander RJ. Blockade of Fc receptor-mediated binding to U-937 cells by murine monoclonal antibodies directed against a variety of surface antigens. J Immunol 1983;131:140–7.

37. Teeling JL, Jansen-Hendriks T, Kuijpers TW, et al. Therapeutic efficacy of intravenous immunoglobulin preparations depends on the immunoglobulin G dimers: studies in experimental immune thrombocytopenia. Blood 2001;98:1095–9.

38. Smith NA, Boughton BJ. The treatment of autoimmune thrombocytopaenic purpura with anti-D immunoglobulin: similar platelet responses in homozygous and heterozygous Rh(D) positive patients. Transfus Med 1991;1:183–5.

39. Soubrane C, Tourani JM, Andrieu JM, et al. Biologic response to anti-CD16 monoclonal antibody therapy in a human immunodeficiency virus-related immune thrombocytopenic purpura patient. Blood 1993;81:15–9.

40. Burdach SE, Evers KG, Geursen RG. Treatment of acute idiopathic thrombocytopenic purpura of childhood with intravenous immunoglobulin G: comparative efficacy of 7S and 5S preparations. J Pediatr 1986;109:770–5.

41. Tovo PA, Miniero R, Fiandino G, et al. Fc-depleted vs intact intravenous immunoglobulin in chronic ITP. J Pediatr 1984;105:676–7.

42. Samuelsson A, Towers TL, Ravetch JV. Anti-inflammatory activity of IVIG mediated through the inhibitory Fc receptor. Science 2001;291:484–6.

43. Crow AR, Song S, Freedman J, et al. IVIg-mediated amelioration of murine ITP via FcgammaRIIB is independent of SHIP1, SHP-1, and Btk activity. Blood 2003;102: 558–60.

44. Crow AR, Song S, Siragam V, et al. Mechanisms of action of intravenous immunoglobulin in the treatment of immune thrombocytopenia. Pediatr Blood Cancer 2006;47:710–3.
45. Bruhns P, Samuelsson A, Pollard JW, et al. Colony-stimulating factor-1-dependent macrophages are responsible for IVIG protection in antibody-induced autoimmune disease. Immunity 2003;18:573–81.
46. Kaneko Y, Nimmerjahn F, Ravetch JV. Anti-inflammatory activity of immunoglobulin G resulting from Fc sialylation. Science 2006;313:670–3.
47. Anthony RM, Wermeling F, Karlsson MC, et al. Identification of a receptor required for the anti-inflammatory activity of IVIG. Proc Natl Acad Sci U S A 2008;105:19571–8.
48. Siragam V, Crow AR, Brinc D, et al. Intravenous immunoglobulin ameliorates ITP via activating Fc gamma receptors on dendritic cells. Nat Med 2006;12:688–92.
49. Crow AR, Brinc D, Lazarus AH. New insight into the mechanism of action of IVIg: the role of dendritic cells. J Thromb Haemost 2009;7(Suppl 1):245–8.
50. Newland AC, Macey MG, Veys PA. Cellular changes during the infusion of high dose intravenous immunoglobulin. Blut 1989;59:82–7.
51. Oksenhendler E, Bierling P, Brossard Y, et al. Anti-RH immunoglobulin therapy for human immunodeficiency virus-related immune thrombocytopenic purpura. Blood 1988;71:1499–502.
52. Ramadan KM, El-Agnaf M. Efficacy and response to intravenous anti-D immunoglobulin in chronic idiopathic thrombocytopenic purpura. Clin Lab Haematol 2005;27:267–9.
53. Malinowska I, Obitko-Pludowska A, Buescher ES, et al. Release of cytokines and soluble cytokine receptors after intravenous anti-D treatment in children with chronic thrombocytopenic purpura. Hematol J 2001;2:242–9.
54. Semple JW, Allen D, Rutherford M, et al. Anti-D (WinRho SD) treatment of children with chronic autoimmune thrombocytopenic purpura stimulates transient cytokine/chemokine production. Am J Hematol 2002;69:225–7.
55. Coopamah MD, Freedman J, Semple JW. Anti-D initially stimulates an Fc-dependent leukocyte oxidative burst and subsequently suppresses erythrophagocytosis via interleukin-1 receptor antagonist. Blood 2003;102:2862–7.
56. Crow AR, Song S, Semple JW, et al. A role for IL-1 receptor antagonist or other cytokines in the acute therapeutic effects of IVIg? Blood 2007;109:155–8.
57. Song S, Crow AR, Siragam V, et al. Monoclonal antibodies that mimic the action of anti-D in the amelioration of murine ITP act by a mechanism distinct from that of IVIg. Blood 2005;105:1546–8.
58. Podolanczuk A, Lazarus AH, Crow AR, et al. Of mice and men: an open-label pilot study for treatment of immune thrombocytopenic purpura by an inhibitor of Syk. Blood 2009;113:3154–60.

Traditional and New Approaches to the Management of Immune Thrombocytopenia: Issues of When and Who to Treat

James B. Bussel, MD[a,b,c,*]

KEYWORDS

• ITP • Platelets • Autoimmunity • Bleeding • Thrombocytopenia

Chronic ITP is currently defined as immune thrombocytopenia (ITP) that has a minimum duration of 12 months, and often longer.[1] ITP, its diagnosis, and definition have been covered in other chapters in this issue and therefore general issues connected with ITP will not be discussed further here except where specific features are particularly relevant to the management of chronic ITP.

In the United States, in addition to steroids, either prednisone and/or dexamethasone, many patients with newly chronic ITP will already have received intravenous immunoglobulin (IVIG) or intravenous (IV) anti-D and rituximab as well before they have reached 12 months from diagnosis. Both high-dose dexamethasone (40 mg/m^2 × 4 days for 3 to 4 cycles 2 weeks apart), especially if used close to the time of diagnosis of ITP,[2,3] and rituximab may have curative-type effects with patients achieving stable normal platelet counts for at least 1 year or longer after treatment, if not indefinitely.[4] It would appear from several studies, including not only those with dexamethasone, but also with IV anti-D,[5,6] that at least 50% of patients improve within 1 to 2 years of diagnosis and no longer require platelet supportive therapy after

[a] Department of Pediatrics, Weill Medical College of Cornell University, 525 E 68th Street, P695, New York, NY 10065, USA
[b] Department of Obstetrics-Gynecology, Weill Medical College of Cornell University, 525 E 68th Street, P695, New York, NY 10065, USA
[c] Department of Medicine, Weill Medical College of Cornell University, 525 E 68th Street, P695, New York, NY 10065, USA
* Corresponding author.
E-mail address: jbussel@med.cornell.edu

Hematol Oncol Clin N Am 23 (2009) 1329–1341
doi:10.1016/j.hoc.2009.09.004
0889-8588/09/$ – see front matter © 2009 Elsevier Inc. All rights reserved.

hemonc.theclinics.com

that time. How much of this effect is the result of a specific treatment or a spontaneous remission in which a particular therapy "buys time" by maintaining a safe platelet count until spontaneous improvement takes place is uncertain. This distinction is complicated by the fact that many patients receive treatments with agents such as prednisone, IVIG, and IV anti-D that are not expected to have lasting effects, but may be used to maintain a safe platelet count. It is uncertain if there are many patients in whom repeated application of therapy such as anti-D or IVIG conveys a lasting benefit.[5,7,8]

Management of chronic ITP is different from that of acute ITP (**Fig. 1**). For acute ITP patients, treatment is initially aimed at rapidly increasing the platelet count and then at maintaining an adequate, safe count while hoping that, whatever therapy is administered, patients will improve and no longer require any treatment. For chronic ITP, the goals and needs are different. On the one hand there may still be further improvement so that short-term therapies may nonetheless be important. On the other hand, improvement and especially attaining remission becomes much less likely after more than 1 year from diagnosis and therefore short-term improvement in the platelet count is not a viable strategy on its own. However, short-term therapies may avoid severe thrombocytopenia while awaiting the response to a "long-term therapy." Also, smaller changes in the count become more significant. A change in the platelet count from 5000 to 10,000/μL to 20,000 to 25,000/μL would likely provide an important impact on the risk and occurrence of bleeding.

Children with chronic ITP are different from adults with chronic ITP in several "less-well-defined ways." There is an anticipation that they will be easier to manage. In fact, children with persistent severe chronic ITP past 1 year may be more difficult to manage than adults and often have subtle underlying immunologic problems. The approach to their care is discussed in the article by Drs Bennett and Tarantino and in the article by Kalpatthi and Bussel 2008.[9] The remainder of this text pertains to adults.

What are the advantages of doing no treatment at all (observation with "emergency" or "rescue" platelet support eg, steroid bolus, IVIG, or IV anti-D or even platelet transfusion) for a patient who has had ITP for more than 1 year without signs of improvement? The obvious advantage is that there is no toxicity of therapy. Virtually all treatments cause some problems. A subtler advantage, but one that is important to patients, is that they no longer have to make frequent appointments with their hematologists, "face up to their condition," and continually decide on the best course of action. Instead typically they come in for follow-up when they feel like it, do not spend "time worrying about their disease" or its treatment, and generally act as if they had been "cured." This frees up time, reduces medical bills, and may also relieve patient anxiety. Much of this depends on the patient however. If they have bruising or especially mouth sores and heavy menses, it may prove impossible to "ignore" their ITP and, even if this approach is tried, the patient may return to the hematologist for management. More serious bleeding may occur in the context of other illness or trauma; a very low platelet count may prevent use of medications to treat other conditions. For these reasons, periodic visits are optimal to maintain a dialog and to further develop the patient-physician relationship and prevent denial, which may have serious consequences.

There are no data on this particular point but one would expect that this would be a time when patients would be most likely to try alternative therapies. Many, possibly most, patients believe that if a substance is "natural" that guarantees that there will be no toxicity and therefore trying anything natural is good, even if realistic expectations of benefit may be very small. This has clearly been proven wrong on a number of

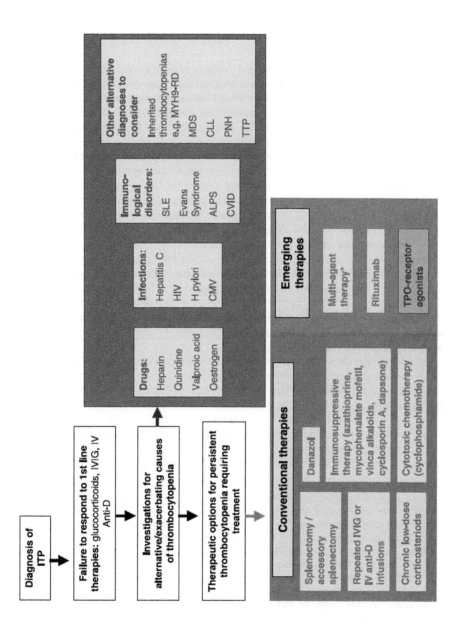

occasions; eg, fatal hepatic failure with herbal teas. Many patients also think that a "Naturopath" saying "this works for my patients with ITP" means that there are sufficient data that a given remedy should reasonably be tried with a reasonable expectation of success. These may be the same patients who would not try an allopathic treatment because they feel the data of a randomized trial were insufficient. In particular, careful reporting in a clinical trial of unrelated adverse events may bias patients who ignore the possibility that adverse events occur with "natural" substances and without treatment.

Therefore "observation and no treatment" may only be no "allopathic" treatment. Patients may decide that certain agents improved their bleeding without changing their platelet counts, which can be very difficult to decide objectively. Nonetheless, it is clear that if the count is low enough (certainly if it is <20,000/μL) and if there is bleeding, then the risk of serious hemorrhage is appreciable. Certain issues need to be considered at this juncture before discussing available treatments. First what if any other reasons exist to treat patients even if they do not appear to be at immediate risk of life-threatening hemorrhage (ICH). Second, what investigations are required to distinguish a case of "refractory" ITP from that of another etiology such as myelodysplasia. Third, where should the balance be between treatment to prevent bleeding, improve health-related quality of life, and a policy of reasonable observation.

The *first* consideration involves Health-Related Quality of Life (HRQoL). Studies of HRQoL in patients have clearly demonstrated that many patients have substantial deficits in this area.[10,11] A discussion of which methods are optimal to define impaired HRQoL, either in general or in ITP, are beyond the scope of this article. However areas in which at least a substantial fraction of patients have reported deficits include libido, cognitive function, time, money required to be used for care of their ITP, and the most universal finding: chronic fatigue. Recent studies with the thrombopoietic agents have suggested that treatment that improves the platelet count may improve complaints in this area across a wide variety of complaints.[12,13] Therefore, this becomes an important impetus to improve HRQoL for the patient, even if one believes that their risk of death or serious impairment from bleeding appears to be small. This approach requires that there be treatments that are sufficiently efficacious, tolerable, and easy to administer that they do not themselves create a substantial impairment in HRQoL. The only ones that have been well demonstrated thus far to fit this category (high response rate, good tolerability, low toxicity) are the thrombopoietic agents. Splenectomy probably would qualify as well, but it and other chronic treatments are largely unstudied and thus more specific comments cannot be made.

Fig. 1. An investigation and treatment algorithm for patients with a diagnosis of ITP who are poorly responsive to first-line therapies. The available therapies are not listed in any suggested order of preference, as there is no consensus on this at present and the choice of agents should be chosen according to the individual patients' clinical needs and preferences. TPO-R agonists are highlighted in red as they still available only in clinical trials. *Multi-agent therapy: IVIG and methylprednisolone plus IV anti-D and/or vincristine for induction and danazol plus azathioprine for oral maintenance therapy.[46] ALPS autoimmune lymphoproliferative syndrome; CLL, chronic lymphocytic leukemia; CMV, cytomegalovirus; CVID, common variable immune deficiency; H pylori, *Helicobacter pylori*; HIV, human immunodeficiency virus; ITP, immune thrombocytopenic purpura; IVIG, intravenous immunoglobulin; MDS, myelodysplastic syndrome; MYH9-RD, May Hegglin anomaly related disorders; PNH, paroxysmal nocturnal hemoglobinuria; SLE, systemic lupus erythematosis; TTP, thrombotic thrombocytopenic purpura; TPO, thrombopoietin. (*From* Psaila B, Bussel JB. Refractory immune thrombocytopenic purpura: current strategies for investigation and management. Br J Haematol 2008;143(1):16–26; with permission.)

Second, if a physician sees a patient with chronic ITP for the first time (or has not "reevaluated" the patient since diagnosis), it is worthwhile to review the items in **Box 1** in deciding how to approach the patient to ensure that this patient really has chronic ITP. The primary considerations are whether this might be a case that resembles ITP, but is not or is a case of secondary ITP in which resolution of the primary, underlying disease would impact on the management of the thrombocytopenia. In this brief overview, there are a number of categories to consider.

One prominent subset is *drug-induced thrombocytopenia* (DIT).[14] It has become clear that ITP occurs frequently in more elderly patients, and therefore the number of medications that patients are on is often not trivial. However, in the absence of diagnostic testing for ITP (which is the current situation) and in the absence of a good way to judge the likelihood of DIT in a given case, the optimal approach appears to be to sequentially change all of a patient's medications to therapeutic equivalents that are biochemically different. In the past this was often arduous, but the increased number of available medications makes this approach currently more feasible.

It is worthwhile commenting briefly on several medications. Heparin-induced thrombocytopenia thrombosis (HITT) is an extremely serious and complex entity and worthy of a separate treatise. It typically occurs in inpatients or those recently discharged. Valproate is almost always a cause of dose-related marrow suppressant and therefore is unusual in that dose reduction to lower the blood level (to less than 100) is usually sufficient and drug discontinuation is not typically required.[15] Diphenylhydantoin is among a small number of drugs known to induce platelet antibodies. In a small number of women, estrogen (whether in oral contraceptives or used unopposed postmenopausally) seems to convert otherwise unexceptional ITP into a refractory state. Discontinuation of estrogen in such a patient (or conversion to only progesterone such as depoprovera) allows the ITP to revert to its "normal" form.[16]

Recent studies have highlighted ITP that is not only "caused" by *infections* but possibly perpetuated by them. The reported infections capable of causing ITP to appear and persist as long as the infection continues unabated are HIV, Hepatitis C, *Helicobacter pylori*, and cytomegalovirus (CMV); there may well be others. HIV-related thrombocytopenia is well known and the thrombocytopenia was first reported in the early 1980's to respond to viral suppression.[17] The "disappearance" of HIV-ITP is a result of the widespread use of HAART.[18] Similarly, hepatitis C has been known to cause thrombocytopenia but the "one-to-one" correlation of viral suppression and amelioration of thrombocytopenia has not been as well demonstrated as in HIV infection.[19] Recent studies have demonstrated the variability of response of thrombocytopenia to *H pylori* eradication, seemingly dependent on geography, which may reflect infection with different strains. For example, platelet response rates to *H pylori*

Box 1

ITP: a diagnosis of exclusion

- Normal complete blood count (CBC) except isolated thrombocytopenia. No other cytopenias (except for possible Fe deficiency).

- Normal peripheral blood smear with some large platelets.

- Normal examination; except signs of bleeding. No splenomegaly.

- *Exclude Secondary ITP*: systemic lupus erythematosus, hypogammaglobulinemia, anti-phospholipid, thyroid disease, Evans syndrome lymphoproliferative disorders, drug-induced.

- Infection: HIV, *Helicobacter pylori*, Hepatitis C, CMV.

eradication in Japan and Italy appear to be far higher than those seen in the United States. Unlike the other infections described and CMV, H pylori infection has not been commonly described as an etiology of "refractory" ITP.[20] A recent report on CMV infection has suggested in four cases that immunosuppression, such as steroids used in the treatment of ITP, may in rare cases result in reactivation of CMV infection, which in turn causes a refractory thrombocytopenia. Platelet counts may improve when immunosuppression is stopped and the CMV treated.[21] Human T-cell lympho-tropic virus (HTLV1) does not appear to have a similar effect.[22] Other infectious agents have not been carefully studied.

ITP associated with lymphoproliferative disorders is well described. The most prom-inent are Hodgkin disease and chronic lymphocytic leukemia (CLL). The former is readily recognized but the latter may smolder and not be immediately noticed in all cases. The diagnosis of early-stage CLL requires recognition of the increased number of small lymphocytes and that these cells are of the B-cell lineage. Recent study of Canale-Smith syndrome (ALPS or autoimmune lymphoproliferative syndrome) has suggested that at least a "forme fruste" of it may underlie a substantial fraction of pediatric autoimmune hemolytic anemia (AIHA).[23] Studies of ALPS, an apoptosis defect in autoreactive T and B cells, in patients with ITP have been very limited, but ALPS pathophysiology may have a role in a small fraction of cases.[24]

Finally, *immune deficiency* is well known to be associated with immune thrombocy-topenia. The commonest form and best understood is common variable immune deficiency (CVID), also known as hypogammaglobulinemia. At least 10% of patients with CVID develop ITP at one time or another; another 10% of CVID patients may develop AIHA.[25] Among patients with CVID, autoimmunity to platelets and red blood cells occurs more frequently in those with mutations in transmembrane activator and calcium modulator and cyclophilin ligand activator (TACI), a B-cell growth factor receptor.[26] Furthermore ITP does not appear to develop in patients with X-linked agammaglobulinemia (Brutons), presumably because there are no abnormal circu-lating B cells and T cells to instigate the autoimmunity.

Third, how does one decide who to treat? This has been considered in depth in "How I Treat ITP" in *Blood* 2005.[27] On the one hand, there is hemorrhagic morbidity and especially mortality in patients with low platelet counts and bleeding symptoms.[28] On the other hand, one study suggested that death as a consequence of infection related to therapy occurs at least as frequently as hemorrhage.[29] Clearly this depends on the treatment in question and in particular the greatest morbidity is related to the persistent use of corticosteroids. As indicated previously, the clinical algorithm has become more complicated by the inclusion of HRQoL into the treatment equation. A surprising example is noted that some students with ITP want treatment to increase their platelet count before examinations because they can "think better when their counts are higher." The issue of treating versus not treating has been best considered in pediatric ITP, but no clear consensus has been reached there.

The rest of this article is devoted to which patients with chronic ITP need to receive treatment because with low platelets, bleeding symptoms and/or HRQoL issues to consider, it may be difficult to judge by the treating physician. For the sake of consensus, this would usually involve a platelet threshold of 20,000 to 30,000/μL, but as discussed in "How I Treat ITP,"[27] it is occasionally appropriate to select a higher target count for a number of reasons. Certain issues discussed earlier in this article affect treatment. If there is secondary ITP, then treating the underlying disease, such as infection or an immune defect, is usually the optimal approach. This section will assume that appropriate evaluation has been undertaken and patients with secondary causes of ITP will have been managed accordingly.

The previous discussion may make it seem as if the identification of secondary ITP is straightforward and clinically obvious; it is often not. One critical issue is the decision in which patient to do which tests. In other words, should certain testing be done "blindly" with no clinical indication? This is an evolving field in which there is not any resolution at this time, in large part because there are no data to inform the decision. Our approach has been to do a battery of tests in all patients with chronic ITP to explore the possibility of CVID, hypothyroidism, Evans syndrome, and other entities even without direct clinical history suggestive of these possibilities. Other centers may advocate hepatitis C testing (as transaminases may be normal in infected patients) and also to look for *H pylori*.

Laboratory testing in a complex patient often requires not only a careful history but often two rounds of testing: a screening set of tests and then follow-up exploration. Testing that depends on IgG antibodies may be false positive for months following IVIG. However CVID can be considered based on IgA and IgM levels and other testing such as *H pylori* done by the breath test and stool antigen, and hepatitis C, HIV, and CMV done by polymerase chain reaction (PCR). Bone marrow evaluation typically requires at least an aspirate, biopsy, and cytogenetics focused on myelodysplasia; flow cytometry is less useful in the absence of a monoclonal population in the marrow, although some investigators have documented small populations of CLL lymphocytes in the marrows of older ITP patients. All of these and other tests are not diagnostic of ITP and are intended to exclude other specific diagnoses linked to apparent ITP. The only specific test that "includes" ITP (although it does not distinguish primary from secondary ITP) is response to ITP-specific therapy (prednisone, IVIG, or IV anti-D). If response is substantial even if transient and if the response is repeated, then this is a strong argument for the presence of immune thrombocytopenia. The issue of diagnostic testing is further delineated in the new International ITP Guidelines scheduled to appear in *Blood* in late 2009.

If a patient has chronic ITP, the utility of repeated IVIG and IV anti-D is usually limited. Further steroids typically are fraught with increasing toxicity and less efficacy. It is "too late" for high-dose dexamethasone to have other than rare curative effects. Therefore other therapies need to be considered.[30]

The gold standard is splenectomy. Unlike what many patients believe based on Internet misinformation, the 5- to 10-year efficacy is approximately 65% for all patients and 85% in the first week after surgery.[31] Laparoscopic splenectomy does not result in additional complications, such as an increased need for accessory splenectomy, or loss in efficacy. The issues deterring at least some patients are:

(1) Knowledge that other patients who have undergone splenectomy have failed to be "cured" of their ITP. This remains active in Internet communication, whereas those who are cured typically do not report this. This means that patients seeking guidance from other patients are often counseled not to undergo the procedure because "splenectomy does not work."
(2) Patients do not wish to undergo an operation without being assured that it will work 100% of the time. There are no good, readily available predictors at this time. Platelet site of destruction studies remain controversial.
(3) The long-term outcome is not known. Specifically 20- to 30-year follow-up data are absent. Concern has been raised about dementia in one small group of patients.[32] A conundrum here is that efficacy decreases as the age of the patient increases above age 45 years.[31] This means that the higher response rates are in the patients with the most potential for late side effects because they are younger and should have the longest lifespan post splenectomy.

(4) Patients are concerned about "post splenectomy sepsis." On the one hand this is quite rare. On the other hand, if or when a fever occurs, it is mandatory to urgently and emergently receive parenteral broad spectrum antibiotics that are effective against pneumococcus. This is true no matter how many years post splenectomy it is when the fever occurs.

Nonetheless the answer to the question *What is the best way to "cure" ITP?* is splenectomy!

Rituximab, anti-CD20 therapy has advantages and disadvantages. It is the answer to the question *"what is the likeliest way to cure ITP if one does not wish to do splenectomy."* It is estimated that approximately one third of patients will have a complete response (CR) (unmaintained normal platelet count) following a standard treatment with 375 mg/m^2 weekly for 4 weeks.[4] Virtually all of these patients in CR will maintain their response for at least 1 year. The current estimate is that after that time approximately one half will lose their response within 4 more years, most by 3 years from initial treatment. Therefore it has high utility to maintain a normal platelet count for 1 to 3 years, but the patient should know that a complete response is not a cure and ITP will often relapse. Repeat treatment for the relapsed complete responder can result in a high rate of repeat response.[33] However, essentially all patients will relapse again after approximately the same time interval, so that one may have to plan on regular repeated treatments. Unfortunately, the optimal approach to patients achieving an initial CR and then relapsing remains to be discovered. The safety of repeated courses of rituximab has not been evaluated. Concerns include development of progressive multifocal leukoencephalopathy (PML)[34] and reactivation of hepatitis B, but the former seems vanishingly rare in patients not receiving multiple chemotherapies with rituximab. Reactivation of hepatitis B does not seem to be very common and will be even less so in the era of hepatitis B vaccination. In addition, it can be monitored so that reactivation could be treated early before serious liver damage occurs. Common but less serious toxicity includes first infusion reactions such as fever and chills, and serum sickness; the latter especially in children.[35] Finally, patients cannot mount humoral responses to vaccines for months after rituximab; but contrary to expectation despite elimination of B cells in the peripheral blood, overall immunoglobulin levels rarely decrease. Newer human or humanized anti-CD20 monclonal antibodies have been and are being developed, but whether their efficacy has been altered by humanizing them or by engineering to affect antigen and/or Fc receptor binding is not clear. Toxicity has been ameliorated by intramuscular injection, which reduces infusion reactions and greatly speeds up administration. This may however lower the dosage because of volume limitation, but it can be argued that the optimal dose of rituximab for the treatment of ITP remains unknown.

The newest development involves thrombopoietin receptor agonists. The rationale for their use, their structure, their biology, and clinical effects in normal volunteers is described in the article by Kuter-Gernsheimer in this issue. There are a series of publications on romiplostim (AMG531) and eltrombopag, which are the first two such agents that are approved for treatment of refractory ITP, at least in the United States. As described by Kuter-Gernsheimer, the current second generation agents were initially evaluated in refractory ITP.

AMG531 (romiplostim, Nplate):
(1) The first study using AMG531 was published in 2006 and had two parts.[36] The first part was a cohort dose increase study that showed a clear dose response in the effective range between 1 and 10 μg/kg. Counts in good responders at the highest dose levels only began to increase on day 5 and peaked after day 8. The second

part of the study was a 6-week, repeated weekly injection study in two groups of 8 patients, one group at 1 μg/kg and the second group at 3 μg/kg. It was demonstrated that at these treatment doses patient platelets counts often increased to higher than 50,000/μL, but with a high degree of fluctuation from one week to the next.

(2) The second publication described two pivotal, randomized, controlled studies that were identical, with one study in splenectomized patients and the other study in nonsplenectomized patients.[37] Both involved slow dose increases week to week depending on the platelet count. There was also the ability to use rescue medication for too low counts and/or bleeding and, after response, to discontinue concomitant prednisone. In both parallel trials, unequivocal efficacy was demonstrated by all efficacy end points: durable response (platelets ≥50,000/μL for 6 of the last 8 weeks and no rescue therapy), overall response (platelet counts ≥ 50,000/μL on 4 of 24 weeks), reduction in the use of concomitant medications such as prednisone; and less use of rescue medications (IVIG, anti-RhD, or prednisone). No tachyphylaxis was seen over the 6 months of the study and no important toxicity emerged such as an increased incidence of thromboembolic events. AMG531 (romiplostim, Nplate) was licensed in August 2008 based on these two studies.

(3) Patients who entered one of the previous studies were eligible to enter the long-term maintenance study, which was recently published representing up to 3 years of follow-up of patients on weekly AMG531.[38] Overall, the study showed that long-term use of AMG531 as a maintenance therapy was feasible from many aspects: platelet counts could be maintained for years; no dose increase was required over time; responses were consistent within most patients; patients could learn to give 3 of 4 weekly injections at home; and no important toxicity developed. This study was the first one to address reticulin fibrosis in the marrow and reported nine cases. Further studies need to be performed to clarify this issue as to whether there is a high potential for important marrow damage or not, although at this time it does not appear to result in permanent injury.

(4) Other studies have been reported in abstract form including a 22-patient study in children preliminarily demonstrating safety and efficacy and a study exploring the utility of presplenectomy use of AMG531 to delay or prevent splenectomy in which splenectomy was performed more often and earlier on the standard-of-care arm.

Eltrombopag (Promacta)
(1) The first study published was a 6-week study at four (daily) doses: placebo, 30 mg, 50 mg, and 75 mg.[39] Responses were seen in 70% to 80% of patients at the two highest doses compared with 11% in placebo. No important toxicity was seen in the study and bleeding decreased as the platelets increased. A second study in the same issue of the New England Journal of Medicine reported similar impressive results for thrombocytopenic patients with hepatitis C infection allowing continued antiviral chemotherapy without dose reduction or interruption.[40]

(2) The second study was a confirmatory 6-week randomized placebo-controlled trial comparing 50 mg of eltrombopag to placebo.[41] The results were again striking with 59% response on the eltrombopag arm to a level higher than 50,000/μL compared with 16% on placebo. Bleeding manifestations again were decreased in responders and increased back to baseline after the medication was discontinued and the platelet counts returned to baseline. In this study, rebound thrombocytopenia was a rare problem on drug withdrawal and no statistically significant specific organ toxicity was seen. However, some patients have developed significant elevations in liver enzymes requiring cessation of medication.

(3) Other eltrombopag studies have been reported only in abstract form. These include a 6-month randomized study with results comparable to the AMG531 pivotal trials described previously and a repeated use study (three cycles of 6 weeks on, 4 weeks off), which showed super-imposable findings for each of the cycles, demonstrating no loss of efficacy with duration of treatment or repeated use.

Single-agent treatment of ITP with agents such as azathioprin, danazol, cyclophosphamide, cyclosporine, and mycophenalate mofetil, to name the most commonly used agents, has been difficult. One review by Berchtold and McMillan[42] suggested that no single agent is effective in more than 30% of cases and this is especially true in chronic cases, particularly those refractory to splenectomy. In the post-splenectomy refractory patients, the higher response rates reported in the patients treated with the thrombopoietin receptor agonists suggest that these would be the drugs of choice for this group of patients (discussed previously). In addition, the use of these agents, by increasing platelet counts in the post-splenectomy patients, allowed for a reduction in the use of concomitant immunosuppressive drugs. This can reduce the infection risk in this high-risk patient population. In general, therefore, single-agent therapy often is ineffective. Even autologous stem cell transplants have only been found to have a 25% to 33% response rate without multiyear follow-up.[43] Individual agents are analyzed and their efficacy and toxicity considered in the soon to be published International Guidelines on ITP.

Combination therapy has been approached in some situations to increase response rate and decrease toxicity of single agents whose dosage must be increased to the maximum to maintain any efficacy. The first report involved a patient with Hodgkin disease and refractory ITP whose thrombocytopenia responded to six cycles of chemotherapy protocol consisting of cyclophosphamide, vincristine, doxorubicin, and prednisone (CHOP). Treatment of further patients resulted in important toxicity, but good responses in certain patients[44] Long-term follow-up showed that all but one responder maintained the response over many years.[45] Boruchov and colleagues[46] tried multiagent therapy with initial IVIG, IV methylprednisolone, and IV anti-D, vincristine, or all four together followed by danazol and azathioprin in combination. The latter was effective in 13 of 17 patients with the only important exclusion being abnormal liver testing before initiation of treatment. Other combinations may be demonstrated to be useful in the future.

Mechanism of therapeutic effect can now be targeted more specifically and this could lead to the development of "intelligent" combinations. The most obvious would be combining an agent that inhibits platelet destruction, such as IVIG, IV anti-D, or the Rigel syk inhibitor,[47] with an agent that stimulates platelet production (AMG531 or eltrombopag). Although this would not be a "curative" approach, it is potentially a highly effective treatment strategy.

SUMMARY

In summary, diagnosis and management of chronic ITP requires experience and the appropriate use of the laboratory despite the absence of a diagnostic test for ITP. The diagnostic test valuable above all others is response to ITP-specific therapy as it is the only test that "includes" ITP, rather than excluding other entities in the differential diagnosis. Consideration of secondary ITP is very important because identification of immunodeficiency or of infections or of lymphoproliferative disorders would change the management approach to a given patient. The development of newer therapies such as rituximab and the thrombopoietic agents have had a major impact on the management of ITP. Further exploration of how to optimize curative effects of any and all therapies remains an important consideration. In the future, additional combinations of agents may be a critical approach although the schedule and dosing remains difficult to establish. Finally, current studies to augment therapy in the newly diagnosed ITP patients to prevent chronic disease may lessen the number of patients in chronic disease category.

REFERENCES

1. Rodeghiero F, Stasi R, Gernsheimer T, et al. Standardization of terminology, definitions and outcome criteria in immune thrombocytopenic purpura (ITP) of adults and children: Report from an International Working Group. Blood 2008;113(11): 2386–93.
2. Cheng Y, Wong RS, Soo YO, et al. Initial treatment of immune thrombocytopenic purpura with high-dose dexamethasone. N Engl J Med 2003;349(9):831–6.
3. Mazzucconi MG, Fazi P, Bernasconi S, et al. Gruppo Italiano Malattie EMatologiche dell'Adulto (GIMEMA) Thrombocytopenia Working Party. Therapy with high-dose dexamethasone (HD-DXM) in previously untreated patients affected by idiopathic thrombocytopenic purpura: a GIMEMA experience. Blood 2007; 109(4):1401–7.
4. Cooper N, Stasi R, Cunningham-Rundles S, et al. The efficacy and safety of B-cell depletion with anti-CD20 monoclonal antibody in adults with chronic immune thrombocytopenia purpura. Br J Haematol 2004;125(2):232–9.
5. Cooper N, Woloski BMR, Fodero EM, et al. Does treatment with intermittent infusions of IV anti-D allow a proportion of adults with recently diagnosed immune thrombocytopenic purpura (ITP) to avoid splenectomy? Blood 2002;99(6): 1922–7.
6. George JN, Raskob GE, Vesely SK, et al. Initial management of immune thrombocytopenic purpura in adults: a randomized controlled trial comparing intermittent anti-D with routine care. Am J Hematol 2003;74(3):161–9.
7. Godeau B, Lesage S, Divine M, et al. Treatment of adult chronic autoimmune thrombocytopenic purpura with repeated high-dose intravenous immunoglobulin. Blood 1993;82(5):1415–21.
8. Bussel J, Pham LC, Aledort L, et al. Maintenance treatment of adults with chronic refractory immune thrombocytopenic purpura using repeated intravenous infusions of gammaglobulin. Blood 1988;72(1):121–7.
9. Kalpatthi R, Bussel JB. Management of refractory immune thrombocytopenic purpura. Curr Opin Pediatr 2008;20:8–16.
10. McMillan R, Bussel JB, George JN, et al. Self-reported health-related quality of life in adults with chronic immune thrombocytopenic purpura. Am J Hematol 2008;83(2):150–4.
11. Mathias SD, Bussel JB, George JN, et al. A disease-specific measure of health-related quality of life for use in adults with immune thrombocytopenic purpura: its development and validation. Health Qual Life Outcomes 2007;5:11.
12. George JN, Mathias SD, Go RS, et al. Improved quality of life for romiplostim-treated patients with chronic immune thrombocytopenic purpura: results from two randomized, placebo-controlled trials. Br J Haematol 2009;144(3):409–15.
13. Cheng G, Saleh MN, Bussel JB, et al. Oral eltrombopag for the long-term treatment of patients with chronic idiopathic thrombocytopenic purpura: results

of a phase III, double- blind, placebo-controlled study (RAISE). [ASH Annual Meeting Abstracts]. Blood 2008;112:400.

14. George JN, Aster RH. Drug-induced thrombocytopenia: pathogenesis, evaluation, and management. ASH Education. Hematology 2009, in press.

15. Acharya S, Bussel JB. Valproate: hematologic toxicities of sodium valproate. J Pediatr Hematol Oncol 2000;22(1):62–5.

16. Onel K, Bussel JB. Adverse effects of estrogen therapy in a subset of women with ITP. J Thromb Haemost 2004;2(4):670–1.

17. Hymes KB, Greene JB, Karpatkin S. The effect of azidothymidine on HIV-related thrombocytopenia. N Engl J Med 1988;318(8):516–7.

18. Marks KM, Clarke RMA, Bussel JB, Talal AH, Glesby MJ. Brief report: risk factors for thrombocytopenia in HIV-infected persons in the era of potent antiretroviral therapy. JAIDS 2009, in press.

19. Rajan SK, Espina BM, Liebman HA. Hepatitis C virus-related thrombocytopenia: clinical and laboratory characteristics compared with chronic immune thrombocytopenic purpura. Br J Haematol 2005;129(6):818–24.

20. Stasi R, Sarpatwari A, Segal JB, et al. Effects of eradication of *Helicobacter pylori* infection in patients with immune thrombocytopenic purpura. A systematic review. Blood 2009;113(6):1231–40.

21. DiMaggio D, Anderson A, Bussel JB. Cytomegalovirus causes refractory immune thrombocytopenic purpura. Br J Haematol 2009;146(1):104–12.

22. Calleja E, Klein R, Bussel J. Is it necessary to test patients with immune thrombocytopenic purpura (ITP) for seropositivity to HTLV-1? Am J Hematol 1999;61: 94–7.

23. Teachey DT, Manno CS, Axsom KM, et al. Unmasking Evans syndrome: T-cell phenotype and apoptotic response reveal autoimmune lymphoproliferative syndrome (ALPS). Blood 2005;105(6):2443–8.

24. Rao VK, Price S, Perkins K, et al. Use of rituximab for refractory cytopenias associated with autoimmune lymphoproliferative syndrome (ALPS). Pediatr Blood Cancer 2009;52(7):847–52.

25. Cunningham-Rundles C. Autoimmune manifestations in common variable immunodeficiency. J Clin Immunol 2008;28(Suppl 1):S42–5.

26. Zhang L, Radigan L, Salzer U, et al. Transmembrane activator and calcium-modulating cyclophilin ligand interactor mutations in common variable immunodeficiency: clinical and immunologic outcomes in heterozygotes. J Allergy Clin Immunol 2007;120:1178–85.

27. Cines D, Bussel J. How I treat idiopathic thrombocytopenic purpura (ITP). Blood 2005;106:2244–51.

28. Cohen YC, Djulbegovic B, Shamai-Lubovitz O, et al. The bleeding risk and natural history of idiopathic thrombocytopenic purpura in patients with persistent low platelet counts. Arch Intern Med 2000;160(11):1630–8.

29. Portielje JE, Westendorp RG, Kluin-Nelemans HC, et al. Morbidity and mortality in adults with idiopathic thrombocytopenic purpura. Blood 2001;97(9):2549–54.

30. Psaila B, Bussel JB. Refractory immune thrombocytopenic purpura: current strategies for investigation and management. Br J Haematol 2008;143(1):16–26.

31. Kojouri K, Vesely SK, Terrell DR, et al. Splenectomy for adult patients with idiopathic thrombocytopenic purpura: a systematic review to assess long-term platelet count responses, prediction of response, and surgical complications. Blood 2004;104(9):2623–34.

32. Ahn YS, Horstman LL, Jy W, et al. Vascular dementia in patients with immune thrombocytopenic purpura. Thromb Res 2002;107(6):337–44.

33. Hasan A, Michel M, Patel V, Stasi R, Cunningham-Rundles S, Leonard J, Bussel JB. Repeated courses of rituximab in chronic ITP: three different regimens. Am J Hematol 2009, in press.

34. Carson KR, Evens AM, Richey EA, et al. Progressive multifocal leukoencephalopathy after rituximab therapy in HIV-negative patients: a report of 57 cases from the Research on Adverse Drug Events and Reports project. Blood 2009; 113(20):4834–40.

35. Wang J, Wiley J, Luddy R, et al. Chronic immune thrombocytopenia purpura (ITP) in children: assessment of rituximab treatment. J Pediatr 2005;146(2):217–21.

36. Bussel JB, Kuter DJ, George JN, et al. Effect of a novel thrombopoiesis-stimulating protein (AMG 531) in chronic immune thrombocytopenic purpura. N Engl J Med 2006;355:1672–81.

37. Kuter DJ, Bussel JB, Lyons RM, et al. Efficacy of romiplostim in patients with chronic immune thrombocytopenic purpura: a double-blind randomized controlled trial. Lancet 2008;371:395–403.

38. Bussel JB, Kuter D, Pullarkat VA, et al. Safety and efficacy of long-term treatment with romiplostim in thrombocytopenic patients with chronic ITP. Blood 2009; 113(10):2161–71.

39. Bussel JB, Cheng G, Saleh MN, et al. Eltrombopag, an oral platelet growth factor, for the treatment of patients with chronic idiopathic thrombocytopenic purpura. N Engl J Med 2007;357(22):2237–47.

40. McHutchison JG, Dusheiko G, Shiffman ML, et al. TPL102357 Study Group. Eltrombopag for thrombocytopenia in patients with cirrhosis associated with hepatitis C. N Engl J Med 2007;357(22):2227–36.

41. Bussel JB, Provan D, Shamsi T, et al. During treatment of chronic idiopathic thrombocytopenic purpura (ITP): a randomized, double blind, placebo-controlled study. Lancet 2009;373(9664):641–8.

42. Berchtold P, McMillan R. Therapy of chronic idiopathic thrombocytopenic purpura in adults. Blood 1989;74(7):2309–17.

43. Huhn RD, Fogarty PF, Nakamura R, et al. High-dose cyclophosphamide with autologous lymphocyte-depleted peripheral blood stem cell (PBSC) support for treatment of refractory chronic autoimmune thrombocytopenia. Blood 2003; 101(1):71–7.

44. Figueroa M, Gehlsen J, Hammond D, et al. Combination chemotherapy in refractory immune thrombocytopenic purpura. N Engl J Med 1993;328(17):1226–9.

45. McMillan R. Long-term outcomes after treatment for refractory immune thrombocytopenic purpura. N Engl J Med 2001;344(18):1402–3.

46. Boruchov DM, Gururangan S, Driscoll MC, et al. Multi-agent induction and maintenance therapy for patients with refractory immune thrombocytopenic purpura (ITP). Blood 2007;110(10):3526–31.

47. Podolanczuk A, Lazarus AH, Crow AR, et al. Of mice and men: an open label pilot study for treatment of immune thrombocytopenic purpura (ITP) by an inhibitor of syk. Blood 2009;113(14):3154–60.

Index

Note: Page numbers of article titles are in **boldface** type.

A

Alternative therapies, for chronic immune thrombocytopenia, 1330, 1332
Anti-D, intravenous, in management of immune thrombocytopenia, **1317–1327**
    activity, 1319–1320
    how it works, 1323–1324
    in pediatrics, 1229, 1321
    in pregnancy, 1320–1321
    in secondary immune thrombocytopenia, 1320
    toxicity and side effects, 1321
Antigen-presenting cells, in pathogenesis of immune thrombocytopenia, 1183–1186
Antiphospholipid syndrome, immune thrombocytopenia in patients with, 1243–1245
Antiplatelet antibodies, in chronic immune thrombocytopenia, **1163–1175**
    as a prognostic factor, 1165–1166
    autoantigens in, 1166–1168
        antigenic repertoire, 1166
        epitopes, 1166
        GPIb-IX, 1168
        GPIIb-IIIa, 1167
    history, 1163–1164
    measurement of, 1164–1166
    production sites, 1168
    role in pathogenesis, 1168–1171
        platelet destruction, 1168–1169
        suppression of platelet production, 1169–1171
Atypical features, of chronic immune thrombocytopenia in children, 1226–1227
Autoantibodies. *See also* Antiplatelet antibodies.
  in chronic immune thrombocytopenia, 1168–1171
    production sites, 1168
    role in pathogenesis, 1168–1171
        platelet destruction, 1168–1169
        suppression of platelet production, 1169–1171
Autoantigens, in chronic immune thrombocytopenia, 1166–1168
    antigenic repertoire, 1166
    epitopes, 1166
    GPIb-IX, 1168
    GPIIb-IIIa, 1167
Autoimmune disorders, antiplatelet antibodies in chronic immune thrombocytopenia,
    1163–1175
Azathioprine, for chronic immune thrombocytopenia, 1338
    in children, 1231

Hematol Oncol Clin N Am 23 (2009) 1343–1350
doi:10.1016/S0889-8588(09)00188-9
0889-8588/09/$ – see front matter © 2009 Elsevier Inc. All rights reserved.

Moving?

Make sure your subscription moves with you!

To notify us of your new address, find your **Clinics Account Number** (located on your mailing label above your name), and contact customer service at:

Email: **journalscustomerservice-usa@elsevier.com**

800-654-2452 (subscribers in the U.S. & Canada)
314-447-8871 (subscribers outside of the U.S. & Canada)

Fax number: 314-447-8029

Elsevier Health Sciences Division
Subscription Customer Service
3251 Riverport Lane
Maryland Heights, MO 63043

*To ensure uninterrupted delivery of your subscription, please notify us at least 4 weeks in advance of move.